Marcella Lawrence

Community Health
and
Nursing Practice

Community Health and Nursing Practice

EVELYN ROSE BENSON, R.N., M.P.H.

Adjunct Associate Professor of Nursing
Widener College
Chester, Pennsylvania

JOAN QUINN McDEVITT, R.N., M.S.N.

Assistant Director
Community Nursing Service
of Chester and Vicinity
Chester, Pennsylvania

Prentice-Hall, Inc., Englewood Cliffs, New Jersey

Library of Congress Cataloging in Publication Data

Benson, Evelyn Rose.
   Community health and nursing practice.

   Includes bibliographical references and index.
   1. Community health nursing. I. McDevitt, Joan
Quinn, joint author. II. Title. [DNLM: 1. Community
health nursing. WY106 B474c]
RT98.B46   362.1'04'25   75-37561
ISBN 0-13-153130-1

Printed in the United States of America

10   9   8   7   6   5

Prentice-Hall International, Inc., *London*
Prentice-Hall of Australia Pty. Limited, *Sydney*
Prentice-Hall of Canada, Ltd., *Toronto*
Prentice-Hall of India Private Limited, *New Delhi*
Prentice-Hall of Japan, Inc., *Tokyo*
Prentice-Hall of Southeast Asia Pte. Ltd., *Singapore*

This book is dedicated to
the Mortons,
the Grandmothers,
the BeckMir Corporation,
Donna,
and all our other loved ones.

Contents

Preface

"People are at the center of nursing's purpose . . . Nursing is a humanistic science dedicated to compassionate concern for maintaining and promoting health, preventing illness, and caring for and rehabilitating the sick and disabled."[1]

Health maintenance organization . . . national health insurance . . . primary health care . . . the expanded role of the nurse . . . patient advocate . . . change agent . . . problem-oriented system . . . professional accountability . . .

These are but a few of the many expressions which have entered the nursing lexicon in recent years. They reflect in a small way the changes which have occurred in the field of health care and the increasing demands upon the nurse. Nursing has a vital role to play in the emerging programs of health care. Ruth Freeman, whose writings in community health nursing are widely quoted here and abroad, has noted that changes in the technical and social nature of health services demand changes in professional practice.[2]

Nurses are being called upon to assume greater responsibility in the operation of the health team. Nursing, while accepting a leadership role, must remain personalized, humane, and nurturing. The nurse is the patient's advocate at all points along the health–illness continuum. In providing comprehensive services to the family/patient, the nurse recognizes the need for increased collaboration among all members of the health team. Together, they combine their unique skills to formulate an overall plan of service to the individual, his family, and the community.

In its report to the Secretary of Health, Education, and Welfare, the Secretary's Committee To Study Extended Roles for Nurses has stated that:

As health care becomes increasingly valued in our society, nurses will be expected to take more responsibility for the delivery of primary health and nursing care, for coordinating preventive services, for initiating or participating in diagnostic screening, and for referring patients who require differential medical diagnoses and medical therapies. Professional nursing is in a period of rapid and progressive change in response to the growth of biomedical knowledge, changes in patterns of demand for health service, and the evolution of professional relationships among nurses, physicians, and other health professions. The role of the nurse cannot remain static—it must change along with that of all other health professionals, which means that the knowledge and skills of nurses need to be broadened. [3]

Dr. Faye Abdellah in commenting on this report has pointed out that "the nursing profession can and must occupy a larger and more effective place in the delivery of health services."[4] She continues by saying that "it will be necessary . . . to prepare nurses in primary health care, including preventive and rehabilitative services; expansion of acute care health services to include the treatment of illness or disability; and expansion of long term care services."[5]

Newly emerging patterns in nursing call for major changes in nursing school curricula. These changes demand the scientific approach to the identification and management of health problems. This book is designed as an introductory text for nursing students who are preparing to function in a variety of health settings in the community. Nursing instructors who are concerned with the integration of community health principles throughout the curriculum should find this book a valuable tool. It may also serve as a guide for the new staff nurse in community health agencies.

In our book, we focus on family health. Our approach is family-centered, and we speak about the family/patient. In referring to the individual "consumer of health care," we use the terms *patient* and *client* interchangeably.

We have organized the textbook into five units. In the first unit, we begin by tracing the development of present-day practice in nursing and public health. Using the terms *public health* and *community health* synonymously, we introduce the basic concepts of health, community health, and community health nursing. In Unit II we elaborate on the community health sciences that we identified in Chapter 2—human ecology, epidemiology, biostatistics, and nutrition. Unit III presents current health problems and trends in the community. Here we describe the health care delivery system and some of the changes which have been recommended to bring about its improvement. Unit IV is concerned with nursing intervention in the community; Unit V is devoted to the problem-oriented system and the nursing process, and shows the interrelationship of these two concepts.

We wish to express our appreciation to the following persons who helped us by reviewing and commenting on selected portions of the manuscript:

Anne Aigner, R.N., Executive Director, Community Nursing Service of Chester and Vicinity, Chester, Pennsylvania.

Norma Dawson, R.N., Assistant Professor of Community Health Nursing, Widener College, Chester, Pennsylvania.

Jessie Glass, R.N., Maternal and Child Health Nursing Consultant, Pennsylvania Department of Health.

Michael Gregg, M.D., Chief, Viral Diseases Branch, Bureau of Epidemiology, Center for Disease Control, United States Department of Health, Education, and Welfare.

Olga Kotalik, R.N., formerly, Associate in Nursing and Chairman of Community Health Nursing Practice, University of Pennsylvania.

Elizabeth W. Lipton, R.D., Associate Professor of Nutrition, Widener College, Chester, Pennsylvania.

Judith Mausner, M.D., Professor of Epidemiology, Medical College of Pennsylvania.

Vivian R. Middleman, R.N., Associate Dean of the Center of Nursing, Widener College, Chester, Pennsylvania.

Marian Miller, R.N., Associate Director of Nursing for Staff Development, Crozer-Chester Medical Center, Chester, Pennsylvania.

Ruth Mrozek, R.N., Assistant Director of Nursing, Inservice Education, Presbyterian-University Hospital, Pittsburgh, Pennsylvania.

Lorraine Nelson, R.N., Nurse Consultant, Pennsylvania Department of Health.

Isadore Rose, M.D., Instructor in Medicine, Presbyterian Hospital-University of Pennsylvania Medical Center, Philadelphia, Pennsylvania.

Jessie Scott, R.N., Assistant Surgeon General, Public Health Service, United States Department of Health, Education, and Welfare.

Dorothy Stewart Thompson, R.N., Dean (retired), Center of Nursing, Widener College, Chester, Pennsylvania.

Betty Weyn, R.N., Associate Professor of Nursing, Widener College, Chester, Pennsylvania.

Elizabeth Zimmerman, R.N., Executive Director, Neighborhood League, Wayne, Pennsylvania.

Elenore Neasham Zinger, R.D., Regional Nutrition Consultant, Pennsylvania Department of Health.

We are grateful to Margaret Kauffman, R.N., Executive-Director, Community Nursing Service of Philadelphia, for permission to use pictures from the Visiting Nurse Society of Philadelphia; to Constance Spicer Johnson, R.N., and Lorraine Martin, R.N., supervising nurses at the Community Nursing Service of Chester and Vicinity, for their help in preparing case material; to our former students Linda Tull, Suzanne Hearne, Shauna Myers, and Kay Simon for their active contribution; and to all the other colleagues and friends who helped us.

For their wisdom and forbearance, we are indebted to the members of the nursing staff of the Community Nursing Service of Chester and Vicinity: Rita Anderson, R.N.; Marjorie Bradley, R.N.; Mary Derrickson, R.N.; Mary Ellen Double, R.N.; Mary Kilson Edwards, R.N.; Patricia Glascoe, L.P.N.; Kathleen Keegan, R.N.; Evelyn Lovett, R.N.; Walter Lumley, R.N.; Sally Mowris, R.N.; Jane Small, R.N.; Darene Wildermuth, R.N.; Nancy Wilson, R.N.; and especially to Roberta ("Bobbi") Pichini, R.N., whose imagination inspired the sketches in the text. We wish to acknowledge the Widener College Center of Nursing classes of 1974, 1975, and 1976, for their enthusiastic participation in various phases of activity involved in the preparation of the manuscript.

We wish to thank the members of the staff of the Wolfgram Memorial Library at Widener College who did so much to help us gather and check our resource materials. We also appreciate the work done by Helen MacArthur, Virginia Novak, and Marcia Zanger, who typed and helped assemble the manuscript. Finally, we have a special word of love and thanks to our families for their boundless patience and support—to Rebecca and Miriam, who checked, typed, and helped in endless ways, and to Dr. Morton Benson for his invaluable editorial assistance.

In closing, we note with sincere gratitude the guidance, support, and encouragement of our friends at Prentice-Hall.

E. R. Benson, R.N.
J. Q. McDevitt, R.N.

REFERENCES

1. Martha Rogers, *The Theoretical Basis of Nursing* (Philadelphia: F.A. Davis Company, 1970), p. vii.

2. Ruth Freeman, *Community Health Nursing Practice* (Philadelphia: W.B. Saunders Co., 1970), p. iii.

3. United States Department of Health, Education, and Welfare, *Extending the Scope of Nursing Practice,* A Report to the Secretary of Health, Education, and Welfare by the Secretary's Committee To Study Extended Roles for Nurses. Reprinted in *Nursing Outlook,* 20 (January 1972) 46–52.

4. *NLN News,* 20 (March–April 1972), 2. Excerpts from a speech prepared for delivery before the National League for Nursing Council of Baccalaureate and Higher Degree Programs, New Orleans, March 22, 1972.

5. *Ibid.*

Community Health
and
Nursing Practice

UNIT I
ORIGINS AND
BASIC CONCEPTS

Chapter 1
Historical Background

"For those who would influence a [profession] to function in a manner relevant to tomorrow as well as to today—two things are essential: an analysis of factors of change in contemporary society and the history of that [profession]."[1]

INTRODUCTION

The best way to comprehend where you are at the moment is to find out how you got there.

A distinctive feature of every profession is an interest in its own history. Recognition of past achievements encourages group pride and a sense of identity, and it helps us develop broader perspectives, providing a barometer for understanding current and future trends. Thus, a brief historical overview of nursing and public health follows. While they are professions of comparatively recent origin, both have elements that can be traced far back into the past. Their development, in many ways, is parallel to the development of medicine and pharmacology.

From the earliest times, human beings, in their fight for survival, devised their own measures to cope with birth, death, and illness. Usually interwoven with mystical, magical, or religious rites, these measures took on special meaning, and the medicine men, who often were also religious leaders or high priests, held a revered place in society. Historical records show that people, even in antiquity, were concerned with disease and had some knowledge of its treatment. A clay tablet inscribed in cuneiform, on display at the University of Pennsylvania Museum (Figure 1-1), describes the remedies used by a Sumerian physician of the third millennium B.C.E. From this tablet, we see that Sumerian pharmacology had made considerable progress and was acquainted

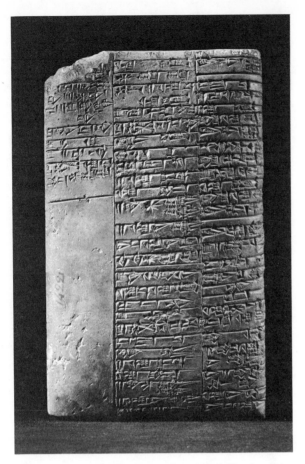

Figure 1-1 Clay tablet with cuneiform inscription describing the remedies used by a Sumerian physician, third millennium, B.C.E.

Source Courtesy of the University of Pennsylvania Museum.

with a large number of rather elaborate chemical operations and procedures.[2] The Babylonians and Egyptians also possessed medical skills that are described in their recorded history. There is also evidence that other ancient civilizations, notably Hebrew, Greek, and Roman, had remarkable knowledge of personal hygiene, community responsibility, and medicine. They had developed some rather sophisticated measures of environmental sanitation, such as water supply and sewage systems, and they also had some understanding of the nature of contagion.

The rise of Christianity had a marked influence on the development of nursing, which flourished as a labor of love and charity among the deaconesses of the early Church. The deaconess Phoebe, often cited as the "first visiting nurse," went out among the people to bring physical and spiritual comfort to the sick and dying. Wealthy Roman matrons, attracted to the teachings of Christianity, often dedicated their homes, fortunes, and personal services to the care of the sick and the poor. Medicine, however, was adversely affected by the Church, which held that disease was the divine punishment for moral wrongdoing.

The knowledge and advances of early civilizations were swept aside when the Dark Ages of history descended. In the Western World, this period was characterized by the decline of the creative spirit, disintegration of society, and the return of political anarchy. Progress in medicine as a science and art was halted. Notable exceptions were the Arabian school of medicine, which flourished between 765 and 1258 C.E., and the medical writings of older civilizations which were preserved in monastery libraries. It was an era marked by great epidemics—leprosy and bubonic plague were the most devastating. The busy ports and commercial centers were especially hard hit, a situation that gave rise to the practice of quarantine. Fourteenth-century Venice banned all travelers suspected of having plague; the port city of Ragusa (present-day Dubrovnik) isolated travelers from plague-ridden countries for thirty days before permitting them to enter; Marseilles adopted this practice and extended the period to forty days, hence the word "quarantine."

Nursing care was provided through the religious orders of nuns and monks (Figure 1–2). Present day vestiges of this period are the nursing caps which identify various schools of nursing, just as various habits identified religious orders. In addition, the use of the term "sister" has survived as a designation for nurse in many languages.[3] A prevailing attitude born in this religious tradition is that nursing is a "calling" that demands dedication, devotion, and sacrifice. Military orders for hospital and nursing care were established at the time of the Crusades, which also left their mark on the future development of nursing: for many years nursing practice in hospitals was characterized by a militaristic, hierarchal system.

Unlike medicine, nursing as a science did not advance in the Renaissance, which began in Italy in the fourteenth century. The Renaissance period, which lasted about three hundred years, was noted for its achievements in scholarship and the arts. This revival of learning spread through the great European universities that had already been established at Bologna, Paris, Oxford, Prague, and Heidelberg. Characterized by the rise of commerce and industry, the Renaissance era was also noted for the growing spirit of humanism, and witnessed progress in science and medicine, including medical education. Education for nursing, however, was not established; nevertheless, nursing continued to exist as a vital human service within the domain of the Catholic religious orders. A significant movement which occurred during the Renaissance era was the Protestant Reformation in the sixteenth century. One of the effects of the Reformation was the suppression of Catholic religious orders, with a concomitant decline of nursing. Both the Renaissance and the Reformation had the effect of influencing political and economic thinking, and paved the way for the Industrial Revolution.

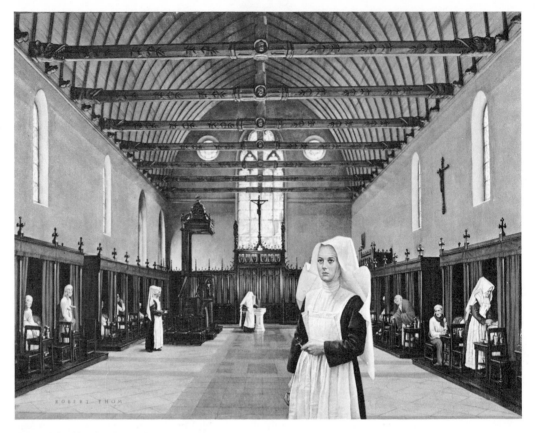

Figure 1-2 Nursing in medieval hospitals. The Great Room of the Poor (La Grand' Chambre des Povres) is believed to be the world's oldest edifice to have been in continuous use as a hospital. Representative of medieval hospitals, it is a part of the Hôtel-Dieu of Beaune, France, founded in 1443. Combined with modern professional hospital service, it carefully preserves the atmosphere of the fifteenth century. Sisters of the Congregation of Sainte Marthe, garbed in habits traditional to their ancient order, have cared for the sick, the aged, and the indigent in this hospital for more than five hundred years, uninterrupted by wars, economic upheavals, or political changes.

Source A History of Medicine in Pictures, a pamphlet accompanying photographs presented by Parke, Davis. ©1958 by Parke, Davis and Company.

The onset of the seventeenth century in England witnessed the passage of the Elizabethan Poor Laws, which provided aid for the "lame, impotent, old, blind, and such others among them being poor and not able to work." The works of John Graunt mark the beginnings of statistical analyses of production and population. With the eighteenth century came England's Industrial Revolution, which resulted in profound changes at every level of society. The concepts characterizing that period include laissez-faire economics, rugged individualism, and the desire for power and profit. Workers were harshly exploited and had no security. They toiled long hours, received scant wages, and lived in squalor. Half of the children of the working class did not reach their fifth birthday.

Against this backdrop, we see modern nursing and public health emerge as developments of the late nineteenth century. They can be viewed as integral parts of an overall social reform movement in Victorian England, which was a humanitarian response to the excesses of the Industrial Revolution. Reform was offered first by the privileged on behalf of the needy and later demanded by all classes on their own behalf. Attention was focused on the weakest groups in society: prisoners, mentally ill, unprotected children, "slaves" of the new industrial conditions, and, finally, the sick poor.

NIGHTINGALE REFORMS

Many of the leaders in the public health movement were social reformers and students of social philosophy rather than medical scientists. Foremost among

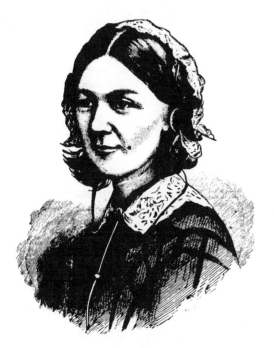

Figure 1-3   Florence Nightingale

Source   From the Australian Town and County Journal, 1875.

the pioneers in the public health movement in England were Edwin Chadwick, William Farr, and Florence Nightingale. Chadwick's 1842 report, "The Sanitary Conditions of the Laboring Population," stimulated the formation of a General Board of Health in 1848. Dr. Farr demonstrated the need to place public health on a sound, statistical basis.

Nightingale's role in bringing about health reforms merits special consideration. Internationally acclaimed as the founder of modern nursing, Miss Nightingale began her work at a time when nursing had reached its lowest point. The tradition of dedicated nursing service established by the religious medieval orders had withered away with the decline of Church power and influence. Earlier hospitals, founded and staffed by religious groups, were replaced by municipal hospitals. These hospitals, when they were unable to recruit nursing nuns and brothers, paid scant wages and attracted thieves, slatterns, drunks, and others equally unfit for responsibility. These undesirables were bitingly satirized by Charles Dickens in his novel, *Martin Chuzzlewit*, in the characters of the Mesdames Sarah Gamp and Elizabeth Prig. Through sheer force of will and an indomitable spirit, Florence Nightingale reversed this trend and created for nursing an atmosphere of dignity and self-respect. She herself was motivated by devout religious feelings and a conviction that she had a "calling" from God. However, she did not care to perpetuate the image of the self-immolating sister of charity that was then fixed in the public mind. Miss Nightingale visualized a radically different kind of nursing career; she saw the nurse as a professional person—trained, efficient, responsible, highly paid. She wrote to Dr. Farr in 1866, "To make the power of serving without pay a qualification is, I think, absurd. *I would far rather than establish a religious order, open a career highly paid."*

The opportunity came when Florence Nightingale was asked to organize and supervise a group of nurses to care for the sick and wounded British soldiers, casualties of the Crimean War. Warfare, once again, was highlighting the crucial need for organized skilled nursing care. The death, illness, and misery generated by this ghastly and senseless military confrontation did not spare either side. The Russians also had their nursing contingent, which had been sent out under the direction of aristocratic women with court connections. However, once the emergency was over, they returned to private life, while Miss Nightingale, upon her return home, pressed on in her mission to create the modern nursing profession.

Miss Nightingale has been recognized for her significant contributions to public health and public health nursing. Her remarkable foresight and practical idealism cut through the barriers of ignorance and apathy. A magnificent organizer, a genius at administration, a keen and analytical thinker, she was also a prolific writer, skillfully using statistics that she herself methodically gathered. Her works include treatises on sanitation, health, hospitals, administration, as well as on nursing. A cost-accounting system she devised for the Army Medical Corps around 1860 proved most efficient and remained in use for over eighty years. She played a conspicuous part in influencing health legislation not only in England, but also in India.

About Florence Nightingale's contribution to health care in England, Cecil Woodham-Smith, in her biography, has written, "Her work for public health in England, for hospitals and the reorganization of nursing, had rapidly expanded and assumed enormous proportions . . . Her enormous energy, her extraordinary history, her capacity to inspire boundless faith, were producing astonishing results."[4] Dr. George Chandler Whipple, Professor of Sanitary Engineering at Harvard, in his *Textbook on Vital Statistics—An Introduction to the Science of Demography*, included among the world's greatest demographers ". . . those who have made important contributions to the study of statistics especially vital statistics: William Farr, Edwin Chadwick, Lemuel Shattuck, Florence Nightingale."[5] Dr. Iago Galdston had this to say in *The Meaning of Social Medicine*, "Florence Nightingale, the real hero of the Crimean War, was not merely or primarily the lady with the lamp, the founder of modern nursing. She was in the deepest sense of the term a pioneer in social medicine. Over and above the skills and techniques which she initiated and cultivated in the care of the wounded and sick she added to the social comprehension of Medicine."[6]

While William Rathbone, a wealthy merchant from Liverpool, was mourning the death of his wife after a lengthy illness, he began to think about the plight of people in poverty faced with long-term illness. He, of course, had provided the best available care for Mrs. Rathbone. However, he wondered, who took care of those who did not have financial means? As a memorial to his wife, he set out to organize a district nursing scheme. Seeking help, he turned to Florence Nightingale, who offered guidance and support from a distance. She encouraged him to organize a training school for nurses in the Liverpool Royal Infirmary. In 1862, the school was opened with a program to provide nurses for hospital, private duty, and district nursing. The function of the district nurse was established and defined by Florence Nightingale; Rathbone consulted her all along the way. The nurses who participated in this program were responsible not only for giving bedside care, but also for teaching principles of health to the families with whom they worked.

BEGINNING OF THE MODERN ERA

In America, the public health movement received its impetus from the work of Lemuel Shattuck, who, in 1850, submitted to the Massachusetts legislature the Report of the Sanitary Commission of the Commonwealth of Massachusetts. A teacher, historian, book dealer, sociologist, and statistician, he set forth detailed, specific recommendations regarding the establishment of: state and local boards of health, a system of sanitary inspection, collection of vital statistics, school health programs, tuberculosis studies, alcohol control, supervision of mental illness, model housing, control of smoke nuisances, health

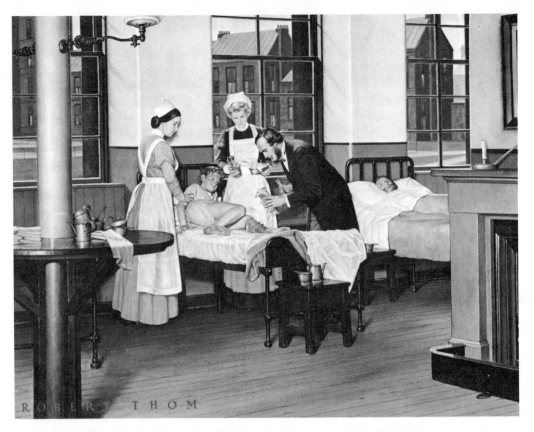

Figure 1-4 Lister introduces antisepsis. When surgeon Joseph Lister (1827-1912) of Glasgow Royal Infirmary removed dressings from James Greenlees' compound fracture, he found that the wound had healed without infection—something unheard of before. For six weeks Lister had treated the boy's wound with carbolic acid. Now Lister had proof of the success of his principle of antisepsis—which was to revolutionize principles of wound care and open new vistas in the practice of surgery, medicine, and environmental sanitation. Hospitals were turned from houses of horror into houses of healing; countless lives were saved.

Source A History of Medicine in Pictures, a pamphlet accompanying photographs presented by Parke, Davis. ©1962 by Parke, Davis and Company.

teaching programs, and nursing schools. The first state Board of Health, in the modern sense, was established in Massachusetts in 1869.

Another milestone was the formation in 1872 of the American Public Health Association (APHA), a national organization of professional community health workers that has consistently striven for the achievement of high standards and the improvement of all public health services. A little more than two decades later, in 1896, the American Nurses Association (ANA) got its start as the Nurses Associated Alumnae of the United States. The ANA is the major national organization of professional nursing and it defines and establishes standards of nursing practice, including community health nursing practice. (See page 34.)

10

Although public health began as part of a larger movement of social reform, it soon moved into the sphere of bacteriology. Capitalizing on the scientific advances made by Pasteur (germ theory), Koch (origin of bacterial infection), Lister (antisepsis), and Ehrlich (chemotherapy), public health concentrated on control of communicable diseases. Community-wide application of the new knowledge from the natural sciences was made possible through the organization of health programs. It became evident that the control of the major fatal diseases—smallpox, diphtheria, tuberculosis—was an attainable goal. That these efforts were successful has been borne out by the overall decline in communicable disease as a major cause of death and disability in the western world.

As these diseases have waned, other serious health problems have emerged. Chronic, degenerative processes, such as heart disease, cancer, stroke, and mental illness, are major concerns today. Social problems, affecting individual, family, and community health, demand attention. Public health has entered a new era. It turns more and more to the behavioral sciences, as the range of health department activities moves beyond the traditional basic seven services: vital statistics, communicable disease control, maternal-child health, environmental services, health education, public health laboratory, and chronic disease control.

All of these changes are reflected in the development of nursing in public health. Community health nursing, as it is more commonly referred to in today's terms, has a rich and highly respected tradition in our country. Basic principles of public health nursing were clearly enunciated in the writings of renowned nursing leaders who blazed the trail through the first half of the twentieth century. The textbooks and other writings of Lillian Wald, Annie Brainard, Mary Gardner, Harriet Frost, and others, reveal great foresight and perceptivity on the part of the authors. Indeed, many so-called innovative ideas of today were envisioned and even advocated by these nurses.

The foundations of district nursing were laid by the turn of the century, largely through private, voluntary, philanthropic efforts. As early as 1877, the Woman's Board of the New York City Mission saw the need for nurses to go into the homes to help the sick poor. The Visiting Nurse Society (Figures 1–5 and 1–6) of Philadelphia, founded in 1886, while caring for the sick poor, extended its services to persons who needed nursing and were able to pay. The Instructive District Nursing Association of Boston, 1886, emphasized the teaching of hygiene and sanitation, along with the care of the sick. The Chicago Visiting Nurse Association was established in 1889. Then in 1893, the Henry Street Settlement, under the direction of Lillian Wald, was founded, and grew into a well-organized health center with visiting nurse services for the surrounding community. Miss Wald, pictured in Figure 1–7, recognized the need for well-prepared nurses, who would lead the way in health promotion, disease prevention, case finding, and follow-up. School nursing, which had already been instituted in England, was introduced in the United States by Miss Wald. One of her nurses, Lina Rogers, was assigned to the

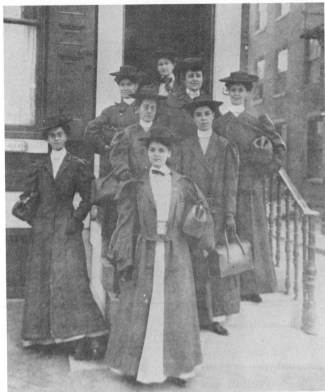

Figure 1-5 Visiting Nurse Society staff nurses, at the turn of the twentieth century, outside the VNS headquarters in Philadelphia.

Source Courtesy of the Visiting Nurse Society of Philadelphia.

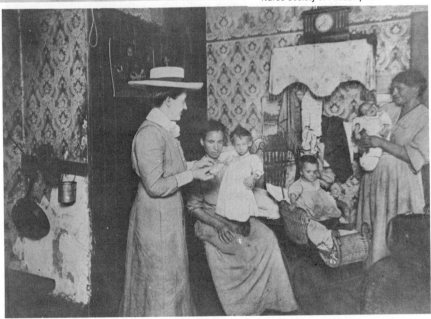

Figure 1-6 A typical home visit by visiting nurses at the turn of the twentieth century.

Source Courtesy of the Visiting Nurse Society of Philadelphia.

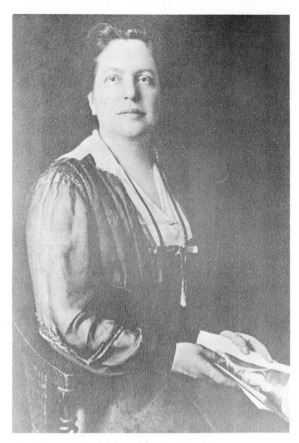

Figure 1-7 Lillian Wald, pioneer in public health nursing, founded the Henry Street Settlement in New York City in 1893.

Source Courtesy of the Visiting Nurse Society of New York.

public schools on a trial basis. Concentrating on communicable disease control, Miss Rogers worked with the children and teachers in the schools and made follow-up home visits to instruct the children and parents in principles of good hygiene. In a very short time, school absences decreased dramatically, demonstrating that nurses could serve effectively in a school setting. With remarkable tenacity and great charm, Miss Wald brought about changes that ensured better, safer, and healthier living for thousands of people.

The health of mothers and children was a matter of great concern to public health and public health nursing pioneers. The maternal and child health (MCH) movement in the United States may be traced back to the end of the nineteenth century when privately-funded milk stations were first established in New York City to provide safe, pasteurized milk for babies and offer health education programs for mothers. The sponsoring private and voluntary groups gathered statistics on infant mortality and presented these facts to the public. The success of these early efforts to bring about a reduction in the infant mortality rate stimulated further action, voluntary and official, for the development of maternal and child health services in the United States. A national event of major importance for the MCH movement was the first White House Conference on Children in 1909, which provided the impetus for the eventual creation of the Children's Bureau. The second White House Conference on Children took place in 1919, and since 1930 they have been held every ten years.

The public health movement and the growth of public health nursing services gathered momentum through stimulation from various sources, private and public. The American Red Cross and private foundations, such as the Rockefeller Foundation, the Commonwealth Fund, the Kellogg Foundation, and others, were very active in the development of community health services. Official agencies, those supported by the government, were growing. By 1919, all states had a board of health, and some local health departments had been established as well (Guilford County, North Carolina; Yakima County, Washington; both in 1911). At the federal level, in 1912, the Public Health and Marine Hospital Service was reorganized into the United States Public Health Service by act of Congress.

At about this same time Congress passed other legislation that had a direct impact on public health:

1912—Congress created the Children's Bureau to draw attention at the highest levels of government to the needs of children. It existed as a separate bureau for nearly sixty years, but has now been integrated into other segments of the United States Department of Health, Education and Welfare.

1918—The Venereal Disease Division of the United States Public Health Service was established by the Chamberlain-Kahn Act.

1921—The Sheppard-Towner Act was passed, providing grants-in-aid, which enabled individual states to create their own bureaus of Maternal and Child Health.

1929—The Narcotics Control Act authorized construction of hospitals for care and treatment of addicts.

In 1912, the National Organization for Public Health Nursing was established. For forty years it functioned as the major professional organization for public health nursing, concerned with the improvement of nursing service for the public. In 1952 it merged with several other national nursing organizations and became a department within the newly formed National League for Nursing (NLN). A major responsibility of the League is the accreditation of community nursing agencies and schools of nursing.

The early part of this century witnessed a marked trend towards specialization in public health nursing. There were specialized nurses, for example, in tuberculosis control, venereal disease control, maternal and child health, communicable disease control, and other fields. This trend was sparked by categorical federal funding, which required such specialization to facilitate cost-accounting. Although categorical funding still exists, the trend towards specialization has not prevailed in community health nursing practice. In today's context, a basic premise is that one public health problem rarely exists alone, and a generalized approach is required in community nursing practice.

After the First World War, nursing began to take a critical look at its system of education, or "nurses' training," which was provided largely in hospital schools and settings. Demands created by the war had led to a lowering of standards, which up to this point had been high. A distinguished panel of experts under the chairmanship of Dr. C.-E.A. Winslow, Professor of Public Health at Yale, set out to examine the educational needs for public health nurses, but in the end their study encompassed nursing education as a whole. The secretary of the committee, Josephine Goldmark, submitted a report, "Nursing and Nursing Education in the United States," in 1923.[7] Usually referred to as the "Goldmark Report," it pointed out the need for including community nursing as a learning experience for well-prepared nurses, and recommended that public health nurses complete special courses to supplement their basic hospital training. It called for the endowment of nursing education and strengthening of university schools for the education of nursing leaders. This was the first major study of nursing education and a direct outgrowth was the establishment of the Yale University School of Nursing. Supported by the Rockefeller Foundation, this school, from its inception, emphasized community health nursing in its curriculum.

What has happened in the intervening half century? On the national scene, we have had a massive economic depression with widespread unemployment and despair, the Second World War, two postwar major military confrontations in Asia, several economic recession periods, a population explosion, environmental decay, a technological boom, educational expansion and subsequent retrenchment, poverty in the midst of affluence, rising taxes, inflation, an energy shortage, and a crisis in the delivery of health care. All of these events have influenced the development of nursing, and, to some degree, have been influenced by the development of nursing.

The end of the twenties saw improvement and expansion in nursing, which had been stimulated, in part at least, by the Goldmark report. But soon after, the effects of the terrible depression of the thirties were felt, with the supply of nurses exceeding the demand. Many nurses were out of work for extended periods of time, and often when they did find employment, they were required to put in long hours of duty for meager salaries. Some progress was noted, with continued efforts to study and upgrade the standards of nursing education, nursing service, and economic security. *The Committee on the*

Grading of Nursing Schools, under the direction of May Ayres Burgess, dealt with the quantity and quality of nursing service, nursing education, and economic status.[8]

Political events of that era and the emergence of the New Deal movement to reform the economy had an impact on health care and nursing. An event of major importance in 1935 was the passage of the Social Security Act, which authorized grants-in-aid to the individual states, to be used for the improvement of state and local public health programs, with the advice and assistance of the United States Public Health Service. Under the Social Security Act, the Children's Bureau was able to revitalize its programs in maternal and child health, crippled children's services, and child welfare. The Social Security Act has served as a basis for additional assistance through subsequent amendments.

The thirties also witnessed a heightened interest in venereal disease control. Dr. Thomas Parran, the Surgeon General of the United States Public Health Service, was a dominant force behind the movement. In 1937 his book, *Shadow on the Land*, created a sensation at a time when syphilis was a topic not discussed openly. He stirred up public interest in the problem, and Congress, in 1938, passed the National Venereal Disease Control Act, which increased the allocations of federal funds to the states on the basis of population, extent of venereal disease problem, and financial need.

With the upsurge of activity in these categorical health programs, which got their impetus from the economic recovery measures of the New Deal, there was an increased need for nursing service. Hard on the heels of this era was the outbreak of World War II. Suddenly, there was a critical shortage of nurses and a tremendous push to recruit students. In 1943, Congresswoman Frances Payne Bolton of Ohio, long a friend of nursing, sponsored legislation bearing her name, which created the United States Cadet Nurse Corps. Students in this program were subsidized by the federal government during their schooling and in their last six months could apply for outside experience in military hospitals, public health hospitals, and community health nursing agencies.

POST-WORLD WAR II

Soon after the war was over, the American Nurses' Association took an important step forward in launching the Economic Security Program for nurses. Through this action, it was hoped that nurses would never again have to face the degrading status of economic helplessness and insecurity that had prevailed during the Depression. Another event of special importance at about that time was the passage of the Hospital Survey and Construction Act (1946), known as the Hill-Burton Act, which provided matching funds up to one-third of the total cost of hospital construction as a stimulus to state and local communities.

The publication of three very significant studies between 1948 and 1950 influenced the course of nursing for the next few decades. *Nursing for the Future*, also known as the "Brown Report," after its director, Esther Lucile Brown, was published in 1948.[9] In developing the central theme of how a basic professional school of nursing should be organized, administered, controlled, and financed to prepare its graduates to meet community needs, the report produced a comprehensive list of recommendations, which touched on nearly every facet of nursing education. It emphasized higher education for nurses, prompted a reexamination of beliefs and attitudes about professional education and practice, and called for an end to discrimination in selection of students based on race, religion, sex, and marital status. Eli Ginzberg's report, *A Program for the Nursing Profession* (1948),[10] in many ways paralleling the Brown study, recommended formalized recognition of two levels of nursing—professional and practical—with the professional nurse prepared in a four-year collegiate program, and the practical nurse in a nine to twelve month program in a school of practical nursing. It also called for changes in nursing service, through the development of nursing teams, better working conditions, an improved system of rewards, and nursing research. *Nursing Schools at the Mid-Century* (1950)[11] established uniform standards regarding organization of schools, cost of nursing education, curriculum content, clinical resources, and student health. It served as the basis for formulating accreditation procedures for professional schools of nursing.

In 1956 the National Health Survey Act was passed, which established an on-going, comprehensive health survey of the entire nation through periodic evaluation of statistically designated population sampling groups. Twenty years earlier a similar attempt had been made, but the program lapsed. The present National Health Survey has continued with periodic reports, which provide a systematic method for measuring health problems in our country. Also in 1956, the Health Amendments Act was passed, providing traineeships for public health personnel and giving nurses an opportunity to obtain advanced preparation for positions in administration, supervision, and teaching.

A five-year program of studies of nursing functions initiated by the American Nurses' Association culminated in the 1958 report *Twenty Thousand Nurses Tell Their Story*. Setting out to effect better care for patients, it revealed what nurses were doing on their jobs, their attitudes, and job satisfactions. It formed the basis for statements on functions, standards, and qualifications of nurses prepared by the American Nurses' Association professional practice sections. In 1959 Mildred Montag's report, *Community College Education for Nursing*,[12] described the overall approach to the two-year associate degree program in nursing education.

Several key events of the sixties and seventies helped to shape the present and future course of nursing and public health. In 1963, the Maternal and Child Health and Mental Retardation Planning Amendments to Title V of the Social Security Act were passed and the Surgeon General's Report *Toward Quality in Nursing: Needs and Goals*[13] was issued. The report cited the shortages of nursing personnel, deficiencies in the present system of educational preparation for nurses, recruitment needs, and the need to augment and support nursing research and improve nursing administration. It pointed out specific areas requiring federal financial assistance and recommended a study of the present system of nursing education. The report inspired the Nurse Training Act of 1964, which provided grants for construction of facilities, improvement of teaching, loans to students, and traineeships for graduate nurses. In the same year Congress also passed the Economic Opportunities Act—an act of historic proportion, which had great implications for community health. It created the Office of Economic Opportunity (OEO), which administered the anti-poverty program. With OEO financial support, creative nurses helped to establish new community health care programs. There have been numerous examples of multidisciplinary health care centers, such as Boston's Columbia Point Health Center and Chicago's Mile Square Health Center, where nurses have been the providers of primary health care (see page 211).

The American Nurses' Association made a historic announcement in 1965 when its Committee on Nursing Education issued its "Position Paper," which declared that "education for those who work in nursing should take place in institutions of learning within the general system of education."[14] It identified the essential components of professional nursing—care, cure, coordination—and recommended three levels of educational preparation, as follows:

(1) baccalaureate degree education in nursing for beginning professional nursing practice;
(2) associate degree education in nursing for beginning technical nursing practice; and
(3) short, intensive preservice programs in vocational education schools for assistants in the health service occupations.

Thus, the ANA endorsed and formalized a position that nursing leaders had been advocating for many years.

The 1965–1966 session of the 89th Congress was responsible for some of the most far-reaching federal health legislation ever passed. The Social Security Act was amended to provide funds for health care of the elderly (Medicare) and for health care of the medically indigent (Medicaid). The Heart Disease, Cancer and Stroke Amendments, authorizing regional medical programs to combat the three "killer" diseases, emphasized the concept of regionalization and gave a boost to professional programs in continuing education. The Comprehensive Health Planning and Public Health Services Act of 1966 created the Partnership for Health program to promote the most efficient use of our health resources and the ready availability of health services to all who need them. It called for planning councils and required that they have consumer as well as provider representation. The Narcotic Addict Rehabilitation Act of 1966 offered treatment and rehabilitation services in lieu of prosecution or sentencing to addicts who have been convicted of federal crimes.

In 1967 the Child Health Act broadened the base of the earlier Maternal and Child Health and Mental Retardation Act, and together they provided the impetus for a network of Maternity and Infant Care Projects and Children and Youth Programs across the nation. Nurses in expanded roles, such as nurse-midwives, pediatric nurse practitioners, and family planning nurse practitioners have made a significant contribution in these programs where, in many instances, they have been responsible for providing primary health care.

In 1968 the Health Manpower Act extended and expanded a number of laws already in effect. It had particular relevance for nursing in that it provided for the Nurse Training Act of 1964 to be amended and continued. Recent federal health legislation includes the following:

1970—Family Planning Services and Population Research Act
1970—Occupational Safety and Health Act
1970—Comprehensive Alcohol Abuse and Alcoholism Prevention, Treatment, and Rehabilitation
1970—The National Environmental Policy Act (established Council on Environmental Quality)
1971—Nurse Training Act (expanded and continued nurse training provisions of the 1964 and 1968 acts)
1971—Comprehensive Health Manpower Training Act
1971—Sickle Cell Anemia Act
1971—National Cancer Act
1972—Communicable Disease Control Amendments Act
1972—Social Security Amendments regarding Medicare and Medicaid
1972—National Heart, Blood Vessel, Lung and Blood Act
1973—The Health Maintenance Organization (HMO) Act
1974—The Health Planning and Resources Development Act
1975—Health Services, Health Revenue Sharing, and Nurse Training Act

With the growth of health programs, stimulated by these federal acts, there was a greater demand for health care personnel. As far as nursing was concerned, there was a need for more nurses and for nurses who could function in expanded or extended roles. Prompted by the recommendations of the 1963 Surgeon General's report *Toward Quality in Nursing,* the American Nurses' Association and the National League for Nursing took the initiative in establishing a National Commission on Nursing and Nursing Education to conduct a comprehensive, nationwide investigation of changing practices and educational patterns in nursing today, as well as the probable requirements in professional nursing over the next several decades.

The survey was carried out under the direction of Dr. Jerome Lysaught. The findings were summarized in the *American Journal of Nursing,* February, 1970, and published under the title, *An Abstract for Action.* [15] The report identified two general fields of nursing practice and recommended that career patterns be developed to parallel them. Termed *episodic* and *distributive,* the fields were described as follows:

> (a) One career pattern (episodic) would emphasize nursing practice that is essentially curative and restorative, generally acute or chronic in nature, and most frequently provided in the setting of the hospital and inpatient facility.
>
> (b) The second career pattern (distributive) would emphasize the nursing practice that is designed essentially for health maintenance and disease prevention, generally continuous in nature, seldom acute, and most frequently operative in the community or in newly developing institutional settings.

It also recommended support for formal, academic education, as well as for continuing education programs. Many of the report's recommendations have stimulated further attempts by state and local nursing groups to examine and evaluate their role in the delivery of health care today.

The report clearly pinpointed the need for better utilization of nursing manpower. In response to this recommendation, a special committee appointed by the Secretary of Health, Education, and Welfare has studied and outlined the potential for extending the contribution of nursing in the delivery of health care. The group's study was published in November 1971 in *Extending the Scope of Nursing Practice—A Report of the Secretary's Committee to Study Extended Roles for Nurses.* [16] The report of this committee calls for nurses to assume greater responsibility in the delivery of primary health care. In endorsing the extended role of nursing, the committee has, in effect, bestowed "official recognition" on practices that have long been within the scope of nursing but have not been universally recognized. The report cites the Family Nurse Practitioner (or *Primex* nurse), the Pediatric Nurse Practitioner, and the Nurse-Midwife as examples of the Extended Role of the Nurse.

In this brief historical review, we can see how the public health movement and the development of nursing have been intertwined and how each has influenced the other. Community health and community health nursing continue to be shaped by the needs, demands, and resources of the community, and in turn are instrumental in shaping the overall structure and function of the community.

REFERENCES

1. V.T. Thayer, *Formative Ideas in American Education* (New York: Dodd, Mead, and Co., 1965), p. ix.

2. Samuel Noah Kramer, *History Begins at Sumer* (New York: Doubleday Anchor Books, 1959), p. 62.

3. In German *Krankenschwester* means "sister who cares for the ill." In Russian *medicinskaya sestra,* "medical sister," has been shortened to *medsestra;* and the term for a man in nursing is *medicinski brat,* "medical brother," now shortened to *medbrat.* In Hebrew *ahot* means "sister"; the Serbo-Croatian *medicinska sestra* translates "medical sister"; and, of course, the British "sister."

4. Cecil Woodham-Smith, *Florence Nightingale* (London: Constable & Company, 1950), pp. 294, 316.

5. George Chandler Whipple, *Textbook on Vital Statistics—An Introduction to the Science of Demography* (New York: Wiley, 1923), p. 6.

6. Iago Galdston, *The Meaning of Social Medicine* (Cambridge, Mass.: Harvard University Press, 1954), p. 105.

7. *Nursing and Nursing Education in the United States.* Report of the Committee for the Study of Nursing Education, Josephine Goldmark, Secretary. (New York: Macmillan Co., 1923), *passim.*

8. The committee issued several reports, "Nurses, Patients, and Pocketbooks" (1928), "Nursing Schools Today and Tomorrow" (1934), and "An Activity Analysis of Nursing" (1934), the latter authored by Ethel Johns and Blanche Pfefferkorn.

9. Esther L. Brown, *Nursing for the Future* (New York: Russell Sage Foundation, 1948), *passim.*

10. The Committee on the Function of Nursing, *A Program for the Nursing Profession* (New York: Macmillan Co., 1948), *passim.*

11. National Committee for the Improvement of Nursing Services, *Nursing Schools at the Mid Century* (New York: Osmond-Johnson, 1950), *passim.*

12. Mildred Montag, *Community College Education for Nursing* (New York: McGraw-Hill, 1959), *passim.*

13. Surgeon General's Consultant Group on Nursing, *Toward Quality in Nursing, Needs and Goals* (Washington, D.C.: Government Printing Office, 1963), *passim.*

14. American Nurses' Association, "A Position Paper: Educational Preparation for Nurse Practitioners and Assistants to Nurses," *American Journal of Nursing,* 65 (December 1965) 106–11, p. 107.

15. "Report of the National Commission for the Study of Nursing and Nursing Education," *American Journal of Nursing,* 70 (February 1970) 279–94. (Published under the title of *An Abstract for Action,* New York: McGraw-Hill, 1970).

16. United States Department of Health, Education, and Welfare, *Extending the Scope of Nursing Practice: A Report of the Secretary's Committee To Study Extended Roles for Nurses* (Washington, D.C.: Government Printing Office, November 1971), *passim.*

ADDITIONAL READINGS

Ashley, Jo Ann, "Nursing and Early Feminism," in *American Journal of Nursing,* 75 (September, 1975) 1465-67.

Austin, Anne L., "Wartime Volunteers—1861-1865," in *American Journal of Nursing,* 75 (May 1975) 816-18.

Brainard, A.M., *Evolution of Public Health Nursing.* Philadelphia: W.B. Saunders Co., 1922.

Bullough, Bonnie, and Vern L. Bullough, *The Emergence of Modern Nursing.* New York: Macmillan Co., 1969.

Christy, Teresa, "Portrait of a Leader: Lavinia Lloyd Dock," in *Nursing Outlook,* 17 (June 1969) 72-75.

———, "Portrait of a Leader: Lillian Wald," in *Nursing Outlook,* 18 (March 1970) 50-54.

———, "The Fateful Decade, 1890-1900," in *American Journal of Nursing,* 75 (July 1975) 1163-65.

Dietz, Lena Dixon, and Aurelia R. Lehozky, *History and Modern Nursing.* Philadelphia: F.A. Davis Company, 1967.

Dolan, Josephine A., "Three Schools—1873," in *American Journal of Nursing,* 75 (June, 1975) 989-92.

———, *Nursing in Society: A Historical Perspective.* 13th ed. Philadelphia: W.B. Saunders Co., 1973.

Ehrenreich, B., and D. English, *Witches, Midwives and Nurses—A History of Women Healers.* Old Westbury, N.Y.: Feminist Press, 1973.

Frost, Harriet, *Nursing in Sickness and in Health.* New York: Macmillan Co., 1939.

Gardner, Mary S., *Public Health Nursing.* New York: Macmillan Co., 1936.

Goodrich, Annie W., *The Social and Ethical Significance of Nursing.* New York: Macmillan Co., 1932.

Griffin, G.J., and H.J.K. Griffin, *Jensen's History and Trends of Professional Nursing.* St. Louis: C.V. Mosby Co., 1969.

Hanlon, John J., *Public Health: Administration and Practice.* 6th ed. St. Louis: C.V. Mosby Co., 1974.

Jamieson, Elizabeth, Mary F. Sewall, and Eleanor B. Suhrie, *Trends in Nursing History.* 6th ed. Philadelphia: W.B. Saunders Co., 1966.

Lambertsen, Eleanor C., *Education for Nursing Leadership.* Philadelphia: J.B. Lippincott Co., 1962.

Nightingale, Florence, *Notes on Nursing.* New York: Appleton-Century-Crofts. 1936.

Nutting, M. Adelaide, "Florence Nightingale as a Statistician," in *Public Health Nurse,* 19 (1927) 207-9.

Rawnsley, Marilyn M., "The Goldmark Report: Midpoint in Nursing History," in *Nursing Outlook,* 21 (June 1973) 380-83.

Roberts, Mary, *American Nursing, History and Interpretation,* New York: Macmillan Co., 1954.

Rosen, George, *A History of Public Health,* New York: MD Publications, Inc., 1958.

Selavan, Ida Cohen, "Nurses in American History: The Revolution," *American Journal of Nursing,* 75 (April 1975) 592-94.

Sigerist, Henry E., *A History of Medicine,* New York: Oxford University Press, 1955.

Wald, Lillian, *The House on Henry Street,* New York: Holt, 1915.

———, *Windows on Henry Street.* Boston: Little, Brown and Co., 1934.

Wilner, Daniel M., Rosabelle Price Walkley, and Lenor S. Goerke, *Introduction to Public Health.* 6th ed. New York: Macmillan Co., 1973.

Wolman, Abel, "APHA in Its First Century," in *American Journal of Public Health,* 63 (April 1973) 319-31.

Chapter 2
Health and
Community Health

"If science and education are the brain and nervous system of civilization, health is its heart."[1]

HEALTH

It is difficult, if not almost impossible, to formulate a clear, concise, universally accepted definition of health. What is health and what is illness? In which category do you place the woman with diabetes, regulated by insulin and diet, who leads a normal life as busy mother and homemaker? Or the well-to-do businessman with adequately treated late latent syphilis whose only symptom is a reactive serologic test? Or the successful college student whose epilepsy is carefully controlled by dilantin or valium? Or the man or woman, suffering from alcoholism, who has been rehabilitated to the point where he or she can lead a productive and effective life? It is not easy to measure health in precise, operational terms which lend themselves to the establishment of specific goals and objectives that can be readily evaluated in service programs.

The Constitution of the World Health Organization (WHO) defines health as a "state of complete physical, mental, and social well-being and not merely the absence of disease or infirmity." To be sure, this definition has been severely criticized on the grounds that the state it describes can neither be attained nor measured. However, the WHO statement must be regarded not as a working definition but rather as a broad, philosophical declaration. It was drafted in the 1940s through mutual agreement by leading international health experts who came from countries with widely varying social and political systems. The statement has helped to publicize an expanded concept that emphasizes the social aspects of health and has implications for positive health promotion.

In formulating a more specific and workable concept of health, we must begin with basic assumptions about the individual person, whom we view within the context of a family in a community. Man is an integrated whole, a biopsychosocial being, who attempts to maintain dynamic equilibrium in the midst of constant change. We may look upon the human being in his totality as an "open social system" interacting with his environment in a process of mutual adaptation (see Chapter 4). He tries to achieve a state of equilibrium that would permit him to function to his fullest potential, reasonably free of undue pain, discomfort, disability, or limitation of activity. Health may be regarded as a person's physical and psychological capacity to establish and maintain this balance. According to Dubos, health or disease are expressions of the success or failure a person experiences in his efforts to respond adaptively to environmental challenges.[2] Therefore, health, as a concept, is best described in relative terms, and may be viewed along a wellness–illness continuum.

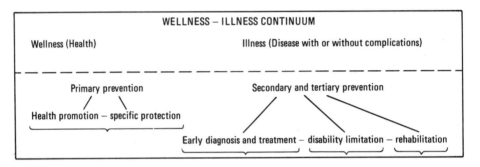

Figure 2-1   Wellness–illness continuum.

Figure 2–1 demonstrates that it is possible to consider the application of various levels of prevention in the maintenance of health and control of disease. Sometimes they are referred to as primary, secondary, and tertiary prevention. Primary prevention measures are those that actively promote optimum health and prevent illness. Secondary and tertiary preventive measures are those which are applied after an illness or disabling condition has occurred. (See Table 2–1.) In differentiating between the last two levels, we might view secondary prevention as consisting of case finding, early diagnosis, treatment, and prevention of complications of illness. Limitation of disability could be considered secondary or tertiary prevention; tertiary prevention also includes rehabilitation as illustrated in Figure 2–2. Leavell and Clark identify five levels of prevention as follows: health promotion, specific protection, early recognition and treatment, disability limitation, and rehabilitation.[3] In looking at these, we see that health promotion and specific protection

Table 2-1   Examples of Preventive Measures

Disease or Condition	Before disease or condition occurs: measures of primary prevention	After disease or condition occurs: measures of secondary and tertiary prevention
Pertussis Diphtheria Tetanus Smallpox Poliomyelitis Measles German measles Mumps	For each of these diseases there are safe, specific, effective measures to produce artificial active immunity.	Early diagnosis and prompt treatment, isolation of contacts where indicated, prevention and/or treatment of complications, restorative and rehabilitative measures.
Diabetes	Genetic counseling, weight control, control of stressful situations.	Early diagnosis, prompt treatment, instructions for administering insulin, nutrition counseling, prevention of infections, care of skin and toenails, self-management in altered life style, emotional support for good mental hygiene.
Rheumatic fever	Maintenance of good general health and nutrition, treatment of predisposing streptococcal infections, prophylactic treatment of contacts.	Early diagnosis and prompt treatment to prevent cardiovascular-renal complications, nutrition counseling, health teaching regarding activities of daily living, postoperative rehabilitation (if heart surgery performed).
Hypertension	Nutrition education, control of stress, regular medical checkup, avoidance of smoking.	Early diagnosis and treatment, antihypertensive medication where indicated, self-management in altered life style, adherence to prescribed dietary regimen, restorative and rehabilitative measures for late manifestations and complications.
Syphilis	Health education, family living and sex education, treatment of pregnant syphilitic women to prevent congenital syphilis, investigation of contacts with treatment where necessary.	Early diagnosis and prompt treatment, case finding and follow-up of patients and contacts, prevention and/or treatment of manifestations of late syphilis (e.g., blindness, heart disease, central nervous system involvement), rehabilitation of patient with late symptomatic syphilis.

correspond to primary prevention; early recognition, treatment, and disability limitation to secondary prevention; and disability limitation and rehabilitation to tertiary prevention.

The effects of specific preventive measures can be demonstrated in controlled epidemiological investigations (for example, the Salk vaccine field trials). It is easy enough to show the results of preventive measures in certain communicable diseases, such as diphtheria and smallpox—we need only com-

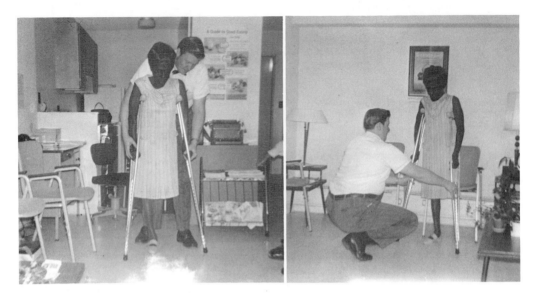

Figure 2-2 Tertiary prevention. A public health nurse instructs a patient following amputation in the correct handling of crutches for optimum mobility and independence.

Source Courtesy of the Community Nursing Service of Chester and Vicinity, Chester, Pennsylvania.

pare disease and death rates today with similar rates at some other point in time. However, the effects of specific preventive measures are not always readily demonstrable. The application of prevention, especially in long-term illness, is often an elusive matter, and results may be difficult to evaluate.

Consequently, it is not always easy to obtain support for public programs aimed at prevention. Similarly, individuals may not be readily persuaded to accept preventive measures. Indeed, you may devote considerable time and energy in planning, preparing, and organizing individual or community health education for prevention without receiving the acknowledgment or recognition that you might get for applying some simple palliative measure.

Example

In the hospital you are assigned to take care of Mr. K., a weary, obese, hypertensive patient who is lying in bed complaining of back pain. He is relieved by a soothing wintergreen rub, which you expertly administer. You have alleviated his discomfort, he is grateful to you, and you have the satisfaction of a job well done. Now Mr. K. has gone home, and you are out in the community, making a home visit to follow up with preventive measures, to do some additional diet teaching, or to invite him to a weight control class. However, he feels well now, and he does not see how any of these measures apply to him; he fails to respond to your efforts at prevention.

How do you evaluate the results of preventive measures? Can you always tell whether, and to what degree, the specific measures you applied have kept a person free of illness? How does that person feel about measures which you apply? To evaluate the efficacy of prevention, the nurse should document her activity with sound statistical data that must include some detailed description of individual cases. The following situation will serve as an illustration.

Example

A nurse was assigned to provide primary health care and to direct a new health maintenance unit in a low-rent, subsidized housing project for the elderly (Figure 2–3). She concentrated on health promotion and disease prevention. After six months she submitted her progress report. She was able to show a growth in the quantity of service through an increased number of clinic visits and home visits, the introduction of group teaching sessions (e.g., on nutrition, control of emphysema, weight control), and the implementation of screening programs (for hearing loss, diabetes, tuberculosis). But how could she show results in the quality of service? In order to do this, she selected specific cases which illustrated her nursing actions. One such case involved a seventy-two-year-old man, whom she heard about soon after the unit opened. This elderly gentleman had spent four weeks in the hospital recovering from a myocardial infarction. Upon discharge, he came home with medication and a copy of a special diet, but with little understanding of either. Furthermore, he lived alone with no friends or relatives nearby, and he slipped into a "post-hospital depression." The nurse called on him to explain the service that was available, and to let him know that she was there to help him. After careful interviewing of the patient and further checking with the physician, she was able to devise a teaching plan to help the patient understand his diet and medication. Before this, he had been quite alone, with no one to turn to. In his state of mind, he probably would have neglected to take his medications or adhere to his diet, and almost certainly would have had to be rehospitalized. The therapeutic intervention and encouragement of the nurse practitioner led the patient to take an active interest in the maintenance of his health. Slowly, his condition improved and he was able to continue to function independently without further deterioration.

The concept of prevention is not new; it has been a recognized part of public health practice for many decades. Recently, it has received renewed attention with the expanded definition of health, and with the growing concern

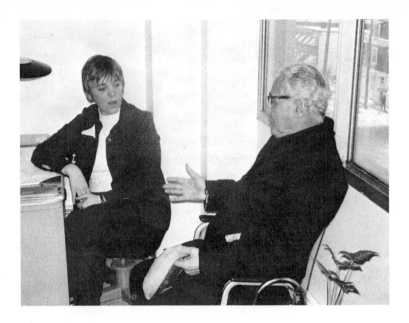

Figure 2-3 Community health nurse counseling a client in a low-rent, subsidized housing project for the elderly.

Source Courtesy of the Community Nursing Service of Chester and Vicinity, Chester, Pennsylvania.

over health care in our nation. Up to now, it has gained only limited acceptance in our total health care system, which, dominated by the medical profession, is steeped in the tradition of curative or therapeutic medicine. Physicians and nurses, unless they have acquired an understanding of health in its broadest sense, often feel more at ease in the curative rather than the preventive realm of practice. And yet, all health practitioners, for now and the future, are expected to develop an appreciation of preventive care and an awareness of health maintenance measures.

COMMUNITY HEALTH

The broad definition of public health, formulated many years ago by Winslow, has withstood the test of time and can be applied to the contemporary scene where it is receiving renewed attention under the designation of community health.

Public health is the science and art of (1) preventing disease, (2) prolonging life, and (3) promoting health and efficiency through organized community effort for (a) the sanitation of the environment, (b) the control of communicable infections, (c) the education of the individual in personal hygiene, (d) the

28

organization of medical and nursing services for the early diagnosis and preventive treatment of disease, and (e) the development of the social machinery to insure everyone a standard of living adequate for the maintenance of health so organizing these benefits as to enable every citizen to realize his birthright of health and longevity. [4]

Hanlon stresses the "multifaceted relationships" of health and public health as follows:

Health is a state of total effective physiologic and psychologic functioning; it has both a relative and an absolute meaning, varying through time and space, in both the individual and in the group; it is the result of the combination of many forces, intrinsic and extrinsic, inherited and contrived, individual and collective, private and public, medical, environmental, and social; and it is conditioned by culture and economy, and by law and government.

Accordingly:

Public health is dedicated to the common attainment of the highest level of physical, mental, and social well-being and longevity consistent with available knowledge and resources at a given time and place. It holds this goal as its contribution to the most effective total development and life of the individual and his society. [5]

The concept of community health was neatly summed up in the title of a book that appeared some years ago, *Public Health Is People.*[6] It means working together to help people help themselves, not to merely survive but to achieve their maximum potential. It is no longer a matter of simply increasing the number of years a person lives, without regard to improving the quality of life. Dr. Paul Purdom, in his presidential address to the American Public Health Association in 1971, cited the following four priorities in public health:

(1) survival of the human species;
(2) prevention of conditions which lead to destruction or retardation of human function and potential in the early years of life;
(3) achievement of human potential and prevention of the loss of productivity of young adults and those in the middle period of life; and
(4) improvement of the quality of life, especially in later years. [7]

In public health practice, the whole community, or a designated component of it, is the "patient." Assessment of the "patient" requires the skills of many different disciplines—nursing, medicine, social work, nutrition, engineering, and others—functioning together as a team. Lines of communication must be kept open. The community health practitioner studies the community, makes a diagnosis and attempts to apply control measures at strategic points. In so doing, he must deal with health problems as well as public problems related to the health problems, examples of which are shown in Table 2-2.

Table 2-2 Examples of Health Problems and Causally Related Public Problems

Health problems	Public problems
Air pollution in cities and industrial centers.	(a) Industries' complaints of high costs to develop pollution control measures, with concomitant loss of corporate profits; (b) lack of public interest for the development of good mass transportation and for the voluntary curtailment of individual automobile use.
Increase in venereal disease incidence and prevalence.	Public attitudes, which, on one hand, condone increasing permissiveness regarding sexual relations but, on the other hand, brand venereal disease with the stigma of immoral behavior, thereby encouraging its victims to conceal their problem and go untreated or delay treatment.
Lead poisoning.	High lead content paint in poorly kept old housing units.
Poor prenatal health related to numerous too-frequent pregnancies.	Religious, political, cultural, and ethnic barriers to the dissemination and acceptance of birth control measures.
Heart disease in the early middle years.	Difficulties involved in attempting to change total life styles in an affluent society—high-cholesterol diets, lack of exercise, use or abuse of alcohol and tobacco, tension in every day living, etc.
Chronic obstructive lung disease; cancer of the lung.	General approval of smoking as a socially acceptable habit; advertising campaigns depicting smoking as a pleasurable activity.
Alcoholism.	Acceptance of drinking as a social amenity.
Arthritis.	Lack of information about the disease.
Drug abuse.	Proliferation of drug advertising through the mass media.

The community health practitioner, in attempting to solve these problems, uses knowledge from the natural sciences and the social sciences. (See Figure 2–4.)

REFERENCES

1. Raymond B. Fosdick, *The Story of the Rockefeller Foundation* (New York: Harper and Brothers, 1952), p. 23.

2. Rene Dubos, *Man Adapting* (New Haven, Conn: Yale University Press, 1965), p. xvii.

3. Hugh R. Leavell and E. Gurney Clark, *Preventive Medicine for the Doctor in His Community,* 3rd ed. (New York: McGraw-Hill, 1965), p. 27.

4. C.-E.A. Winslow, "The Untilled Field of Public Health," *Modern Medicine,* 2 (March 1920) 183.

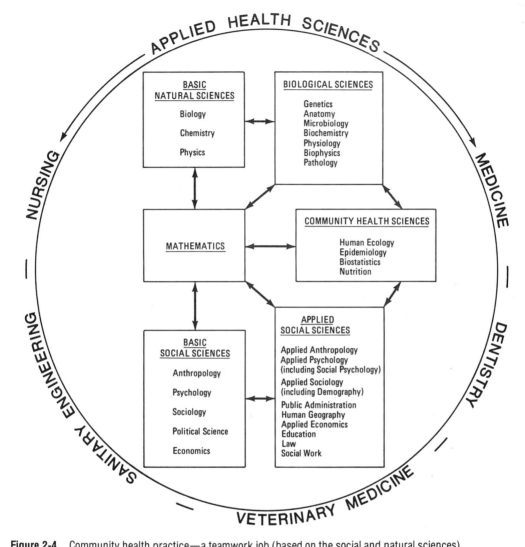

Figure 2-4   Community health practice—a teamwork job (based on the social and natural sciences).

Source   Adapted from Hugh R. Leavell and E. Gurney Clark, Preventive Medicine for the Doctor in his Community, 3rd ed. (New York: McGraw-Hill Book Co., 1965), p. 614. By permission of the publisher.

5. John J. Hanlon, *Principles of Public Health Administration,* 5th ed. (St. Louis: C.V. Mosby Co., 1969), pp. 23–24.

6. Ethel Ginsburg, *Public Health Is People* (New York: The Commonwealth Fund, 1950), *passim.*

7. Paul Purdom, "The Shape of a National Health Program," *American Journal of Public Health,* 62 (January 1972) 12–15.

ADDITIONAL READINGS

Anderson, C. L., *Community Health.* 2nd ed. St. Louis: C. V. Mosby, Co., 1973.

Apple, Dorrian, *Sociological Studies of Health and Sickness.* New York: McGraw Hill, 1960.

Breslow, I., "Research in a Strategy for Health Improvement," in *International Journal of Health Service,* 3 (Winter 1973) 7–16.

Burton, Lloyd E., and Hugh H. Smith, *Public Health and Community Medicine.* Baltimore: Williams and Wilkins, 1970.

Dubos, Rene, *So Human an Animal.* New York: Charles Scribner's Sons, 1968.

Duff, Raymond S., and August B. Hollingshead, *Sickness and Society.* New York: Harper and Row, 1968.

Dunn, Halbert L., *High-Level Wellness.* Washington D. C. : Mount Vernon Printing Co., 1961.

Folta, Jeanette, and Edith S. Deck, *A Sociological Framework for Patient Care.* New York: Wiley, 1966.

Freeman, Howard, S. Levine, and G. Reeder, *Handbook of Medical Sociology.* Englewood Cliffs, N. J.: Prentice Hall, 1963.

Gordon, Gerald O., *Role Theory and Illness: A Sociological Perspective.* New Haven, Conn.: College and University Press, 1966.

Grant, Murray, *Handbook of Preventive Medicine and Public Health.* Philadelphia: Lea and Febiger, 1967.

Hart, Sylvia, "An Overview of Health-Health: A Conceptual Model." As reported in *Maintaining Health, An Adventure in Transition* (proceedings of the Fourth Mid-Atlantic Regional Conference) Mid-Atlantic Regional Assembly, National League for Nursing, New York, 1972.

Jaco, E. Gartley, ed. *Patients, Physicians and Illness.* 2nd ed. New York: The Free Press, 1972.

Katz, Alfred H., and Jean Felton, *Health and the Community.* New York: The Free Press, 1965.

Kluckholn, Clyde, *Mirror for Man.* New York: McGraw-Hill, 1949.

Mechanic, David, *Medical Sociology: A Selective View.* New York: The Free Press, 1968.

Paul, Benjamin, *Health, Culture, and the Community.* New York: Russell Sage Foundation, 1965.

Polgar, Steven, "Health and Human Behavior: Areas of Interest Common to the Social and Medical Sciences," in *Current Anthropology,* 3 (April 1962) 159–205.

Rogers, Martha, *An Introduction to the Theoretical Basis of Nursing.* Philadelphia: F. A. Davis, 1970.

Sartwell, Philip E., ed., *Maxcy-Rosenau Preventive Medicine and Public Health.* 10th ed. New York: Appleton-Century-Crofts, 1973.

Sellew, Gladys, *Sociology and Its Use in Nursing Service.* 5th ed. Philadelphia: W. B. Saunders Co., 1965.

Skipper, James K., Jr., and Robert C. Leonard, *Social Interaction and Patient Care.* Philadelphia: J. B. Lippincott Co., 1965.

Spero, Jeanette R., "An Overview of Health-Health: A Community Regional Conference) Mid-Atlantic Regional Assembly, National League for Nursing, New York, 1972.

Wilner, Daniel M., Rosabelle Price Walkley, and Lenor S. Goerke, *Introduction to Public Health.* 6th ed. New York: Macmillan Co., 1973.

Chapter 3
Community Health Nursing

"The role of the nurse cannot remain static—it must change along with that of all other health professionals, which means that the knowledge and skills of nurses need to be broadened."[1]

INTRODUCTION

Nursing is a universal response to a human need. The essence of nursing is caring. Nursing began because somebody cared. Somebody had compassion for his fellow human being. The word *nurse* itself has come down to the present by way of Middle English, through Old French, from the original Latin (feminine of *nutritius* or 'nourishing'). The concept of caring has been reiterated officially by the American Nurses' Association in the 1965 Position Paper, which identified the three essential components of nursing as care, cure, and coordination (see page 18).

Traditionally, nurses have been prepared in sick-care settings. The image of the nurse in the hospital as the provider of care, the "ministering angel of mercy," is worldwide. But what about the nurse who works in the community, outside of the institutional setting, the nurse whose primary focus is family and community health, and whose basic concern is health maintenance, health promotion, and prevention of illness? You might like to conduct an interesting little experiment. Select eight or ten nonnurse friends, relatives, neighbors, or acquaintances, and pose any of the following questions: "What is a public health nurse?" "What does a community health nurse do?" "What are some of the settings outside the hospital where nursing is performed?" Try it on yourself. Before you came into nursing how much did you know about the nurse in the community? Do you remember ever having received service from a public health nurse? If so, do you recall any of your impressions?

Another revealing experience is the reaction you get when you ask someone from a foreign country to give you the word in their language for public health nurse. Usually they know the word for "nurse who works in a hospital or clinic," but hesitate when they try to express the term for "nurse who works in the community," "public health nurse," "visiting nurse," or "district nurse." This is true in spite of the fact that in most of the developed countries, and even in some of the lesser developed countries, public health nursing is well established and highly esteemed, often having greater prestige than nursing in the hospital.

What does all of this signify? For one thing, it may signify that while we may understand among ourselves what we mean by public health nursing, community health nursing, or, for that matter, the newly coined terms—*"nurse practitioner," "family nurse practitioner," "pediatric nurse practitioner"*—we have not been wholly successful in communicating these various roles to the public. Public health nursing[2] has been an integral part of health care delivery service for decades and yet, outside of professional circles, many people are not fully aware of its unique role and contribution.

WHAT IS COMMUNITY HEALTH NURSING?

How, then, might we describe community health nursing? The American Nurses' Association, Division on Community Health Nursing Practice, in formulating a definition, has made the following statement:

> Community health nursing is a synthesis of nursing practice and public health practice applied to promoting and preserving the health of populations. The nature of this practice is general and comprehensive. It is not limited to a particular age or diagnostic group. It is continuing, not episodic. The dominant responsibility is to the population as a whole. Therefore, nursing directed to individuals, families or groups contributes to the health of the total population. Health promotion, health maintenance, health education, coordination and continuity of care are utilized in a holistic approach to the family, group and community. The nurse's actions acknowledge the need for comprehensive health planning, recognize the influences of social and ecological issues, give attention to populations at risk and utilize the dynamic forces which influence change.[3]

This statement summarizes the following concepts of community health nursing practice, also issued by the ANA:[4]

> (1) The primary focus of community health nursing practice is on health promotion. The community health nurse has a greater contact with people who are seeking health care—to "reach" the community—and has more opportunity and responsibility for evaluating the health status of such persons and groups and relating them to practice.
>
> (2) Although the primary concern and initial contact with a family may be with

or in relation to an individual, community health nursing practice is extended to benefit the whole family and community.

(3) The community health nurse is a generalist in terms of her practice throughout life's continuum—its full range of health problems and needs.

(4) Contact with patient and/or family may continue over a long period of time—include all ages and all types of health care.

(5) The nature of community health nursing practice requires that current knowledge derived from the biological and social sciences, ecology, clinical nursing, and community organization be utilized.

(6) The dynamic nursing process of assessing, planning, implementing and intervening, periodic measurements of progress, evaluation, and a continuum of the cycle until termination of nursing is implicit in the practice of community health nursing.

While we still speak of nursing in hospitals, nursing in community health, and nursing in other settings, the National Commission for the Study of Nursing and Nursing Education has set forth a description of career patterns for nursing in accordance with the goals rather than the setting where it takes place. Two career patterns are identified—episodic and distributive (see page 20). Community health nurses are essentially concerned with distributive practice.[5]

The health of the community is the major goal of nursing in public health. In community health practice, the nurse focuses on the individual as a member of a family unit, and thereby offers a family-centered service. (See Figure 3-1.) Nursing has an invaluable contribution to offer at all levels of prevention—it goes beyond the purely physical problems of patients, and attends to the psychosocial needs of individuals and families. The public health nurse, through her unique relationship with families, is usually accepted by them as a supportive, helpful person to whom they can turn in times of stress and difficulty. She is the liaison between the family and the community with all of its resources.

The nurse working in the community is removed from the formalized structure of the therapeutic institution. She is called upon to exercise independent judgment and take action on her own initiative without the built-in network of supervision available to the hospital nurse. As a practitioner of nursing the community health nurse must test and evaluate various concepts and theories drawn from behavioral sciences, microbiology, physics, chemistry, and economics to devise a framework for action. Data must be collected and systematized to formulate the health and social profile. On the basis of this profile, family health problems are defined, priorities are set, and a nursing care plan is developed. Implementation of this plan is based on (1) the nurse's ability to coordinate needed services through direct care and/or appropriate referral to community agencies; and (2) the family's ability to understand the need for the plan and their willingness to participate in achieving the health goals (see units 4 and 5).

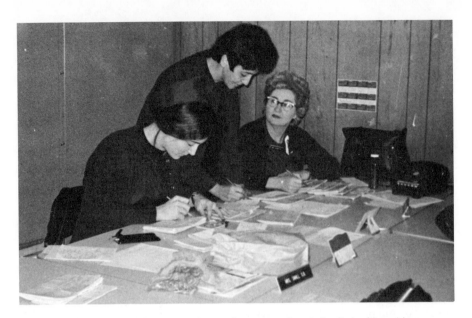

Figure 3-1 Staff nurses in a community nursing agency discuss family health problems.

Source Courtesy of the Community Nursing Service of Chester and Vicinity, Chester, Pennsylvania.

Essential to the establishment of a sound working relationship between the nurse and the family are a basic sense of trust and mutual respect. In actuality, although there is no written agreement, a contractual arrangement exists between the nurse and the family, just as there is a general contract between society as a whole and the nursing profession. Society permits a fair amount of autonomy and in return the profession is expected to act responsibly. In the individual case, the family will have certain expectations of the nurse by virtue of her professional education, her license to practice, the agency's policies, and her expertise and personal interest. How this is expressed will depend on the nurse's interpretation of her role and the family's ability to comprehend what the nurse can do. The nurse has certain expectations of the family which are determined by our culture, by the individual family's capability for coping, its socioeconomic and educational background, and other factors. The nature of the contract may differ from family to family, but in each case, the contract must be mutually acceptable to the family and to the nurse for nursing intervention to be successful.

THE NURSE PRACTITIONER—EXPANDING/EXTENDING THE NURSING ROLE

It is essential to point out that the term *nurse practitioner* has taken on a special meaning in contemporary nursing practice. The expression has come to imply an "expansion" or "extension" of the traditional nursing role. The

Commission on Nursing Education of the American Nurses' Association has described the responsibilities of the Nurse Practitioner referred to in the Nurse Training Act of 1971.[6] According to the ANA, the term Nurse Practitioner refers to one who has completed a program of study leading to competence as a registered nurse in an expanded role whose responsibility encompasses:

(1) Obtaining a health history;

(2) Assessing health–illness status;

(3) Entering a person into the health care system;

(4) Sustaining and supporting persons who are impaired, infirm, ill and during programs of diagnosis and therapy;

(5) Managing a medical care regimen for acute and chronically ill patients within established standing orders;

(6) Aiding in restoring persons to wellness and maximum function;

(7) Teaching and counseling persons about health and illness;

(8) Supervising and managing care regimens of normal pregnant women;

(9) Helping parents in guidance of children with a view to their optimal physical and emotional development;

(10) Counseling and supporting persons with regard to the aging process;

(11) Aiding people and their survivors during the dying process; and

(12) Supervising assistants to nurses.

In reviewing these skills, one finds that they have long been incorporated into nursing practice. The extent to which they have been accepted as part of nursing (by the nurse, by others on the health team, and/or by the public) has often depended on time and place as well as on the individual nurse and how she perceives her role. Nursing in hospitals and institutions, by nature of its setting, has been more strictly limited than nursing in the community. Nurses in public health agencies, as is pointed out in the Report of the Secretary's Committee to Study Extended Roles for Nurses,

> . . . have traditionally functioned relatively independently, but with physician collaboration, in patients' homes, in remote, isolated rural and ghetto areas, and more recently in clinics, hospitals, and community care centers where they have: assessed problems of individuals and families; treated minor illnesses; referred patients for differential medical diagnosis; arranged for referrals to social service agencies and organizations; given advice and counsel to promote health and prevent illness; supervised health regimens of normal pregnant women and of children; and worked with health-related community action programs.[7]

Traditionally the established public health nursing system includes those nurses who are employed in health departments or other official agencies, visiting nurse associations or other voluntary health agencies, combined official and voluntary agencies, as well as school health and occupational health programs. In many of these programs, nurses have always functioned relatively independently in a way that corresponds to the current concept of the "expanded" or "extended" role. In recent years numerous health programs have been created outside the established public health nursing system, for example, health maintenance organizations (HMOs), neighborhood health centers, home care services, emergency health programs, and others (see chapter 11). In quite a few of these programs, a major input has come from nursing in an expanded role and as the source of primary health care. Nurses have moved in as primary care practitioners, and have assumed responsibility for family health care in a variety of settings, for example, the Cambridge-Council clinics, Idaho; the Terrace Village Health Center, Pittsburgh; the Thacher Project, Albany; the Harvard Community Health Plan, Boston; and others.[8, 9, 10, 11] In these situations, nursing has forged ahead in many ways that had been envisioned, and, indeed, practiced in an earlier day. The "expanded" role of the nurse, while it is receiving wide attention as something innovative, is not really new. An outstanding example of a well-established and ongoing program is the Frontier Nursing Service of Kentucky, in existence over fifty years, where the nurse has always been accepted as the primary care practitioner.[12]

Situations requiring the expanded role of the nurse are challenging and stimulating. A recent graduate of a collegiate nursing program, writing to the Dean of her alma mater, describes her whole new way of life. After working for several years in a large city hospital in New England, during which time she had taken a course preparing her to be a geriatrics nurse practitioner, she accepted a position as a nurse practitioner in a rural setting of Appalachia. She writes as follows:

Dear Dean,

Greetings from down here in the hill country! The _____ Health Program consists of three clinics in a county of 5500 people. There are four practicing physicians at the far end of the county. _____ _____ Clinic with X-Ray, EKG, and laboratory facilities is the main branch. The other two clinics are located in small renovated homes. The nurse practitioners handle all sorts of problems, taking calls on weekends. We are called out all the time, at all hours, for all sorts of problems. At times it has been necessary for us to perform the tasks of X-Ray, EKG, and laboratory technicians. In addition, we are expected to be able to identify, through nursing assessment, conditions such as congestive heart failure, pneumonia, hepatitis, digitalis toxicity, sprains, strains, pregnancy, otitis media, upper respiratory infections, etc. It's a fun game, but it's no game—a myocardial infarction always manages to slip in—so far we have been fortunate enough to recognize the symptoms before complications set in.

We have hopes of getting a lot more involved with community action things, but with the limited number of staff it's difficult. To start with, we are teaching two American Red Cross Basic First Aid Classes—one to a group of eighteen Girl Scouts, the other to a group of six adults, including the two local ambulance drivers.

By the way, this handsome, stylish stationery is from the X-Ray film coverings—that's all I can find down here so I acquired a bunch, cut it, and began writing. I'm roughing it too—my outside shower makes the mornings even crisper. My oil stove is broken—I've rigged up all sorts of strings to keep the oil flowing into it. My mother says that Tom, my brother, has it softer in Alaska—I think she's right.

Peace,

Linda

NURSING AS A SOCIAL AND POLITICAL FORCE

"More than they realize, nurses are respected as caring and giving professionals. The nursing profession, historically, has taken positions more socially valid than other health professions."[13] As an example, nurses were among the first to require racial integration in their professional organization. Similarly they took a stand in favor of health insurance, financed through Social Security legislation, for the disabled, retired, and aged as early as 1958. Nevertheless, nurses, as a whole, have not been very aggressive in creating social change. Indeed, patterns of training in earlier generations encouraged passive roles. Nursing, however, has taken on a new look in recent years.

As the largest single group of health-care providers, nurses today are beginning to recognize their potential for wielding tremendous political force. Nurses now are encouraged more than ever before to take an active role and become involved in community problems. Helping patients and families find their way through our complex health care delivery system has become a major responsibility of the nurse. The nurse serves as the patient's advocate, and must learn to speak out, to knock on doors, to write letters, to become interested and active in civic affairs, and to never let up until the needs are met. Nursing is not a nine-to-five job. The modern community health nurse can be inspired by the work of those exceptional, dedicated, and creative nurses of an earlier day—Florence Nightingale, Lillian Wald, Lavinia Dock, Mary Breckinridge. Dynamic, energetic, demanding, and persuasive in their approach, they have all made a lasting mark on society.

The concept of the "nurse as a change agent" has gained widespread recognition. Even in their beginning experiences in nursing school, students can seek and use opportunities to help bring about desired change in a community. For example, in a liberal arts college located on the borderline of a poverty area, some nursing students participated in health teaching and follow-up of families in the community. They became greatly concerned about the fact that through lack of funding, health services had been discontinued to the elderly residents in a federally subsidized, low-rental housing unit (the "Towers"). Looking for some way to be of help, they sought guidance from members of the faculty and other nurses active in the community. They then proceeded to arm themselves with facts, and they wrote letters to the local newspaper and to leaders in the community. One of these letters is presented, in part, as follows:

Dear Editor:

I am writing to express my concern over the discontinuation of nursing service at the Towers. I first became familiar with the Towers and its health maintenance unit early last fall. As part of our curriculum, we were encouraged to become involved in the program for the elderly. This we did, participating in home visits to Towers residents, observing the walk-in clinic, and assisting with the screening and health teaching programs.

Through our contact with the Towers program, we gained an appreciation of the valuable contribution made by the nursing and social services to Towers residents as well as the community at large. By making available to these people an easily accessible source of health counseling, the nursing service was able to help avoid medical crises and hospitalizations. The value of the Towers nursing service goes beyond the health maintenance of its residents. It provides a feeling of emotional security to these senior citizens, who know that there is a "place to turn" for comfort and guidance for any problem.

Unfortunately, only a year after its inception, and despite a thoroughly documented record of success, the Towers nursing service has been discontinued due to a cutback of federal funding. In expressing my concern to you, it is my hope that you will bring this matter to the attention of other members of the community and initiate appropriate action in an attempt to find some source of funding to continue this primary health care program.

Shortly thereafter the students were gratified to learn that their action had borne fruit. Funds were made available, the service was resumed, and the students were credited with helping to educate the community to bring about desired change. A valuable lesson was learned, namely, the importance of mobilizing reasoned and informed collective action to put pressure on the community's power structure. In this way they gained an awareness of the need for community health nurses to be knowledgeable, articulate, and able to act within the political system. They also reaped the satisfaction of having waged a successful campaign to bring about change.

One of the major consequences of the emerging emphasis on "extending" or "expanding" the nursing role is the need to review and reform present Nurse Practice Acts. In many states existing laws do not reflect current nursing practice and often pose legal barriers. Efforts to create new legislation require the interest, support, and participation of all nurses. A united nursing profession can be a powerful political force to bring about change, as illustrated in Figure 3–2, when over 3500 nurses marched to the state capitol in Harrisburg, Pennsylvania, in 1973. Individually and collectively they demonstrated their support for the passage of a new Nurse Practice Act, designed in response to the contemporary health needs of the citizens of the Commonwealth. Nurses, singly and in groups, called on their legislators, many of whom expressed their appreciation. One of them, a young woman serving her first term in the House of Representatives, commented to the nurse who called on her, "Your mass demonstration as well as your personal visit to my office have convinced me to vote favorably on this issue. Without such action, I

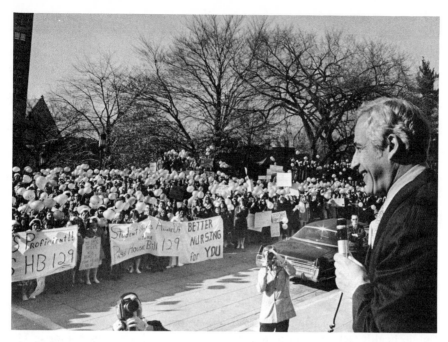

Figure 3-2 Pennsylvania nurses march on the state capitol in Harrisburg, December 1973. Collective action by Pennsylvania nurses effectively influenced political action by state legislators for passage of H.B. 129, modernizing the Nurse Practice Act. Nursing students played a prominent role in this demonstration.

Source Reproduced with permission of the Pennsylvania Nurses Association. Photographer: Ed Hoffman, Capitol Films.

might have voted against the bill, because the mail I received was sparse, and, what I did get, expressed opposition to the proposed law. You are to be congratulated on such an effective show of collective action.'' The bill was voted on and passed by the State House of Representatives that day.

NURSING MANPOWER

The American Nurses' Association 1972 Inventory of Registered Nurses estimated that there were 1,127,657 registered nurses in the United States. Of these, about 800,000 were employed, with a ratio of 380 nurses per 100,000 population.[14] Although the number of men actively engaged in nursing has grown, only 1.4 percent of employed registered nurses were men. The median age of employed nurses was 39.4 years old, which represents a slight decline from 39.8 in 1966.[15]

According to the 1972 Inventory, the overall number of nurses, the percentage of nurses who are actively employed, and the ratio of nurses to the population consistently increased over the last two decades. Why, then, do we continue to hear about a nursing shortage? The above figures do not reveal the total picture—for example, they do not take into account the factors related to the maldistribution of nurse supply. Some states greatly exceed the national average; others fall far below—Massachusetts, Vermont, and the District of Columbia have over 600 nurses per 100,000 population, while Arkansas has less than 200.[16]

A major drain on the nursing manpower supply is caused by many nurses withdrawing from their profession each year. "At any given time, almost two out of every four nurses in the United States are totally inactive. Of those who are working, almost one out of three is a part-time nurse. Thus, we can begin to see why we have a shortage of nurses to provide direct patient care at the same time that we do not truly have a shortage of nurses in the literal sense."[17] There is a need for a greater number of active, dedicated, inspired, and creative nurses, who are willing to devote themselves to improving the health care of the people and to strengthening the nursing profession.

Hospitals continue as the predominant place of employment for registered nurses—nearly two-thirds of all employed nurses work in hospitals. Public health, school health, and occupational health nurses comprise 11.5 percent of the total number of employed nurses.[18] The number of nurses employed in public health agencies has risen. With continued population growth, increasing availability of public and private health insurance coverage, growing consumer involvement, and the movement of care out of the hospital into the community, we can expect an increased demand for nursing manpower in community health.

NURSING EDUCATION

Nursing education today, just as education in general, is in a state of ferment. Many schools throughout the country are experimenting with new approaches, as for example, offering individualized experiences, recognizing past achievements, granting transfer credits or offering challenge examinations, and setting up revised curricula in response to current problems. Efforts are being made to recruit more men. Special projects have been initiated to encourage, assist, counsel, and tutor disadvantaged students.

Increasing emphasis is being placed on the need for continuing education in nursing. There are many who feel that it should be mandatory for relicensure though others are opposed to the compulsory element and feel that it has a place in nursing, but only on a voluntary basis.

Most nurses practicing today are graduates of hospital schools of nursing, that is, diploma schools. Collegiate nursing programs include both the two-year (junior college) associate degree program and the four-year baccalaureate program. The greatest growth in nursing education has been in the associate degree program, where the enrollments have multiplied more than 17 times from 3,860 in 1961 to 67,543 in 1972. Enrollments in baccalaureate programs more than tripled the 1961 total of 22,546 so that in 1972 with 73,890, they had more students than either of the other two types of programs. Diploma program enrollments have decreased from 96,606 in 1961 to 71,694 in 1972.[19]

NURSING RESEARCH

Nursing today stands at the threshold of fulfilling its responsibility as a scientific discipline with respect to conducting research. Systematic inquiries into the study of nursing as a profession, or nursing education, or attitudes of nurses, or economic problems, were made even in the early days of modern nursing. However, only recently have nurses been accorded recognition and support for the basic premise that their unique field of inquiry is problems in patient care. The issue has been crystallized in the report of the National Commission for the Study of Nursing and Nursing Education, which calls for greater support for research efforts, such as the one shown in Figure 3-3, to determine the "relative effectiveness of various forms of nursing intervention, and the impact of particular innovations in nursing practice."

In nursing research, one must pose the question, "what are the kinds of things that nurses do that make a difference for patients?" The current demand is for research in nursing practice in clinical settings. Diers points out that although it is difficult to study nursing problems in so complicated a place as a hospital, an outpatient service, an agency, office, or community, it is nevertheless possible to do good clinical research if " . . . one is deeply enough involved in practice to know what can be controlled and how. The real blending of research knowledge and practice skill occurs in the field, not in the research office."[20]

Example

To illustrate this "real blending of research knowledge and practice skill" occurring in the field, we can describe the experience of two senior students in a baccalaureate program who became intensely interested in a young paraplegic patient with severe decubitus ulcers. The ulcers, which had not responded to any previous treatment, were so debilitating that the young man could not be accepted for enrollment in a vocational rehabilitation program. One of the students had worked with this patient and his family during her clinical assignment in a community nursing agency. Realizing that rehabilitation plans would be delayed until the ulcers healed, she sought guidance from her instructor and consulted with staff nurses at the agency. At that time staff members were doing

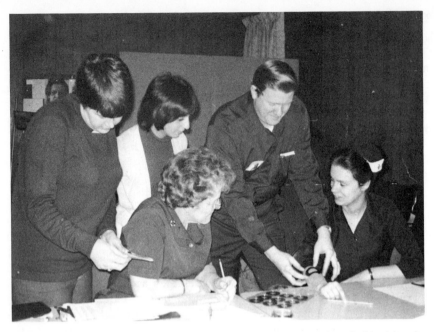

Figure 3-3 A group of staff nurses collaborate in an agency research project to determine the effectiveness of a new treatment.

Source Courtesy of the Community Nursing Service of Chester and Vicinity, Chester, Pennsylvania.

preliminary work with the testing of the karaya gum treatment regimen for decubitus ulcers (Figure 3-3). The student and one of her fellow classmates, in collaboration with the staff nurses and with the approval of the medical advisory board, set up a plan of treatment with the cooperation of the patient and his family. The treatment, which was based on findings reported in nursing literature, soon began to show encouraging results. Within six months, the ulcers had healed to the point where the patient was again evaluated for a rehabilitation program, and a date was set for his admission to the program.

A research problem always begins with perception of a discrepancy between two states of affairs—an uncomfortable feeling about things as they are, rather than as they could be or should be, and thus demands study of the operative factors in the situation. The problems that will result in really relevant research will begin with observations in practice. Research forces one to consciously plan, predict, test, and evaluate the results. This process is not alien to nursing; indeed, it is the essence of thoughtful practice. In fact, clinical research should draw nurses closer to an examination of their practice—systematically, consciously, thoroughly—and allow planned instead of random change. (See chapters 5, 14.)

REFERENCES

1. United States Department of Health, Education, and Welfare, *Extending the Scope of Nursing Practice: A Report of the Secretary's Committee To Study Extended Roles for Nurses* (Washington, D.C.: Government Printing Office, November 1971), cited in *Nursing Outlook,* 20 (January 1972) 46–52, p. 46.

2. Just as we equate public health with community health, so do we consider public health nursing and community health nursing to be synonymous, and we use the terms interchangeably.

3. American Nurses' Association, *Standards of Community Health Nursing Practice* (Kansas City: ANA Publications CH-2 5M, 1973), unnumbered pages.

4. American Nurses' Association, *Report of the Standards Committee,* 1970 Business Meeting, reissued June 1972.

5. "Report of the National Commission for the Study of Nursing and Nursing Education," *American Journal of Nursing,* 70 (February 1970) 279–94.

6. Commission on Nursing Education of the American Nurses' Association's Stand was endorsed by the National League for Nursing's Council of Baccalaureate and Higher Degree Programs, March 24, 1972.

7. United States Department of Health, Education, and Welfare, *Extending the Scope of Nursing Practice: A Report of the Secretary's Committee To Study Extended Roles for Nurses* (Washington, D.C.: Government Printing Office, November 1971), cited in *Nursing Outlook,* 20 (January 1972) 46–52, p. 46.

8. John A. Edwards, Jane Curtis, Kay Ortman, and Phoebe Lindsey, "The Cambridge-Council Concept, or Two Nurse Practitioners Make Good," *American Journal of Nursing,* 72 (March 1972) 460–63.

9. Susan Gerberding Sheedy, "Medical Nurse Practitioner in a Neighborhood Center, *American Journal of Nursing,* 72 (August 1972) 1416–19.

10. Gloria Levinger and Holly Billings, "Nursing in a Low-Rent Housing Project," *American Journal of Nursing,* 71 (February 1971) 315–18.

11. Doris L. Wagner, "Nursing in an HMO," *American Journal of Nursing,* 74 (February 1974) 236–39.

12. Helen Tirpak, "The Frontier Nursing Service—Fifty Years in the Mountains," *Nursing Outlook,* 23 (May 1975) 308–10.

13. Howard J. Brown, "National Health Insurance—Some Vital Issues," *Nursing Outlook,* 19 (January 1971) 24–25.

14. American Nurses' Association, *The Nation's Nurses: 1972 Inventory of Registered Nurses,* ANA Statistics Department, 1974, p. 4.

15. Ibid., p. 11.

16. Ibid., p. 4.

17. "National Commission for the Study of Nursing and Nursing Education: An Abbreviated Summary," *Abstract for Action* (New York: McGraw-Hill, 1970).

18. American Nurses' Association, *The Nation's Nurses,* p. 7.

19. American Nurses' Association, *Facts About Nursing, 72–73* (Kansas City: ANA, 1974), p. 101.

20. Donna Diers, "This I Believe . . . About Nursing Research," *Nursing Outlook,* 18 (November 1970) 50–54.

ADDITIONAL READINGS

Anderson, Eva Mae, Barbara Leonard, and Judith A. Yates, "Epigenesis of the Nurse Practitioner Role," in *American Journal of Nursing,* 74 (October 1974) 1812–16.

Andrews, Priscilla M., and Alfred Yankauer, "The Pediatric Nurse Practitioner, Parts I and II," in *American Journal of Nursing,* 71 (March 1971) 504-8.

Archer, Sarah Ellen, and Ruth P. Fleshman, "Community Health Nursing: A Typology of Practice," in *Nursing Outlook,* 23 (June 1975) 358-64.

Armiger, Sister Bernadette, "Nursing Shortage or Unemployment?" in *Nursing Outlook,* 21 (May 1973) 312-16.

———, "Scholarship in Nursing," in *Nursing Outlook,* 22 (March 1974) 160-64.

Auld, Margaret E., and Linda H. Birum, *The Challenge of Nursing—A Book of Readings* (Unit One—Introduction to Nursing). St. Louis: C. V. Mosby Co., 1973.

Bean, Margaret, "The Nurse-Midwife at Work," in *American Journal of Nursing,* 71 (May 1971) 949-52.

Bowar-Ferres, Susan, "Loeb Center and Its Philosophy of Nursing," in *American Journal of Nursing,* 75 (May 1975) 810-15.

Bowman, Rosemary Amason, and Rebecca Clark Culpepper, "Power: RX for Change," in *American Journal of Nursing,* 74 (June 1974) 1053-56.

Brown, Esther L., *Nursing Reconsidered: A Study of Change* (Part II, The Professional Role in Community Nursing). Philadelphia: J. B. Lippincott Co., 1970.

Brunetto, Eleanor, and Peter Birk, "The Primary Care Nurse—The Generalist in a Structured Health Team," in *American Journal of Public Health,* 62 (June 1972) 785-94.

Cady, Louise, "Extending the Role of Public Health Nurses," in *Nursing Outlook,* 22 (October 1974) 636-40.

Cooper, Signe, and Ella Allison, "Mandatory Continuing Education?" in *American Journal of Nursing,* 73 (March 1973) 442-43.

Davis, Fred, *The Nursing Profession: Five Sociological Essays.* New York: John Wiley, 1966.

Fagin, Claire M., and Beatrice Goodwin, "Baccalaureate Preparation for Primary Care," in *Nursing Outlook,* 20 (April 1972) 240-44.

Flynn, Beverly C., "The Effectiveness of Nurse Clinicians' Service Delivery," in *American Journal of Public Health,* 64 (June 1974) 604–11.

Freeman, Ruth, *Community Health Nursing Practice.* Philadelphia: W. B. Saunders Co., 1970.

French, Jean, "This I Believe . . . About Community Nursing in the Future," in *Nursing Outlook,* 19 (March 1971) 173–75.

Gortner, Susan R., "Research in Nursing: The Federal Interest and Grant Program," in *American Journal of Nursing,* 73 (June 1973) 1052–55.

Hall, Lydia E., "A Center for Nursing," in *Nursing Outlook,* 11 (November 1963) 805-6.

Henderson, Virginia, "Excellence in Nursing," in *American Journal of Nursing,* 69 (October 1969) 2133–37.

Hohle, Beth, Jane McInnis, and Almyra Gates, "The Public Health Nurse as a Member of the Interdisciplinary Team," in *Nursing Clinics of North America,* 4 (June 1969) 311.

Jordan, Judith D., and Joseph C. Ship, "The Primary Health Care Professional Was a Nurse," in *American Jounal of Nursing,* 71 (May 1971) 922–25.

Kalisch, Beatrice, "Creativity and Nursing Research," in *Nursing Outlook,* 23 (May 1975) 314–19.

Kallins, Ethel. L., *Textbook of Public Health Nursing*. St. Louis: C. V. Mosby Co., 1967.

Kelly, Lucie Young, "Institutional Licensure," in *Nursing Outlook*, 21 (September 1973) 566-72.

Kibrick, Anne, "NLN: Nursing's Voice in Community Health," in *Nursing Outlook*, 19 (July 1971) 455.

King, Imogene, *Toward a Theory for Nursing: General Concepts of Human Behavior*. New York: John Wiley and Sons, 1971.

Kosik, Sandra Henry, "Patient Advocate, or Fighting the System," in *American Journal of Nursing*, 72 (April 1972) 694-98.

Kramer, Marlene, *Reality Shock*. St. Louis: C.V. Mosby Co., 1974.

Leahy, Kathleen, Marguerite Cobb, and Mary C. Jones, *Community Health Nursing*. 2nd ed. New York: McGraw-Hill, 1972.

Levine, Myra E., "Holistic Nursing," in *Nursing Clinics of North America*, 6 (June 1971) 253-64.

Munier, Sandra K., and Aldean Richardson, "Development of New Nursing Roles in a Comprehensive Health Center," (A Nursing Service and Education Project) in *Journal of Nursing Administration*, 4 (July–August 1974) 44-49.

Murphy, Juanita, *Theoretical Issues in Professional Nursing*. New York: Appleton-Century-Crofts, 1971.

Murphy, Marion I., "Health Maintenance—Implications for Nursing," as reported in *Maintaining Health, An Adventure in Transition*, proceedings of the Fourth Mid-Atlantic Regional Conference, Mid-Atlantic Regional Assembly, National League for Nursing, New York, June 1972.

Newman, Margaret A., "Nursing's Theoretical Evolution," in *Nursing Outlook*, 20 (July 1972) 449-53.

"The Nurse Practitioner: Preparation and Practice," (collection of articles on the expanded role of the nurse), in *Nursing Outlook*, 22 (February 1974) 89-127.

"The Nurse Practitioner Question," in *American Journal of Nursing*, 74 (December 1974) 2188-91.

"Nursing at the Crossroads," (collection of articles on issues involved in extending the scope of nursing practice), in *Nursing Outlook*, 20 (January 1972) 21-63.

Rogers, Martha, *The Theoretical Basis of Nursing*. Philadelphia: F. A. Davis, 1970.

Schaefer, Marguerite J., "The Political and Economic Scene in the Future of Nursing," in *American Journal of Public Health*, 63 (October 1973) 887-89.

Schlotfeldt, Rozella M., "This I Believe . . . Nursing Is Health Care," in *Nursing Outlook*, 20 (April 1972) 245-46.

Scott, Jessie M., "The Changing Health Care Environment: Its Implications for Nursing," in *American Journal of Public Health*, 64 (April 1974) 364-69.

———, "Federal Support for Nursing Education, 1964 to 1972," in *American Journal of Nursing*, 72 (October 1972) 1855-61.

Skrovan, Clarence, Elizabeth Anderson, and Janet Gottschalk, "Community Nurse Practitioner: An Emerging Role," in *American Journal of Public Health*, 64 (September 1974) 847-53.

Snyder, Lilja A., " 'We Care Enough To Come to You,' " in *Nursing Outlook*, 22 (March 1974) 168-71.

Thurston, Hester I., "Education for Episodic and Ditributive Care," in *Nursing Outlook*, 20 (August 1972) 519-23.

Tinkham, Catherine, and Eleanor F. Voorhies, *Community Health Nursing Evolution and Process.* New York: Appleton-Century-Crofts, 1972.

Toms, Kathleen, and Sister Frances M. Walker, "A Free Clinic for the Working Poor," in *Nursing Outlook,* 21 (December 1973) 770–72.

Vaillot, Sister Madeline, *Commitment to Nursing: A Philosophic Investigation.* Philadelphia: J. B. Lippincott Co., 1962.

Wagner, Doris L., "Issues in the Provision of Health Care for All," in *American Journal of Public Health,* 63 (June 1973) 481–85.

UNIT II
SCIENCES RELATED TO
COMMUNITY HEALTH

Chapter 4
Human Ecology

"Man does not and cannot live separately from his environment. Each influences the other."[1]

NATIONAL AND INTERNATIONAL CONCERN

Landscapes littered with cans and bottles, lakes transformed into stagnant pools, the air we breathe a mass of impurities—environmental problems continue to grow. Ecology, a household word in recent years, has become a political issue as environmental problems have increased. By 1970 the byproducts of postwar abundance and technology were seen in the uncontrolled pollution of the earth's air, land, and water. Waste products from gas and electricity pollute the atmosphere; no-deposit, no-return soft drink bottles, pop-top cans, and plastic containers build up unsightly mountains of refuse in our urban and suburban centers; nonbiodegradable effluent fouls our streams and waterways—even the oceans in their vastness have not been spared. Thor Heyerdahl crossing the sea in his papyrus boat discovered plastic bottles, traces of oil, and other waste products adrift on large areas of the ocean far away from ships and shore.[2]

While the menace of pollution has been growing over the years, dedicated members of conservationist movements—"voices crying in the wilderness"—have been trying to sound the alarm. It was not until 1970 that Congress enacted legislation creating an overall national agency, the Environmental Protection Agency (EPA), to coordinate activities earlier spread over a number of governmental bureaus. This agency, along with the Council on Environmental Quality, is concerned with environmental control—including control of air, water, pesticides, solid wastes, and radiation hazards, and has authority over all states, industries, and municipalities in

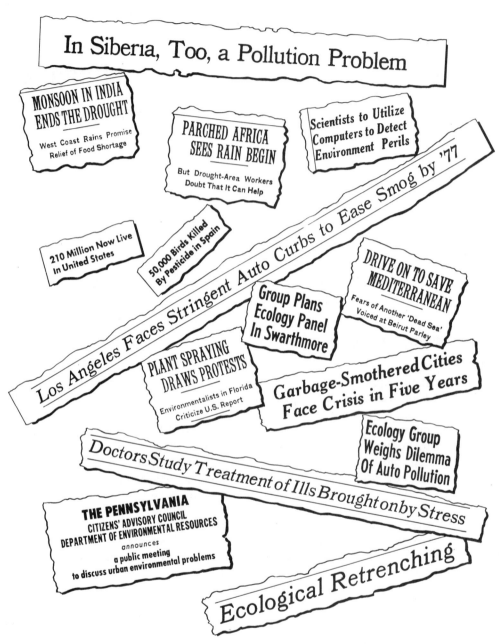

In Siberia, Too, a Pollution Problem

MONSOON IN INDIA ENDS THE DROUGHT

West Coast Rains Promise Relief of Food Shortage

PARCHED AFRICA SEES RAIN BEGIN

But Drought-Area Workers Doubt That It Can Help

Scientists to Utilize Computers to Detect Environment Perils

210 Million Now Live In United States

50,000 Birds Killed By Pesticide in Spain

Los Angeles Faces Stringent Auto Curbs to Ease Smog by '77

DRIVE ON TO SAVE MEDITERRANEAN

Fears of Another 'Dead Sea' Voiced at Beirut Parley

Group Plans Ecology Panel In Swarthmore

PLANT SPRAYING DRAWS PROTESTS

Environmentalists in Florida Criticize U.S. Report

Garbage-Smothered Cities Face Crisis in Five Years

Ecology Group Weighs Dilemma Of Auto Pollution

Doctors Study Treatment of Ills Brought on by Stress

THE PENNSYLVANIA
CITIZENS' ADVISORY COUNCIL
DEPARTMENT OF ENVIRONMENTAL RESOURCES
announces
a public meeting
to discuss urban environmental problems

Ecological Retrenching

Figure 4-1.

controlling pollution. Essentially, EPA is responsible for conducting research, establishing and enforcing standards, and monitoring pollution in the environment. Perhaps, its most important task is to assist state and local governments in their own environmental control efforts.

For several years, ecology has taken on the air of a popular crusade around which many persons and special interest groups have rallied. However, it has begun to lose some of its momentum under the impact of energy and economic problems that have emerged. Suddenly environmentalists are no longer popular heroes, and their message has lost some of its appeal. Measures they have promoted to help decrease environmental pollution are seen as incompatible with existing fuel shortages and inflationary problems. For example, clean air regulations limiting the use of high-sulfur coal and oil have created hardship because "clean" fuels, such as natural gas, are in great demand and short supply. The federal government has begun to reverse some of its earlier stated positions on strict standards in environmental control. Indeed, federal government consideration of environmental matters has shown signs of weakening, with indications of fiscal cuts in the EPA budget for 1976.

International recognition of environmental problems, such as those shown in Figure 4-2, culminated in the United Nations Conference on the Human Environment held in Sweden in the summer of 1972. The theme of the conference—"Only One Earth"—was chosen to emphasize that all animate and inanimate things in man's environment are part of a single interdependent system, and that man is without recourse if he destroys his surroundings through thoughtlessness and carelessness.[3] From the outset, the conference was faced with the harsh realities of international political dissension—the Soviet Union and most other Eastern European countries did not attend; every participating country found something in the resolutions that they planned to ignore; China hurled charges of imperialism and aggression at the United States; racist feelings surfaced.

Nevertheless, the 1200 delegates from 110 countries persisted and approved a plan of international action to protect man's habitat on earth, and established a fund to support the plan. The Action Plan consists of the following:

> (1) a global assessment program, known as Earthwatch, through a network of 110 specially equipped monitoring stations, to identify and measure environmental problems of international importance and to warn against impending crises;
>
> (2) environmental management activities to use what is known or learned about the environment, so as to preserve what is desired and prevent what is feared; and
>
> (3) supporting measures, such as education and training, public information, and organizational and financing arrangements.

World Health Organization scientists, in their international monitoring,

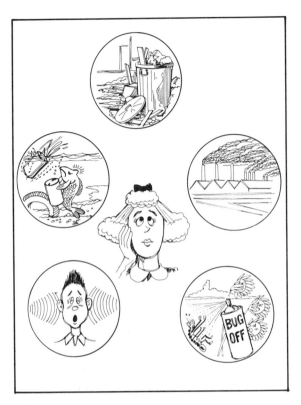

Figure 4-2 Environmental hazards.

are using computers to develop an "early warning system" for the detection of environmental health hazards. Through computer analysis, they are watching the physical, chemical, biological, and social factors that affect health, such as disease-bearing insects and malnutrition. They are continually studying and doing research on community health problems related to air pollution, water, food, and climate.

Food and population—two issues that are intimately bound up with environmental problems—have also commanded international attention. In August 1974 the first intergovernmental World Population Conference was convened in Bucharest, Rumania, followed in November of that same year by the World Food Conference in Rome. Both conferences—attended by the majority of the world's countries—were marked by stormy debate and harsh exchanges among the delegations. The Population Conference issued a Plan of Action, which, while placing strong emphasis on social and economic development as a prerequisite for population control, affirmed the right of couples to decide on the number and spacing of their children, and urged that family planning services be made fully available to all persons to prevent unwanted pregnancy. The World Food Conference emphasized the urgency of adopting a world food plan that would help alleviate famine and starvation in many parts of the world. During this conference, many of the same nations that had rejected responsibility for curbing populations they cannot feed were looking to the United States and a handful of other nations for food supplies.

WHAT IS HUMAN ECOLOGY?

Ecology has been defined as the science that studies environmental problems and examines the relations of organisms with each other and with their surroundings. It deals with the effect of the environment on living things and the effect of living things on each other and on their environment. Embracing the scientific study of plants, animals, and humans, ecology has some features in common with other sciences, such as plant ecology and botany, animal ecology and zoology. Ultimately, plants, animals, and humans are intimately bound together, and the ecologist must look at all of them. The total complex of their interactions makes up what is known as the ecosystem.

Human ecology is concerned with plant and animal ecology at common points within the ecosystem. As a scientific discipline developed in this century, human ecology examines the ways in which human beings adapt to their environment. In this process of adaptation, man alters the ecosystem, thereby affecting plants and animals, as he clears land for agriculture, cuts down trees for paper products, or sprays insect vectors for disease control.

Man shares many biological traits with the other primates. He is a social animal, that is, he lives in groups, as do other animals. However, a characteristic that distinguishes man and makes his group life different from that of other social animals is *culture*. Culture is a shared and organized body of skills, customs, and values that are transmitted socially from one generation to the next. Culture influences population, technological progress, the standard of living and ultimately the environment. Various parts of a culture are interrelated; if one part of a culture changes, other parts will be affected. Any single behavior pattern or value derives meaning from its associations with other behavior patterns and values. When we ask people to change one behavior or shift one value, we must realize that other, sometimes unexpected changes, will occur.

The desire for survival is inherent in man's nature. It gives force and direction to what he does to promote his own well-being and to postpone his death. A person can do much to enhance survival; society, through collective action, can help the individual to survive. In so doing, society is benefited because its greatest resource is its members. For its own preservation, society must conserve its human resources.

Man is the most restless of all life forms, the most widely dispersed over the face of the earth, and the most adaptable. He is capable of exerting some measure of control over nature and of solving problems of survival created by environmental conditions, though often at the expense of creating another problem. For example, DDT, the chemical that destroys disease-bearing and crop-damaging insects, does not break down quickly into harmless substances, but persists in the environment and accumulates into harmful concentrations within organisms. It upsets the ecosystem by contaminating the food chain and natural habitat of many fish, birds, other animals, and ultimately man. With a change in one element in the system, there will be a resultant change in another part of the system, sometimes unexpected. Survival is a constant struggle for man, and unfortunately one in which his solutions to today's problems contain the seeds of tomorrow's.

HEALTH AND HUMAN ECOLOGY

Man's environment is more than physical surroundings. Environment is the world in all its aspects as it affects the life system of man; it has physical, biological, and social components. The more complex life becomes, as civilization and industrialization progress, the more complex must be the environment, and therefore the more complex the adjustment. Good public health is good ecology; persons concerned with health matters keep this principle in mind at all times. The diseases of the day are strikingly man-made, commonly through inept adaptation, often through willful error. Examples are emphysema, cancer of the lung, heart disease, and obesity. The chance of survival in the kind of world man is creating requires awareness that his health is related to that of all living things in a common environment. Man must find his place in nature.

Jamann points out, in "Health Is A Function of Ecology," that man is an integrated entity whose "state of health is multidimensional and there are no simple solutions to the problem of maintaining, or restoring, this state."[4] She identifies several ecological factors that bear on individual and community health, as follows:

(1) Environmental pollution—air pollution and water pollution are threats to health. If the quality of the air we breathe continues to deteriorate, life cannot be sustained. Air pollution is especially severe in our major cities—Chicago, Los Angeles, Philadelphia, Washington, Cincinnati, San Francisco, New York, Cleveland, Pittsburgh, Boston, Newark, Detroit and St. Louis. Water pollution poses a serious threat to the biological, psychological and aesthetic health of mankind. Uncontrolled dumping of organic wastes, detergents, pesticides, and industrial wastes have threatened man's food chain, his drinking water, and his recreational activities.

(2) Food and nutrition—faulty nutrition is the largest single cause of disease in the world today.

(3) Man-microbe interaction—microbes are not necessarily good or bad in themselves; it is their relationship with other living things which determines their detrimental or beneficial effects.

(4) Drugs—when used wisely, they are a boon to man's health and survival both in short-term and long-term needs; but in their misuse they pose a threat to man's biopsychosocial system.

(5) Population expansion—overpopulation affects health in relation to food supply, other natural resources, housing and territorial limitations, cultural and economic development.

(6) Sensory stimulation—"sound deprivation" as well as "sound overload" can be detrimental to health. Sensory stimulation is essential to development. Lack of such stimulation leads to stunted biopsychosocial growth. Over-stimulation—or noise pollution from such things as jet airplanes, electronic amplification, domestic and industrial machines—can be related to impairment of hearing.

(7) Creativity and life style—human beings, through a balance of work, play, and rest and sleep, develop individual life styles and tastes. These influence one's ability to handle stress and ultimately affect health.[5]

These ecological factors must be taken into consideration in nursing practice when we assess the health of individuals, their families, and communities. We must identify those conditions within the environment that contribute to the causes of death, disease, injury, and disability. In formulating nursing plans with realistic goals for health promotion, prevention of illness, and rehabilitation or restoration, we dare not ignore the dynamic forces of the environment that affect and are affected by the patient and family.

It is essential to view the human being as an integrated whole person. This "whole person," in his totality may be regarded as an open social system, continuously interacting with his environment. We cannot limit our concern to specified disease processes, anatomical malformations, or physical malfunctioning. We observe the individual and the family. We look for the kinds of adaptive mechanisms they employ to maintain the "dynamic equilibrium" that reflects the state of health or illness, as described on page 24. Human ecology provides a theoretical base upon which we may develop this holistic approach.

REFERENCES

1. A. Hunter Dupree, "History Inscribed on the Land," *National Parks and Conservation Magazine* (September 1971), p. 24.

2. Thor Heyerdahl, *The Ra Expeditions* (Garden City, New York: Doubleday & Co., 1971), p. 209.

3. "U.N. Conference on the Human Environment," *U.N. Monthly Chronicle,* Vol. 9, No. 7 (July 1972), 50-54.

4. Joann S. Jamann, "Health Is a Function of Ecology," *American Journal of Nursing* 71 (May 1971) 970-73.

5. Ibid.

ADDITIONAL READINGS

Anderson, C. L., *Community Health.* St. Louis: C. V. Mosby Co., 1969.

Berelson, Bernard, et al., *World Population: Status Report 1974. A Guide for the Concerned Citizen.* Reports on Population/Family Planning, The Population Council, New York, January 1974.

Blowers, Jay H., "The United States' Position on Environment," in *American Journal of Public Health,* 62 (May 1972) 634–38.

Chanlett, Emil, Donald W. Rogers, and Grant Hurst, "The Necessity for Environmental Health Planning," in *American Journal of Public Health,* 63 (April 1973) 341–44.

Cook, C. Sharp, "Energy: Planning for the Future," in *Nursing Digest,* 1 (October 1973) 59–66.

Cropp, G. J., "Effects of Air Pollution on Health," in *Nursing Digest,* 1 (October 1973) 32–35.

Dubos, Rene, "The Genius of the Place," in *American Forests,* 76 (September 1970) 9, 16 ff.

———, *Mirage of Health.* New York: Harper and Row, 1959.

———, *Man Adapting.* New Haven, Conn.: Yale University Press, 1965.

———, "Human Ecology." *WHO Chronicle,* 23 (1969) 499–504.

Gordon, John E., and T. H. Ingalls, "Ecological Interplay of Man, Environment and Health," in *American Journal of the Medical Sciences,* 252:3 (September 1966) 341–56.

Harrison, James T., Emil Paul DeJan, and Lewis E. Hackett, "Environmental Protection—A Local Administrative Dilemma," in *American Journal of Public Health,* 62 (May 1972) 642–44.

Kilbourne, Edwin D., and Wilson G. Smillie, *Human Ecology and Public Health.* 4th ed. New York: Macmillan Co., 1969.

Levine, Myra E., "The Pursuit of Wholeness," in *American Journal of Nursing,* 69 (January 1969) 93–98.

Parrish, Henry M., "Animal-Man Relationships in Today's Environment," in *American Journal of Public Health,* 63 (March 1973) 199–200.

Phillips, John, *Environmental Health: A Paradox of Progress.* Dubuque, Iowa: Wm. C. Brown Co., 1971.

Revelle, Roger, "Food and Population," in *Scientific American,* 231 (September 1974) 161–71.

Rogers, Martha E., *An Introduction to the Theoretical Basis of Nursing.* Philadelphia: F. A. Davis, 1970.

Sargent, Frederick, "Man-Environment—Problems for Public Health," in *American Journal of Public Health,* 62 (May 1972) 628–33.

Savage, Eldon P., John D. Tessare, and Laurier P. Couture, "Pesticides Sold in Grocery Stores Are Potential Health Hazards," in *Health Services Reports,* 87 (October 1972) 734–36.

Swan, James A., "The Environment, the Citizen, and the Environmental Health Professional," in *American Journal of Public Health, 62 (May 1972)* 639-41.

Chapter 5
Epidemiology

"It is not a divine moral purpose, or a satanic punitive ingenuity that connects syphilis with genital activities, but a mere biologic accident no more significant in the last analysis than the fact that potatoes grow in sandy loam."[1]

WHAT IS EPIDEMIOLOGY?

Ecology, applied to health and illness, lays the foundation for epidemiology. Epidemiology is more than the study of epidemics. It has been defined in the broadest sense as a "field of science which is concerned with the various factors and conditions that determine the occurrence and distribution of health, disease, defects, disability and death among groups of individuals."[2]

Epidemiology Is Concerned With

(1) mass phenomena of disease—effect of diseases or conditions on groups of individuals, as small as a family unit or as large as a whole community, nation or group of nations;
(2) distribution and causes of human health problems;
(3) multiple factors of causation; and
(4) measures of prevention and control.

Epidemiology draws from many other disicplines and uses the problem-solving approach to investigate disease causation. Steps in problem solving are compared with the epidemiologic process in Table 5-1.

Table 5-1   Who, What, When, Where, Why, How?

Steps in Problem Solving	Epidemiologic Process
Title: What is the problem?	Define the problem

Objectives:
    What are the objectives?
	Design the investigation
	    Formulate hypothesis
	    Identify population
	    Determine instruments

Material or tools: What resources are available?	Collect data
Method of procedure: What approach can be taken?	Process and analyze data
Treatment of results: What do the results show?	State conclusions
Discussion: What do the results mean?	
Conclusion: What conclusions can be drawn?	

Historically, epidemiology began with the study of the great epidemic diseases—leprosy, plague, cholera, smallpox, yellow fever, and typhus. The techniques that were developed became applicable to the study of all infectious diseases—diphtheria, scarlet fever, measles, diarrheal disease, syphilis, tuberculosis, and so forth. And now we apply these methods to the study of cancer, hypertension, coronary artery disease, accidents, diabetes, arthritis, and other noninfectious diseases which have emerged as the major chronic cripplers and killers of today.

METHODS OF EPIDEMIOLOGIC STUDY

The methods of epidemiologic study include description, formulation of hypotheses, and testing of hypotheses, which may be presented as follows:

Descriptive Method

The epidemiologist seeks an accurate description of a specific disease phenomenon that has already occurred. He gathers pertinent data regarding time (year, season, day) and place of occurrence (geographic, political subdivision, rural/urban). He investigates characteristics of persons affected (age, sex, ethnic group, occupation, family history).

Examples:

(1) case information registries maintained by health agencies (state or local, voluntary or official, community nursing) for diseases or conditions such as tuberculosis, cancer, lead poisoning, congenital defects, and so forth;

(2) investigations of communicable disease outbreaks, such as the 1972 smallpox epidemic in Yugoslavia.

Formulation of Hypotheses

Clues to disease causation are sought from descriptive data. Tentative theories regarding causal association are proposed. These lead to the formulation of hypotheses that can be tested. Acceptable hypotheses must be consistent with known facts regarding disease occurrence.

Examples:

(1) John Snow's classic study of the outbreak of cholera in which he hypothesized that the disease could be traced to specific agents discharged in the feces of cholera patients;

(2) hypotheses regarding causal associations between heart disease and diet, cancer of the cervix and age at initiation of intercourse, and so forth.

Testing of Hypotheses

Analytic studies, which may be either observational or experimental, are designed to test hypotheses. In such studies the investigator seeks to demonstrate an association between disease occurrence and an antecedent factor or factors. Observational studies may be retrospective (looking back) or prospective (looking forward). Experimental studies, of course, can only be done prospectively. For ethical reasons experimental studies in human populations are limited to attempts at preventing disease.

Examples:

(1) analytic study (retrospective)—N. M. Gregg of Australia, observing an unusual occurrence of congenital cataracts and cardiac defects in children born in 1941, hypothesized some underlying prenatal factor; he interviewed mothers of affected children, discovered that many of them had had rubella early in pregnancy, and hypothesized a causal relationship between rubella in the mothers and congenital defects in the children.

(2) analytic study (prospective)—based on Gregg's analysis, a prospective study

was designed; women with a history of rubella during pregnancy were sought and the results of their pregnancies were investigated; the findings of this study and subsequent studies supported Gregg's hypothesis.

(3) experimental study—the 1954 field trial of Salk vaccine involving nearly two million children, which documented an efficient method of preventing poliomyelitis and demonstrated the efficacy of this vaccine.

Proceeding from the known to the unknown, the epidemiologist begins with a curiosity about an event which cannot be explained by chance, that is, why a particular illness strikes a particular individual out of a whole population of apparently equally eligible individuals. Our environment is so complex that the study of the circumstances relating to illness in a single person is just the beginning. The epidemiologist is like a detective. Examining numbers of cases of a disease as they occur throughout a population, he tries to discover what it is that makes the victims different from the rest of the population. He seeks out the essential determinants of disease. His aim is to identify those factors that are essential or contributory to disease occurrence so that they may be intercepted or altered in some way, and the disease prevented.

Because opportunities for experimentation are limited, epidemiology is generally regarded as an observational science in which comparison is the essential element. The characteristics of a group having a specific disease or health problem are compared with the characteristics of a group without that disease or health problem. From knowledge of the similarities and the differences between the two groups, hypotheses are formulated about the processes that are causally related to the disease or health problem. Facts are collected concerning the problem under investigation—incidence, prevalence, and other statistical indices are recorded.

In epidemiologic investigations, the community may be likened to a laboratory where data on health-related phenomena are collected under controlled conditions. The epidemiologist seeks to elucidate risk factors in disease and to identify etiologic agents. Epidemiological investigation is best conducted on subjects from clearly defined populations in order to insure the validity of inferences drawn from the experimental findings. The systematic and objective collection of health information relating to defined populations may be considered to have its roots in the social and sanitary survey movements of the eighteenth and nineteenth centuries, beginning perhaps with John Howard's studies of conditions in English prisons in 1777. The sanitary surveys made by Chadwick (1842) and Shattuck (1850) in a later era were essentially epidemiological studies. (See pages 8 and 9.)

THE EPIDEMIOLOGIC TRIAD

In determining the natural history of a disease or condition, one looks at the basic elements which comprise the "epidemiologic triad"—the host, the agent, and the environment (see Figure 5-1).

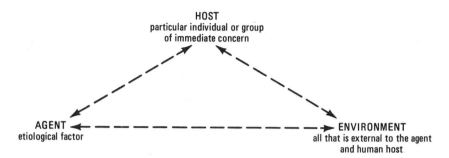

HOST
particular individual or group
of immediate concern

AGENT
etiological factor

ENVIRONMENT
all that is external to the agent
and human host

Figure 5-1   The epidemiologic triad.

These three elements are closely bound together and each affects the other. The interaction of host, agent, and environment determines the mode of transmission, the natural history, occurrence, and control of disease, illness, or other condition. The health of an individual or community depends upon the state of equilibrium maintained within this triad of elements.

Sometimes the characteristics of these basic elements are clearly understood and can be cited when one is identifying causal relationships. For example, syphilis is transmitted only through close, intimate contact because of a specific biological property of the agent, the treponema pallidum, which is very fragile and dies as soon as it dries. In other instances causal relationships could be identified although the basic factors were not altogether clear. For example, the Surgeon General's Committee ascribed a causal relationship to cigarette smoking in lung cancer in 1964, even though not as much was known then as is known today about mechanisms in the host-agent-environment interrelationships by which cigarette smoking may produce disease.

Measures of prevention and control can be successfully applied even though causal mechanisms are not understood in their entirety. Recognition of even one small component can result in some degree of prevention. For example, long before there was any knowledge of vitamin C, it was known that citrus fruits could be used to prevent scurvy (Figure 5-2). A more recent example was the introduction of a federal regulation requiring that cigarettes be labelled a health hazard, even though the exact disease mechanism was not completely clear. Probably one of the most dramatic examples of applying preventive measures on the basis of only limited understanding is seen in the work of Dr. Ignaz Semmelweis, a nineteenth century Hungarian physician, portrayed in Figure 5-3.

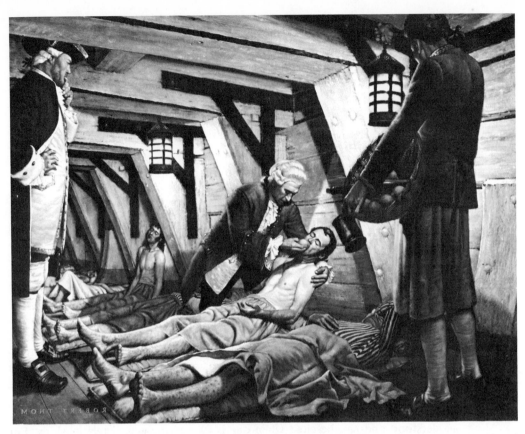

Figure 5-2 In the mid-eighteenth century—long before the discovery of vitamins and their role in health and disease—James Lind, a surgeon in Britain's Royal Navy, demonstrated the effectiveness of citrus fruits in the treatment and prevention of scurvy, a dread dietary deficiency disease that killed thousands of seamen.

Source *A History of Medicine in Pictures,* a pamphlet accompanying photographs presented by Parke, Davis. © 1959 by Parke, Davis and Company.

Observing patients in two of the wards in his maternity hospital, Dr. Semmelweis had noticed a difference in the number of deaths from puerperal sepsis (a major cause of mortality among women in those days). In one ward, where the student midwives worked, there were fewer deaths than in the other ward, where the medical students worked. From his observations he concluded that medical students coming directly to the patients' quarters from the dissecting room might be carrying the infection on their hands. He instituted the practice of thorough handwashing before the students were permitted to examine their patients. The results were dramatic, with a marked decline in maternal mortality from child-bed fever. However, many of his colleagues would not accept his findings. They were unable to understand his rationale, and they felt that his ideas were a

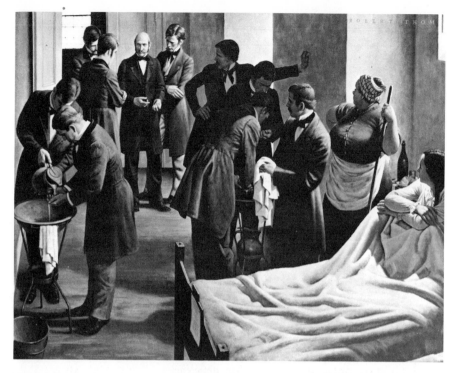

Figure 5-3 In 1847 the great Hungarian physician Ignaz Philipp Semmelweis discovered that childbed fever could be prevented when hand-washing was consistently and carefully practiced by physicians and other attendants. He insisted on the use of strict hand-washing techniques in his obstetric wards. These techniques were resented at first by many of his colleagues, but his stringent rules saved the lives of hundreds of mothers.

Source A History of Medicine in Pictures, a pamphlet accompanying photographs presented by Parke, Davis. ©1961 by Parke, Davis and Company.

rebuke to their own methods of practice. Semmelweis' contribution to health care went unrecognized for many years, and was brought to light only with the advent of antisepsis under Lister.

APPLYING EPIDEMIOLOGY TO COMMUNITY HEALTH

The epidemiologist views the whole community as his patient. In making his diagnosis, he calls upon the principles of clinical medicine and laboratory diagnosis, as well as his own special observational skills and techniques. His findings should be utilized in determining the best course of action for prevention and control to promote community health. The epidemiological approach to establishing a control program for a health problem involves several steps, as follows:

65

STEP ONE—DETERMINING THE NATURAL HISTORY OF THE DISEASE, CONDITION, OR HEALTH PROBLEM

Host

(1) demographic characteristics—age, sex, ethnic group, marital status;

(2) general health status—anatomical structure, physiologic state, nutrition, genetic determinants, reaction to stress;

(3) body defenses—skin and mucous membranes, lymphatic system;

(4) state of immunity and immunological response—natural immunity, artificial immunity (active, passive); and

(5) human behavior—diet, food handling, personal hygiene, forms of personal contact, household hygiene, occupation, recreation.

Agent

(1) biological—bacteria, viruses, fungi, helminths, protozoa, and determination of their life cycle: morphology, chemical composition, multiplication, virulence, viability, vulnerability;

(2) physical—temperature, noise, radiation;

(3) chemical—gases, dusts, vapors, liquids; and

(4) absence of a substance—nutrient deficiencies.

Environment

(1) physical—weather, climate, season, soil, terrain, geology, geography;

(2) biological—animal reservoirs, arthropod vectors, food supply;

(3) social—family and community structure, population density and mobility, occupations, role and status, activities, cultural values (customs, beliefs, political and economic realities, attitudes), technological developments, transportation, schools, housing, provisions for health services.

STEP TWO—DETERMINING THE EXTENT OF THE PROBLEM

(1) What proportion of the people are affected?

(2) How serious are the effects on the host?

(3) How serious are the effects on the community?

(4) What is the geographic distribution?

(5) What are the time relationships?

STEP THREE—PLANNING THE STRATEGY OF CONTROL

(1) Strategic points at which control measures may be applied are determined through knowledge of the natural history of the condition.

(a) Identification of the vulnerable population groups in which the problem is centered, and on which the program should focus—for example, measures could be taken to immunize the population at risk to increase host resistance and herd immunity.

(b) Identification of points at which the agent is most vulnerable to attack, and control measures available for use—for example, steps could be taken to eliminate the agent through water purification, milk pasteurization, and food sanitation. Another example would be attempts to render an infected host noninfectious, as in drug treatment for tuberculosis.

(c) Identification of strategic points at which changes of environment may affect the health problems favorably for man, and selection of appropriate control measures—for example, environmental measures to eliminate vectors, such as mosquitoes, flies, and other insects, would help in the control of infectious diseases.

(2) Priorities are determined on the basis of the relative importance of the problem to the community as a whole in comparison with other problems the community must face.

(3) Application of appropriate control measures must be determined on the basis of available community resources and other factors in the total situation.

STEP FOUR—ESTABLISHING A CONTROL PROGRAM

After determining the strategy of control, the health department, or other agency responsible for coordinating the program, seeks community approval and cooperation from the public, the government, and other health agencies. A workable plan is formulated with clearly defined objectives. The control program will include services directed at the applicable levels of prevention, that is, promotion of health, specific protection, early diagnosis and treatment, disability limitation, and rehabilitation.

STEP FIVE—EVALUATING THE RESULTS

(1) to see how well the objectives of the program were met;

(2) to compare the new situation with the original situation;

(3) to present to the whole community the results of responsible action by an agency that is held accountable for the health of the people; and

(4) to provide a basis for future action.

STEP SIX—PROMOTING RESEARCH

(1) to learn more about the natural history of the health problem;

(2) to find improved control measures; and

(3) to seek better ways of applying these measures.

REFERENCES

1. John Stokes, Herman Beerman, and Norman Ingraham, *Modern Clinical Syphilology* (Philadelphia: W.B. Saunders Co., 1945), p. 11.

2. Hugh R. Leavell and E. Gurney Clark, *Preventive Medicine for the Doctor in His Community,* 3rd ed. (New York: McGraw-Hill, 1965), p. 40.

ADDITIONAL READINGS

Austin, Donald F., and S. Benson Werner, *Epidemiology for the Health Sciences: A Primer on Epidemiologic Concepts and Their Uses.* Springfield, Ill.: Charles C. Thomas, 1974.

Benenson, Abram S., ed., *Control of Communicable Diseases in Man.* 12th ed. New York: American Public Health Association, 1975.

Cassel, John M., "Potentialities and Limitations of Epidemiology," in Alfred Katz and Jean Felton, *Health and the Community.* New York: The Free Press, 1965.

Fox, John P., Carrie E. Hall, and Lila R. Elveback, *Epidemiology: Man and Disease.* London: Macmillan & Co., 1970.

Gehlbach, Stephen, Wilton A. Williams, Jimmie S. Woodall, and John I. Freeman, "Pesticides and Human Health—An Epidemiologic Approach," in *Health Services Reports,* 89(May–June 1974) 274-77.

Hrehorovich, Victor, William W. Dyal, and William D. Schrack, "Influenza Epidemic in Pennsylvania," in *Health Services Reports,* 87 (November 1972) 835-44.

Kark, Sidney L., *Epidemiology and Community Medicine.* New York: Appleton-Century-Crofts, 1974.

Kessler, Irving I., and Morton L. Levin, eds., *The Community as an Epidemiologic Laboratory—A Casebook of Community Studies.* Baltimore: The Johns Hopkins Press, 1970.

MacMahon, Brian, Thomas F. Pugh, and Johannes Ipsen, *Epidemiologic Methods.* Boston: Little, Brown and Company, 1960.

Mausner, Judith, and Anita Bahn, *Epidemiology: An Introductory Text.* Philadelphia: W.B. Saunders Co., 1974.

Roueche, Berton, *Eleven Blue Men.* Boston: Little, Brown and Company, 1953.

———, *The Orange Man and Other Narratives of Medical Detection.* Boston: Little, Brown and Company, 1971.

Slaughter, Frank Gill, *Immortal Magyar: Semmelweis, Conqueror of Childbed Fever.* New York: Schuman, 1950.

Terris, Milton, "The Epidemiologic Revolution," in *American Journal of Public Health,* 62 (November 1972) 1439-41.

Wilner, Daniel M., Rosabelle Price Walkley, and Lenor S. Goerke, *Introduction to Public Health.* 6th ed. New York: Macmillan Co., 1973.

Winslow, C.-E.A., Wilson G. Smillie, James A. Doull, and John E. Gordon, *The History of American Epidemiology.* Edited by Franklin H. Top. St. Louis: C.V. Mosby Co., 1952.

Appendix
Glossary of Terms Commonly Used in Epidemiology

Agent The specific factor without which a disease or condition cannot occur. It may be an animate or inanimate substance, or it may be the lack of a particular essential substance.

Antibody A protein substance produced in response to either naturally or artificially introduced antigenic stimulation, which tends to neutralize the antigen.

Antigen A substance that stimulates the production of antibodies when it gains entrance to the blood or body tissues.

Carrier A person (or animal) who harbors a specific disease-causing agent, in the absence of clinical manifestations, and who serves as a potential source of infection to others.

Contact A person (or animal) who has been in association with an infected person or animal or a contaminated environment.

Disinfection Destruction of pathogenic microorganisms by physical or chemical means.

Droplet nuclei Small airborne residues that result from evaporation of droplets emitted by an infected host.

Endemic Prevailing, or continuously present, in a community—as distinguished from epidemic.

Environment The entire surroundings external to the human host.

Epidemic Prevalence of a disease in a community in excess of normal expectancy. It affects many in a community at once, but not prevailing continuously.

Herd immunity Resistance of a group to invasion and spread of an infectious agent, based on the immunity of a high proportion of individual members of the group.

Host Vertebrate or invertebrate species capable of being infected (or in the case of noninfectious agents, affected) by an agent.

Immunity The state of being immune, i.e., possessing specific antibodies as a result of previous infection, immunization, or other specific experience that causes an adequate response of antibody production (active immunity), or as a result of receiving antibodies produced elsewhere (passive immunity).

Incidence Frequency of occurrence of new cases of a disease in a population over a stated period of time expressed as a rate.

Incubation period   Time interval between exposure to an infectious agent and appearance of the first sign or symptom of disease.

Isolation   Limitation of movement of a person having a communicable disease or of a carrier who harbors an infective agent.

Pandemic   Denoting a disease affecting or attacking all, or a large portion of the population; extensively epidemic, with wide geographic distribution.

Prevalence   The number of cases of a disease existing at a particular time within a given population.

Quarantine   Restriction of movement of those who have been in contact with a communicable disease for the period of time during which they may be potentially infectious to others.

Reservoir   Animate or inanimate matter in which an infectious agent normally lives and multiplies and on which it depends primarily for survival, reproducing itself so that it can be transmitted to a susceptible host.

Suspect   A person whose medical history and symptoms suggest that he may have or be developing a particular disease.

Vector   An arthropod or other invertebrate that transmits an infectious agent from an infected to a susceptible host.

Chapter 6
Biostatistics

"Statistics tell the story of how people live and die, and help us to understand some of the important causes of health and long life and of disease and death."[1]

INTRODUCTION

In measuring the health status of a patient, the nurse and physician who work in the hospital or private office make use of certain tools—for example, thermometers, sphygmomanometers, X-ray machines, electrocardiograms, laboratory tests, and other devices. In measuring the health status of their "patient"—that is, the community—the public health nurse and physician use statistics as their basic tool. Statistics are facts that are systematically selected and compiled in numerical form. They serve as the essential ingredients for the process which has been called poetically "the bookkeeping of humanity."[2]

As we have seen, the rise of the modern public health movement is fairly recent. The scientific application of statistical methods is also recent, although certain aspects of statistical usage have long been known. Man and society have made "head counts" from the earliest times. The practice of enumerating the population was an integral part of government administration even among ancient civilizations. Often an unwelcomed and imposed feature, census taking in those days usually had the purpose of gathering information for tax assessments or military conscriptions. In the United States, the Constitution provided for an official census to be made every ten years. The chief reason was to give a basis for apportionment of congressional representatives. The first census was carried out in 1790.

Recording of births and deaths can be traced back to compulsory ecclesiastical registration in the late medieval period in Europe. Registration of birth and death information was related to the church in early colonial America. Massachusetts Colony in 1639 ordered that all births and deaths be recorded. Prior to 1850 only six states had adopted laws requiring birth and death registration. The annual collection of mortality statistics for the national death registration area began in 1900. Included were ten states and the District of Columbia where model laws had been adopted and where registration was at least 90 percent complete. The national birth registration area was established in 1915 and included ten states and the District of Columbia. By 1933, the national birth and death registration areas included all states in the union.

Statistics need not be regarded as impersonal; often they are more revealing than any descriptive writing. Systematic statistical procedures are indispensable to the practice of nursing. What is needed is an intelligent grasp of what figures stand for and what they can be used to express. Statistics are essential for the study and practice of epidemiology, which measures and evaluates the health problems of a community. How does a community measure its health problems? Through mandatory and voluntary sources, a community gathers demographic, vital registration, and health information. Tabulated in workable units, these demographic data, vital statistics, and health statistics are components of biostatistics, the branch of statistics that measures biological phenomena. (See Table 6-1.)

Vital statistics are concerned with people. They describe events related to individuals entering or leaving life or changing their civil status. Registration of vital events in the United States is a state and local function, and is one of the basic services of a qualified health department. The laws of every state provide for a continuous and permanent birth and death registration system. Each system requires accuracy in reporting and depends upon the conscientious efforts of the persons who prepare or certify the information needed to complete the original records. In many states local registrars collect records of events occurring in their areas and transmit them to the health department in the state office. (See Figure 6-1.) The state vital statistics office inspects the records for promptness, completeness, and consistency. The state is responsible for issuing official copies of certificates to individuals in need of such records and verifying the facts of birth and death for agencies requiring legal evidence of such facts. (For specimens of birth, fetal death, and death certificates, see Appendix.)

At the federal level, the National Center for Health Statistics in the Public Health Service is the major coordinating body in matters dealing with vital and health statistics. Universal guidelines for gathering and analyzing vital and health data have been established by international agreement under the auspices of the World Health Organization. The WHO publishes the *International Statistical Classification of Diseases, Injuries, and Causes of Deaths* in the form of a manual, which is periodically reviewed and revised.

Table 6-1

	Demographic Data	Vital Statistics	Health Statistics
Description	Specific information regarding the population, e.g., the number of inhabitants, age, sex, race, marital status, number and makeup of households, condition of housing, migration, income, education, occupation, distance traveled to and from work, etc.	The vital events that occur over a period of time within a population—such as birth, death, marriage, divorce, adoption, annulment, and separation—often called the "bookkeeping of public health."	(a) measurements of the state of health, i.e., morbidity data that relate to the distribution of illness (incidence and prevalence), as distinct from mortality; (b) measurement of factors closely related to health, e.g., sanitation, nutrition, poverty; (c) measurements of health programs, services, activities.
How Gathered	Nationwide census enumeration every ten years as decreed by the Constitution—first census was taken in 1790; for each state a census report is published with four sections—the number of inhabitants, general population characteristics, general social and economic characteristics, detailed characteristics.	Facts, systematically selected and compiled in numerical form, are derived from official records; compulsory reporting of births and deaths is a function of state and local governments; standard recommended certificates are provided by the National Center for Health Statistics, but must be approved by state legislatures (the right to privacy must be preserved); facts of reporting life and death have been classified and standardized by international agreements through WHO (International Classification of Diseases, Injuries, and Causes of Death).	Morbidity data are gathered from official sources (such as the reports of notifiable diseases, the National Health Survey, state and local health registries, other health surveys) as well as voluntary sources (such as industry, mass screening, insurance companies); other health data are derived from surveys, agency reports, peer review groups, etc.
How Applied in Public Health	Census data, expressed in statistical terms such as averages, percentages, and ratios, offer information relevant to public health, e.g., (a) age distribution of a population, (b) dependency ratio, related to the age distribution, (c) socioeconomic characteristics (income, education, employment); all of these factors are considered in community health planning.	Data are expressed in vital rates—a vital rate is the number of occurrences of a vital event that take place during a given period of time (usually a calendar year) divided by the average population "at risk" to the event (usually the estimated mid-year population); examples of vital rates are crude birth rate, crude death rate, infant mortality rate, perinatal mortality rate, maternal mortality rate, cause-specific death rate; these facts are helpful in identifying health needs, establishing priorities, determining allocation of funds, planning and evaluating health programs.	Health statistics serve as the basis for assessing specific health needs and planning public health programs; incidence and prevalence rates help in determining priorities for prevention and control of disease; health data provide information for allocation of funds, evaluation of health programs, and research.

FLOW OF VITAL RECORDS AND STATISTICS IN THE UNITED STATES

RESPONSIBLE PERSON OR AGENCY	BIRTH CERTIFICATE	DEATH CERTIFICATE	FETAL DEATH CERTIFICATE (Stillbirth)	NOTIFIABLE DISEASE REPORT	REPORTING OFFICIALS	MARRIAGE RECORD	DIVORCE OR ANNULMENT RECORD
Physician or Other Professional Attendant	Completes entire certificate in consultation with parent(s). Files certificate with local registrar of district in which birth occurs.	1. Completes medical certification and signs certificate. 2. Returns certificate to funeral director.	Certifies to the cause of fetal death and signs certificate. Returns it to funeral director.	Reports each case by telephone or by mail on special form to local or State health department.	Clerk of Local Government	1. Receives application for marriage license. 2. Verifies information from serological tests. 3. Issues marriage license. 4. Sends completed record of marriage to State registrar.	
Funeral Director		1. Obtains personal facts about the deceased. 2. Takes certificate to physician for medical certification. 3. Delivers completed certificate to local registrar and obtains burial permit.	1. Obtains facts about the fetal death. 2. Takes certificate to physician for entry of causes of fetal death. 3. Delivers completed certificate to local registrar and obtains burial permit.		Marriage Officiant	1. Performs the marriage ceremony. 2. Certifies to facts of marriage and sends the record to license clerk.	
Local Registrar of Vital Statistics	Verifies completeness and accuracy. Makes copy, ledger entry, or index for local use. Sends certificates to local health department or to State registrar.	1. Verifies completeness and accuracy. Makes copy, ledger entry, or index for local use. Sends certificates to local health department or to State registrar. 2. Issues burial permit to funeral director. 3. Verifies returns of burial permits.	1. Verifies completeness and accuracy. Makes copy, ledger entry, or index for local use. Sends certificates to local health department or to State registrar. 2. Issues burial permit to funeral director. 3. Verifies returns of burial permits.		Clerk of Court		1. Provides form for report to petitioner or attorney, or uses petition for decree to make entries on such form. 2. Verifies entries on returned form. 3. Enters final decree facts. 4. Sends completed report to State registrar.
City or County Health Department	1. Uses certificates in allocating medical and nursing services, follow up of infectious diseases, planning programs, and measuring effectiveness of activities. 2. Forwards certificates and case reports to State registrar.				Attorney for Petitioner		1. Enters personal facts relative to spouses. 2. Returns form to clerk of court.
State Health Department Bureau of Vital Statistics	1. Queries incomplete or inconsistent information. 2. Maintains files for permanent reference and source of certified copies. 3. Compiles statistics for State and civil divisions of State for use of the health department and other interested agencies or groups. 4. Prepares transcripts or microfilm copies of birth, death, and fetal death certificates, and summary reports of marriage, divorce, and notifiable disease records for transmission to National Office of Vital Statistics.						
Public Health Service National Office of Vital Statistics	1. Prepares and publishes national statistics of births, deaths, fetal deaths, marriages, divorces, and notifiable diseases for official and voluntary consumers. 2. Publishes analyses of data as they relate to public health and social problems. 3. Provides services needed to foster more complete and uniform registration.						

Figure 6-1 Note: In some states certificates of birth, death, and fetal death, and reports of notifiable diseases are not routed through local health departments; in others, there is no central file for marriage and divorce records at the state level.

Source U.S. Department of Health, Education, and Welfare, National Vital Statistics Needs, A Report of the U.S. National Committee on Vital and Health Statistics. National Center for Vital Statistics, 1965.

The eighth revision appeared in 1965, in a two-volume report. WHO member nations are currently making recommendations for the ninth revision, which will be released for use in 1978.

PRESENTATION OF DATA

After information has been gathered in numerical counts, it must be classified in an orderly manner, so that emerging data can be readily analyzed and effectively utilized. Beginning with an unsorted mass of raw material, the public health worker must first consider what answers the material can provide. Then he must determine the form of presentation that brings out the answers most clearly. We shall now discuss ways in which data may be presented. An important first step is the categorical grouping of data and the calculation of certain measures so that meaningful relationships can be demonstrated as follows:

Basic Mathematical Approach

(1) Grouping of Data

Frequency distribution A statistical table constructed from grouped data, showing the number of observations in each one of several classification groups, which are established at equal intervals.

(2) Measures of Central Tendency

Average A value that is typical or representative of a set of data. Such typical values tend to lie centrally within a set of data arranged according to magnitude. Averages are also called measures of central tendency. Several types of averages can be defined, the most common in public health reporting being arithmetic mean, median, and mode.

Arithmetic mean The sum total of values recorded in a series of observations, divided by the number of observations. The term "average" is often used synonymously with "mean."

Median The value in a set of observations that neither exceeds nor is exceeded by more than half of the observations. The median is often said to be the "middle" observation, or the value above which half of the observations lie and below which half lie. When there is an odd number of observations, the median is the value of the middle observation after the individual items have been ranked in order. With an even number of events, e.g., one hundred cases, the median is the value obtained by averaging observations fifty and fifty-one. The median is a useful average when the mean is greatly affected by extremely large or small outlying observations.

Mode The value that occurs most frequently in a series of observations.

(3) Measures of Dispersion

Range   The distance between the lowest and highest values recorded in a series of observations.

Standard deviation   A measure of variability that reflects the scatter or dispersion of the observations around their mean. The value is obtained by setting out all the observations, determining the difference of each from the mean, squaring this difference, totalling these squares, dividing the total thus obtained by the number of observations, and taking the square root of this number. It is customary to present the mean with the standard deviation attached.

To illustrate the above terms, the following example may be used. There is a group of twenty-five eight-year-old girls whose individual heights in centimeters are recorded as follows: 114, 117, 118, 119, 119, 120, 121, 121, 122, 122, 124, 124, 125, 126, 127, 127, 127, 127, 127, 127, 128, 129, 129, 130, 130. The frequency distribution could be expressed as it is in Table 6-2.

Table 6-2   Frequency of measurements of height of twenty-five eight-year-old girls

Height (to nearest centimeter)	Number of girls
114	1
115	0
116	0
117	1
118	1
119	2
120	1
121	2
122	2
123	0
124	2
125	1
126	1
127	6
128	1
129	2
130	2

The range for this distribution would be the distance between the lowest value (114 centimeters) and the highest value (130 centimeters), or 16 centimeters. The average height expressed as the arithmetic mean would be the sum total of the heights in centimeters (3100) divided by the number of observations (25), or 124 centimeters. The median height in this series of observations (total 25, an uneven number) falls at 125 centimeters, which is the middle observation. The mode, or the value that occurs most frequently, is 127 centimeters. The standard deviation is 4.35 centimeters.

Conversion of Absolute Numbers to Relative Numbers

In presenting data, the health worker may find that the use of gross figures is pertinent for the description of certain health-related facts, for example, the total number of cases of a reportable infectious disease over a given period of time (see page 121), the number of motor vehicle accidents resulting in death or disability (see page 136), the daily fluctuations of bed occupancy in a hospital. Such data may be usefully presented in absolute numbers, without any further computation.

When it is necessary to show relationships between given sets of events, absolute numbers must be converted to relative numbers and may be expressed as percentages, ratios, or rates.

Percentages   The general function of percentage figures is to clarify relationships between numbers. One of the numbers (the base) is translated into 100, which is easily divided into and by other numbers. The use of percent figures makes it easy to see the precise relationship of the part to the whole. The base of 100 may be raised to a higher figure, for example, 1000, 10,000, or 100,000, in expressing particular ratios or rates that have been established through international agreement in reporting health data.

Percentages are used in describing the characteristics of a population, for example, the United States census of 1970 shows that of the 203,200,000 persons counted:

149,300,000 or 73.5 percent lived in urban areas (it is interesting that only 1.5 percent of the total land area is classified as urban, thus in the United States, nearly three-fourths of the population lives on less than 2 percent of the land);

177,748,975 or 87.5 percent were white;

22,580,289 or 11.1 percent were black;

2,882,662 or 1.4 percent were other races (Indian, Japanese, Chinese, Filipino, and others).

Ratios and Rates   Ratios and rates express values in relative terms, rendering them useful in the analysis of vital events. It is difficult to make a rigid distinction between the terms "ratio" and "rate." All rates are ratios, but not all ratios are rates. We will attempt to clarify the difference by citing examples.

In simplest terms a ratio is a relative number obtained by dividing one number by another. For example, when a population is described, the sex ratio is often cited. The 1970 census shows 98,910,000 males as compared with 104,290,000 females, or a ratio of 94.8 males to 100 females.

Rates, on the other hand, are always based on the population defined as "at risk." The population at risk may be the total population as in the crude birth rate, crude death rate (see below), or the population at risk may be only a segment of the population indentified for a specific rate as in a specific death rate for age or sex. Rates imply a time period, for example, birth rates, death rates, marriage and divorce rates are usually cited in terms of a given year.

The rates and ratios commonly used to describe the health status of a community are listed below. For the most part, they are generally accepted and widely applied terms, which, once defined, can be readily interpreted.

Rates and Ratios Commonly Used in Community Health

$$\text{Crude birth rate} = \frac{\text{number of live births in a given year}}{\text{estimated mid-year population}} \times 1000$$

The crude birth rate shows the number of live births in relation to the total population expressed in multiples of 1000. It measures the rate at which additions are being made to the entire population through childbirth. All states in the U.S. follow, with minor variations, the definition of live birth recommended by the World Health Organization. Essentially this provides that all births that show any evidence of life after being completely outside the mother's body are live births regardless of duration of gestation or birth weight.

$$\text{Crude death rate} = \frac{\text{number of deaths in a given year}}{\text{estimated mid-year population}} \times 1000$$

The crude death rate measures the resultant of all the various forces acting on a population that will lead to death, in a given year. It represents, within broad limits, the average chance of death for persons in a given group, and it expresses the expected toll against the population by death. The crude death rate does not differentiate the various types of forces and the various parts of the population affected by these forces. Taken alone, this rate must be used with utmost caution in comparisons of one locality with another or of one time period with another.

$$\text{Specific death rate} = \frac{\text{number of deaths in a specified group [e.g., by age or sex] in a given year}}{\text{mid-year population of the specified group}} \times 1000$$

The death rate specific for any defined class of the population measures the risk of dying in that class. It is computed from the number of deaths occurring in the defined class and the total number of persons in that class.

$$\text{Infant mortality rate} = \frac{\text{number of deaths of infants under one year of age in a given year}}{\text{number of live births during the same year}} \times 1000$$

The infant mortality rate relates the number of deaths under one year of age to the number of live births. When based on accurate data and complete birth and death registration, this rate is universally recognized as a most sensitive index, and perhaps the best single index, of the health status of a community. A high infant mortality rate in a community is often associated with inferior living and sanitary conditions, poor nutrition, low educational levels and inadequate health care resources. Children in their first year of life are highly vulnerable. The death rate during this period is about equal to that for ages one to twenty-nine combined, and is not exceeded until age sixty-five and over.[3]

$$\text{Neonatal mortality rate} = \frac{\text{number of deaths under 28 days of age in a given year}}{\text{number of live births during the same year}} \times 1000$$

The neonatal mortality rate measures the risk of death during the first few weeks of life, a most vulnerable period for the infant.

$$\text{Fetal mortality rate} = \frac{\text{number of fetal deaths of specified period of gestation in a given year}}{\text{number of live births plus number of fetal deaths of specified period of gestation during that same year}} \times 1000$$

The World Health Organization's definition of fetal death states essentially that death of a product of conception must occur prior to complete expulsion or extraction from its mother, as indicated by the fact that after separation the fetus shows no signs of life. (Fetal death may be early—less than twenty weeks of gestation; intermediate—more than twenty but less than twenty-eight weeks; or late—twenty-eight weeks and over.) Such an event is defined as a fetal death regardless of the duration of pregnancy. Some states have adopted this definition while others have included in their definition a specified minimum gestation period. Thus, each state varies in its requirements for registering fetal deaths. The policy of the National Center for Health Statistics has been to collect and publish data only on fetal deaths with a gestation age of twenty weeks or more. Reporting of fetal deaths is often incomplete—a serious gap is the lack of reporting of the abortion component of fetal deaths. For all these reasons, the fetal mortality rate is recognized as a limited measure of the risk of fetal death.

$$\text{Perinatal mortality rate} = \frac{\text{fetal deaths plus neonatal deaths in a given year}}{\text{fetal deaths plus live births in that same year}} \times 1000$$

The perinatal mortality rate measures the risk of death prior to, during, and soon after the birth process. This rate was developed after it was recognized that the problems of the late fetal period and neonatal period are closely interwoven, and any attempt to study these problems must include both periods. The perinatal period is of utmost importance to the life and health of the child; the risk of death is greater at that point than at any other time until old age.

$$\text{Maternal mortality rate} = \frac{\text{number of deaths attributed to maternal conditions in a given year}}{\text{number of live births in that same year}} \times \begin{array}{c} 10,000 \\ \text{or} \\ 100,000 \end{array}$$

The maternal mortality rate measures the risk of death from deliveries and complications of pregnancy, childbirth, and the puerperium. For purposes of statistical reporting, the post partum period extends to ninety days. The maternal mortality rate is another sensitive index to the health status of a community, and to the priority that is given to the care of its citizens.

$$\frac{\text{Cause-of-death}}{\text{rate}} = \frac{\text{number of deaths from a stated cause in a given year}}{\text{estimated mid-year population}} \times 100{,}000$$

This rate measures the loss of population due to stated causes, and is reflected in the oft-cited lists of the "ten" or "five" or "three leading causes of death."

$$\frac{\text{Incidence}}{\text{rate}} = \frac{\text{number of newly reported cases of a particular disease or condition during a given time period}}{\text{total population exposed to the risk of the disease or condition during that time}} \times \begin{array}{c} 1000 \\ \text{or} \\ 10{,}000 \\ \text{or} \\ 100{,}000 \end{array}$$

The incidence rate measures the frequency of new cases of a specified disease or condition that occur in a population (see also p. 69). Incidence rates refer to a given time interval rather than a single date in contrast with prevalence. The incidence rate also marks the beginnings of epidemics and helps to analyze their course, extent, and control. It is subject to errors of interpretation as a result of faulty diagnosis or deficient reporting, and must be based on carefully conducted investigations.

$$\frac{\text{Prevalence}}{\text{rate}} = \frac{\text{number of cases of a particular disease, injury, or condition existing at a stated time}}{\text{total population at that time}} \times \begin{array}{c} 1000 \\ \text{or} \\ 10{,}000 \\ \text{or} \\ 100{,}000 \end{array}$$

The prevalence rate measures the amount of a given disease or condition existing in a population at a particular point in time, regardless of when that illness or condition began (see also p. 70).

$$\frac{\text{Case}}{\text{fatality}} = \frac{\text{number of deaths from a specific condition}}{\text{number of cases of that same condition}} \times 100$$

The case fatality rate measures the fatality among persons who have a specified disease or condition. It is usually expressed in percent terms. The rate is reliable and useful in connection with clinical studies of disease, that is, under clinical conditions where one can observe a definite number of cases in a well-defined category.

Use of Tables and Graphs

Tables and graphs are indispensable tools for the presentation of statistical data. These tools, in order to be useful, must be clear and concise, properly labeled, and identified as to their source. They must be entirely self-explanatory without reference to the text. Somewhere—in the title, label, or legend—they should explain what, where, when, and how. If we need to ask why, they should be discarded immediately.

PRIVACY AND CONFIDENTIALITY OF HEALTH DATA

All thoughtful health practitioners are concerned about the issue of privacy and confidentiality in collecting and using health data. They must be sensitive to the feelings of individuals who might regard any kind of questioning or information gathering as an invasion of privacy and a violation of personal rights. People worry about computers, case registers, data banks, and other repositories of detailed personal information.

As nurses, we need to understand how we are perceived, and we need to communicate a broader understanding of what we are doing when we gather information for assessment or statistical tabulation. We should be ready to explain why we are doing this, and point out that the privacy of the individual is protected in several ways. First of all, there are legal safeguards—controls, checks, and conformance requirements—for the statistical files where data are stored. More importantly we can offer assurance through our own personal conduct, with guidance from the Code of Ethics adopted by our profession.

Nursing has a professional obligation to maintain the confidentiality of the people it serves, as reflected in the following statements:

> The nurse holds in confidence personal information and uses judgment in sharing this information.[4]

> The nurse safeguards the individual's right to privacy by judiciously protecting information of a confidential nature, sharing only that information relevant to his care. . . . The nurse participates in research activities when assured that the rights of individual subjects are protected.[5]

REFERENCES

1. C. Fraser Brockington, *The Health of the Community,* 3rd ed. (London: J.A. Churchill, 1965), p. 6.

2. Wilson G. Smillie, *Preventive Medicine and Public Health* (New York: Macmillan Co., 1953), p. 29.

3. Helen C. Chase, "The Position of the United States in International Comparisons of Health Status," *American Journal of Public Health,* 62 (April 1972) 581-89.

4. International Council of Nurses, "1973 Code for Nurses—Ethical Concepts Applied to Nursing," *American Journal of Nursing,* 73 (August 1973) 1351.

5. American Nurses' Association, "Code for Nurses," (adopted 1950; revised 1960 and 1968), *American Journal of Nursing,* 68 (December 1968) 2581-85.

ADDITIONAL READINGS

Goldsmith, Seth B., "The Status of Health Status Indicators," in *Health Services Reports,* 87 (March 1972) 212–20.

Hill, A. Bradford, *Principles of Medical Statistics.* 9th ed. New York: Oxford University Press, 1971.

Levine, Eugene, "The ABCs of Statistics," in *American Journal of Nursing,* 59 (January 1959) 71–75.

———, "Interpreting Statistical Data," in *American Journal of Nursing,* 59 (February 1959) 230–33.

Miller, Arthur R., *The Assault on Privacy: Computers, Data Banks, and Dossiers.* Ann Arbor, Mich.: University of Michigan Press, 1971.

National Center for Health Statistics, *Annual Report of the United States National Committee on Vital and Health Statistics, 1973.* Available from the United States Department of Health, Education, and Welfare.

———, *Health Statistics Today and Tomorrow.* (4,15) Washington, D.C.: Government Printing Office, 1973.

———, *Hospital Handbook on Birth and Fetal Death Registration, 1973.* Available from the United States Department of Health, Education, and Welfare.

———, *Medical Examiners' and Coroners' Handbook on Death and Fetal Death Registration, 1971.* Available from the United States Department of Health, Education, and Welfare.

———, *National Vital Statistics Needs: A Report of the United States National Committee on Vital and Health Statistics.* (4,2) Washington, D.C.: Government Printing Office, 1965.

———, *Report of the Twentieth Anniversary Conference of the United States National Committee on Vital and Health Statistics.* (4,13) Washington, D.C.: Government Printing Office, 1970.

———, *Proceedings of the Public Health Conference on Records and Statistics.* (12th national meeting) Washington, D.C.: Government Printing Office, 1968.

———, *Vital Statistics Rates in the United States, 1940-1960.* Washington, D.C.: Government Printing Office, 1968.

The Philadelphia Inquirer, 1973 World Almanac. New York: Newspaper Enterprise Association.

Phillips, Jeanne S., and Richard F. Thompson, *Statistics for Nurses.* New York: Macmillan Co., 1967.

Puffer, Ruth R., *Practical Statistics in Health and Medical Work.* New York: McGraw-Hill, 1950.

Schor, Stanley S., *Fundamentals of Biostatistics.* New York: G. P. Putnam's Sons, 1968.

Swaroop, Satya, *Introduction to Health Statistics.* Edinburgh and London: E. & S. Livingstone, Ltd., 1960.

Terris, Milton, "Desegregating Health Statistics," in *American Journal of Public Health,* 63 (June 1973) 477–80.

Tokuhata, George K., Virginia C. Colflesh, Krishnan Ramaswamy, Linda A. Mann, and Eaward Digon, "Hospital and Related Characteristics Associated with Perinatal Mortality," in *American Journal of Public Health,* 63 (March 1973) 227–37.

Trauger, Donald A., "What is a Good Statistical Report?" in *Health Services Reports,* 87 (October 1972) 693–96.

WHO Manual of the International Statistical Classification of Diseases, Injuries, and Causes of Death. 8th rev. Geneva: World Health Organization, 1965.

Wilner, Daniel, Rosabelle Price Walkley, and Lenor S. Goerke, *Introduction to Public Health.* 6th ed. New York: Macmillan Co., 1973.

Appendix
Sample Copies of Live Birth, Fetal Death, and Death Certificates

H105. 142 REV. 3-72
500M 3-72

Local Registrar's No. ____________

Primary Dist. No. ____________

COMMONWEALTH OF PENNSYLVANIA
DEPARTMENT OF HEALTH
VITAL STATISTICS

CERTIFICATE OF LIVE BIRTH

SPECIMEN FORM ONLY

1. PLACE OF BIRTH a. County
b. City, borough, or township
c. Name of hospital or institution

2. MOTHER'S MAILING ADDRESS a. Street address, R.D. or box number
b. Post office, state, and zip code

3. INFORMANT

CHILD

4. THIS CHILD'S NAME a. (First) b. (Middle) c. (Last)

5. THIS CHILD'S SEX

6 a. THIS BIRTH WAS Single ☐ Twin ☐ Triplet ☐

6 b. If TWIN or TRIPLET. This child was born: 1st ☐ 2nd ☐ 3rd ☐

7. DATE OF BIRTH (Month) (Day) (Year)

FATHER

8. FATHER'S FULL NAME a. (First) b. (Middle) c. (Last)

9. HIS AGE Years

10. HIS BIRTHPLACE (State or foreign country)

11. a. HIS USUAL OCCUPATION

11. b. KIND OF BUSINESS OR INDUSTRY

MOTHER

12. MOTHER'S FULL MAIDEN NAME a. (First) b. (Middle) c. (Last)

13. HER AGE Years

14. HER BIRTHPLACE (State or foreign country)

15. WHERE DOES MOTHER ACTUALLY LIVE? a. State b. County

16. CHILDREN Previously Born to This Mother (DO NOT include this child)
a. How many are NOW living?
b. How many were born alive but are NOW DEAD?
c. How many were delivered dead after sixteen weeks pregnancy?

c. Does Mother Live in a Township? (NOT within the limit of a city or borough)
☐ YES, she lives in ____________ Township.
☐ NO, she lives within the actual limits of ____________ City or Borough.

17. I hereby certify that this child was born alive on the date stated above at ____________ m., E. T.
Signed ____________ ☐ M.D. ☐ D.O. ☐ Other (Specify) Certifier's Address ____________
Date Signed ____________

18. DATE RECEIVED FOR FILING

19. LOCAL REGISTRAR'S SIGNATURE S.S. No.

CONFIDENTIAL medical report below MUST be completed for MEDICAL and HEALTH use

20. FATHER'S RACE

21. MOTHER'S RACE

22 a. LENGTH of PREGNANCY in ____________ COMPLETED WEEKS

22 b. WEIGHT OF CHILD AT BIRTH ______ grams or ______ lbs. ______ oz.

23. LEGITIMATE? Yes ☐ No ☐

24. IN WHAT TRIMESTER WAS FIRST VISIT PRENATAL CARE? 1st ☐ 2nd ☐ 3rd ☐ No visit ☐ Unknown ☐

25. SEROLOGIC TEST for SYPHILIS Yes ☐ No ☐ Date

26. METHOD OF DELIVERY

27. DESCRIBE ANY CONGENITAL MALFORMATION

28. DESCRIBE ANY COMPLICATION OF LABOR

29. DESCRIBE ANY BIRTH INJURY

30. DESCRIBE ANY COMPLICATION OF PREGNANCY

A ____________
B ____________
C ____________
D ____________
E ____________
F ____________
G ____________
H ____________
I ____________

NOTICE

Make certain that the appropriate Letter "D" or "S" is inserted in the Time Element in Item 17.

Figure 6-2

Source Figures 6-2 through 6-4 reproduced courtesy of the Pennsylvania Department of Health.

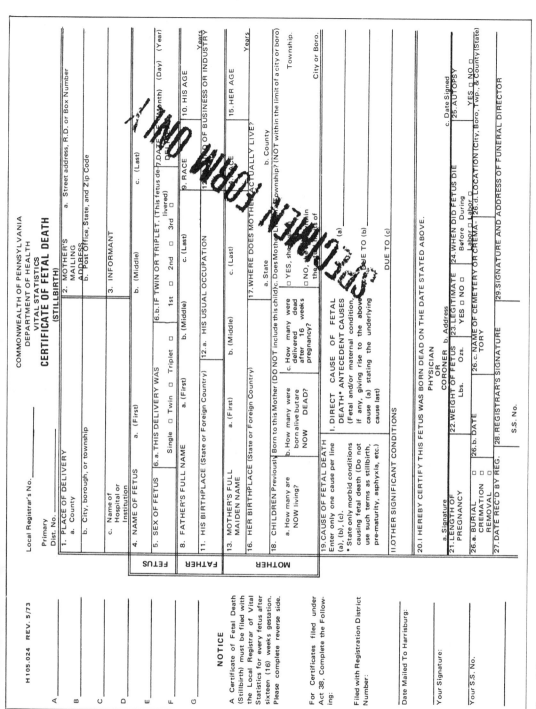

Figure 6-3

250M 3-72

COMMONWEALTH OF PENNSYLVANIA
DEPARTMENT OF HEALTH
VITAL STATISTICS
CERTIFICATE OF DEATH

H105.143 REV. 3-72
LOCAL REG. NO. _____
PRIMARY
DIST. NO. _____

1. DEATH OCCURRED IN:
   a. County
   b. City or borough
   a. Street address, R.D., or Box Number

2. DECEASED'S MAILING ADDRESS
   b. Post Office, State and Zip Code

   c. If death did not occur in City or borough, give name of township (Do not use R.D. or Box Number)

3. VETERAN   Yes ☐   No ☐
   a. Which War   b. Serial No. _____

d. Full Name of Hospital or institution (if not in hospital, give street address)

4. NAME OF DECEASED (Type or print)
   a. (First)   b. (Middle)   c. (Last)

5. DATE OF DEATH   (Month) (Day) (Year)

6. WHERE DID DECEASED ACTUALLY LIVE?
   a. State
   b. County
   c. Did deceased live in a township?
   ☐ Yes, deceased lived in _____ township.
   ☐ No, deceased lived within actual limits of _____ city or borough.

7. SEX 8. RACE

9. MARRIED ☐ NEVER MARRIED ☐
   WIDOWED ☐ DIVORCED ☐

10. DATE OF BIRTH

11. AGE (years last birthday) If under 1 year If under 24 hours
    Months Days Hours Min.

12. USUAL OCCUPATION (even if retired)

13. SOCIAL SECURITY NO.

14. BIRTHPLACE (State or foreign country)

15. CITIZEN OF WHAT COUNTRY?

16. FULL NAME OF SPOUSE

17. MOTHER'S MAIDEN NAME

18. FATHER'S NAME

19. INFORMANT'S NAME, ADDRESS AND ZIP CODE

20. CAUSE OF DEATH: Enter only one cause per line for (a), (b) & (c).

MEDICAL CERTIFICATE (Items 20 through 23 must be completed by physician only)

PART 1. Death was caused by:
   IMMEDIATE CAUSE (a) _____

Conditions, if any, which gave rise to above cause (a) stating the underlying cause last.
   DUE TO (b) _____
   DUE TO (c) _____

INTERVAL BETWEEN ONSET AND DEATH

PART II. OTHER SIGNIFICANT CONDITIONS: contributing to death but not related to the immediate cause given in Part I (a)

21. WAS AUTOPSY PERFORMED   Yes ☐ No ☐

22. a. ACCIDENT Yes ☐ No ☐
    b. DESCRIBE HOW ACCIDENT OCCURRED

22. c. TIME OF ACCIDENT   Month Day Year
    Hour   m. E.   T.

22. d. ACCIDENT OCCURRED
    While at work ☐ Not while at work ☐

22. e. PLACE OF ACCIDENT (e.g., home, farm, street, etc.)

22. f. CITY, BOROUGH, TOWNSHIP   COUNTY   STATE

23. I hereby certify that I attended the above named deceased and that death occurred from the causes and on the date stated above at _____ m., E. _____ T.

   a. Signature
   M.D. or D.O.
   b. Address
   c. Date signed

24. a. BURIAL ☐ CREMATION ☐ REMOVAL ☐
    b. DATE
    c. NAME OF CEMETERY OR CREMATORY

24. d. LOCATION (City, Boro., Twp., & County) (State)

25. DATE REC'D BY REG.

26. REGISTRAR'S SIGNATURE
    S.S. No. _____

27. SIGNATURE AND ADDRESS OF FUNERAL DIRECTOR

A _____
B _____
C _____
D _____
E _____
F _____
G _____

NOTICE

Make certain that the appropriate Letter "D" or "S" is inserted in the Time Elements in Items 22c and 23.

For Certificates filed under Act 38, Complete the Following:

Filed with Registration District Number: _____

Date Mailed To Harrisburg: _____

Your Signature: _____

Your S. S. No. _____

Figure 6-4

88

Chapter 7
Nutrition

"Undoubtedly, the desire for food has been, and still is, one of the main causes of great political events." [1]

INTRODUCTION

Looking back to your days in elementary or secondary school, you may recall those lists of "Rules for Good Health," which nearly always started with "Eat a balanced diet." Such lists might have included explanations that a balanced diet provides the essential nutrients—proteins, carbohydrates, fats, vitamins, minerals, water—in amounts adequate to create the energy we need to work, play, think, read, laugh, and cry. You may remember nutrients being described as the food elements required for the physiological and biochemical body processes involved in energy and heat production, growth and development, tissue repair and maintenance, and reproduction. Your basic health courses probably included guides for a balanced diet through the proper selection of items from established food groups. For many years, the accepted guide has been one that classifies foods into four basic food groupings — breads and cereals, milk and milk products, vegetables and fruits, and meat (see Figure 7-1).

In our activities of daily living, food plays a vital role that most of us take for granted; it provides the nourishment essential to the life and health of every human being. But the matter does not rest there, for we eat not only to live. Food influences almost every facet of life. It is a psychosocial and economic vehicle. Going out for dinner is often a social occasion, or it may be an opportunity to discuss business. The practice of dining together daily at home may provide the only setting for family togetherness, a time for sharing experiences, seeking mutual support, and strengthening bonds of affection, in an otherwise hectic and stress-filled existence. Food has also been used as a

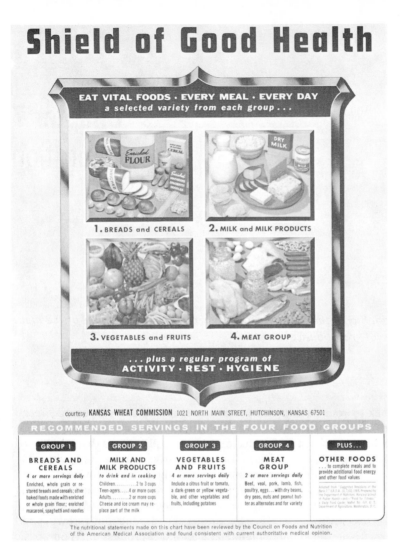

Figure 7-1

Source Courtesy of the Kansas Wheat Commission.

political weapon. For want of food, nations have warred against each other. Throughout history, the great migrations of people can often be traced to their efforts at finding new supplies of food. It has served as an offering in humanitarian gestures, whether through individual hospitality, community disaster relief, food basket distribution during holiday seasons, or worldwide shipments of food from the more affluent nations to the less fortunate people of the world.

The science of nutrition, occupying a special place in community health and nursing, has been defined as the study of food and food nutrients in relation to health and disease. Nutrition may be regarded as the sum total of all processes by which the body receives and utilizes food nutrients necessary for maintaining its functions. Nutrition is the most important single factor affecting health. It plays a vital role in the prevention and control of many diseases and conditions. This is true at any age and at every stage of development. Good nutrition implies the right amounts and kinds of food to meet the needs of all body cells. Good nutritional status is a condition of the body which results from proper utilization of all essential nutrients.

FACTORS WHICH INFLUENCE NUTRITIONAL STATUS

There are many overt and subtle influences on nutritional status. Genetic factors—sex, age, race, anatomical structure, and physiological functioning—are well recognized. Of equal importance are environmental and cultural influences, including geographic location, agricultural practices, technology, communication, transportation, social and economic conditions, political policies, poverty, affluence, education, ethnic background, habits, customs, mores, prejudice, superstition, and religion. Tradition and intense feelings are often tied up with food. Food habits are deeply ingrained and are slow to change even when people are confronted with a major health crisis. A thorough understanding of this concept is basic to any type of nursing or medical intervention. Health teaching that effects desired change is the nurse's major contribution to good nutrition.

Scientific and technologic advances, which inevitably affect food production, have not been equally available throughout the world; hence food supplies are inadequate in many areas. Malnutrition has been and continues to be the major global health problem. Famine and near-starvation are a way of life for large segments of the world's population. Other peoples who "enjoy" the affluent life are afflicted with an overabundance of foodstuffs and an excessive intake of calories. Malnutrition, whether manifested as undernutrition or obesity, includes those conditions related to diet deficiencies and irregularities, as well as those related to defects in absorption and utilization of foods. Common forms of malnutrition are summarized as shown in Table 7-1.

Malnutrition is causally related to other acute and chronic, infectious and non-infectious diseases and conditions. For example, diarrheal disorders increase and tuberculosis mortality rises in periods of famine or other serious food restrictions. In many cases of heart attack and stroke, a causal relationship has been demonstrated with diets too high in saturated fats. Diabetes is frequently associated with obesity, and in many instances can be treated or prevented through diet therapy aimed at weight control.

Another group of disorders that are related to diet and respond to diet therapy are those classified as inborn errors of metabolism. One of these diseases, phenylketonuria (PKU), is characterized by the inability to

Table 7-1 Some Common Forms of Malnutrition

Nutrient Irregularity	Clinical Condition or Disease	Treatment
Lack of adequate calories	General undernutrition or chronic partial starvation, ranging from slight impairment of vital functions and underweight to extreme malnourishment and debility	Increased intake of highly nutritious, easily digested foods
Protein-calorie malnutrition	Kwashiorkor (caloric intake may be sufficient but protein is lacking) and marasmus (both calories and protein are deficient)—conditions which occur when infants, after they are weaned, must subsist on diets inadequate in protein	A protein-rich diet with plenty of milk (and added calories for the more extreme condition of marasmus)
Iron-deficiency	Anemia, microcytic, hypochromic	Adequate diet with iron supplements
Vitamin B-12 deficiency (related to lack of intrinsic factor in gastric juice)	Pernicious anemia	Adequate diet with vitamin B-12 by injection
Lack of folic acid	Macrocytic anemia in pregnancy and infancy	Additional folate therapy
Riboflavin deficiency	Cheilosis (lesions at corners of mouth); skin lesions; corneal vascularization and opacities	Diet rich in milk and organic meats - natural sources of riboflavin
Thiamine deficiency (vitamin B-1)	Beriberi; polyneuritis; emaciation; circulatory failure	Vitamin B-1 daily, orally or by injection
Niacin deficiency	Pellagra (dermatitis, diarrhea, dementia)	Niacin daily; supplements of yeast; liver injections
Vitamin A deficiency	Night blindness; xerophthalmia	Diet therapy with vitamin A supplement
Vitamin D deficiency	Rickets; bone deformities; osteomalacia	Diet therapy with vitamin D supplement
Lack of ascorbic acid (vitamin C)	Scurvy	Daily administration of ascorbic acid in large doses
Iodine deficiency	Endemic goiter	Preventive measures are most effective—iodine added to table salt
Excess of calories	Obesity	Diet therapy; exercise; emotional support

metabolize the amino acid, phenylalanine. PKU can be detected through urine screening in infancy. Galactosemia and maple syrup urine disease are two other genetically determined metabolic disorders. All of these are similar in that they begin to produce harmful effects at birth, and unless diet therapy is started early, they may result in irreversible brain damage and mental retardation.

NUTRITION IN GROWTH AND DEVELOPMENT

Nutrition as a factor in primary prevention is seen at every level of the life cycle. Even prior to conception, the outcome of pregnancy and the subsequent growth and development of a child are greatly affected by the nutritional status of the mother. From the very beginning of intrauterine life, the course of fetal development is heavily dependent on the mother's nutritional state.

Pregnancy

Pregnancy is a period when dietary needs are especially crucial and when diet counseling is of utmost importance. Research in recent decades has shown a relationship between maternal nutrition and the baby's condition at birth. Current concepts in dietary management during pregnancy are described below.

NEW CONCEPTS IN DIETARY MANAGEMENT DURING PREGNANCY

(1) An average weight gain during pregnancy of 24 pounds is commensurate with a better than average course and outcome of pregnancy. There is no scientific justification for routine limitations of weight gain of lesser amounts.

(2) The pattern of weight gain is of greater importance than the total amount—a sudden, sharp increase after about the 20th week of pregnancy may indicate water retention and possible onset of pre-eclampsia.

(3) Severe caloric restriction, which has been very commonly recommended, is potentially harmful to the developing fetus and to the mother and almost inevitably restricts other nutrients essential for growth processes.

(4) The young adolescent (i.e., under 17 years of age) poses special problems during pregnancy. Her own growth requires an adequate diet, with particular reference to calories, protein and calcium, and she tolerates caloric deprivation poorly.

(5) Special attention should be paid to the dietary intake and food habits of women who enter pregnancy in a poor nutritional state. When modification of the customary diet is indicated during pregnancy, it should be undertaken in accordance with the principles of good nutrition.

(6) The widespread practice of routinely restricting salt intake and at the same time prescribing diuretics is of doubtful value in preventing pre-eclampsia and is potentially dangerous.

(7) Except for iron and folic acid, the routine supplementation of diets of pregnant women with vitamin and mineral preparations is of uncertain value.

Source National Research Council, Committee on Maternal Nutrition. Maternal Nutrition and the Course of Pregnancy. Summary Report, 1970. In this report, the National Research Council calls for ''a single standard of high-quality maternity care, including nutrition, for all pregnant women'' and recommends that ''public health agencies and the health professions should assume greater responsibility for disseminating sound nutrition information, thus minimizing the influence of food faddists and charlatans.''

Infancy

There is growing evidence that the adequacy of nutrition during fetal life and early infancy may affect intellectual and behavioral development as well as physical growth. The first year of a baby's life marks the period of most rapid growth, and it is essential to provide him with a good start nutritionally. In infancy, milk is the basic source of the nutrients essential to normal growth. Nutrients not provided by milk, for example, iron and vitamin C, must be supplemented for optimum growth and health. There is a critical need for iron in infancy, greater than at any other period of life. There is a need also for vitamins A, C, and D: vitamin A for healthy skin and vision, vitamin C for resistance to infection, vitamin D for developing bones and teeth. Nutritional deprivation in infancy, unless corrected very early, can have long-term adverse effects on physical and mental growth and development. According to one report, "current scientific opinion is that nutritional deprivation incurred before four months of life can often be speedily and permanently remedied by a proper diet. After the child is four months of age, the more severe the malnutrition and the earlier it occurs, the more marked, and perhaps permanent, appear to be the adverse effects produced on any system in the body (including the nervous system)."[2] By contrast, overfeeding poses another kind of problem. Obesity in many children has its origin in infancy. One theory is that the excess calories stimulate an overabundance of fat storage cells that could trigger a lifelong overweight problem. Salt intake is being studied as another instance of potential overnutrition in infancy. The use of commercially prepared pureed infant foods has been found to increase the sodium intake above the amounts required for normal growth. Research efforts are concerned with the potential effects of this increased salt in infancy on renal function and blood pressure. A suggested health teaching guide for nutrition in infancy is presented in Table 7-2.

Childhood

The rapid growth of infancy continues through the second year of life, leveling off between the ages of two and six when children grow more slowly than in their first two years. In the preschool period, children develop the food likes and dislikes which will be the basis for their attitudes and food habits during later years. They like to serve themselves and they begin to show their independence with definite food preferences, which may change from time to time. Reinforcing desirable eating habits at this stage of development will help to establish good nutrition for the rest of the child's life. Throughout childhood, nutrition continues to play an important role, not only for growth and development but also for optimum physical and mental performance as the child enters into a wide range of activities outside of the home. During this period, food likes and dislikes are influenced by contacts with other children in

Table 7-2 Health Teaching Guide for Nutrition in Infancy

	Birth to 3 Months	Three to Six Months	Six to Nine Months	Nine to Twelve Months
Milk and Milk Products	Breast milk or formula recommended by your doctor.	Breast milk or formula recommended by your doctor.	Milk—give some by cup. Start with small amount. Doctor may advise pasteurized milk without sugar.	Milk—baby may take all by cup, except bedtime bottle. Pudding, custard and ice cream occasionally — if baby is not drinking enough milk.
Cereals	About 2 or 3 months, or when the doctor advises, start one of the following baby cereals: barley, corn, rice, oatmeal.	Gradually *add* other kinds of baby cereals. Soon your baby will have developed a liking for many kinds.	*Add*—at 6 to 7 months, dry toast, crackers, or biscuits (not cookies) to chew on after other foods are eaten. Continue to give baby cereals or Enriched Cream of Wheat.	All cereals listed before. Cereals prepared for the family may be given. But they do not contain as much iron as baby cereals. Be sure your baby is getting at least two iron-rich foods daily.
Vegetables		Try one and let baby get used to it. Then try another. *Dark-green and deep-yellow for vitamin A*—strained carrots, squash, spinach, sweet potatoes. *Other vegetables*—strained beets, peas, string beans, tomatoes.	*Add*—potatoes (baked or boiled) and made "soupy" with milk. Give other vegetables to help baby learn to like different kinds.	All vegetables listed before. Give coarser foods, mashed instead of strained. Give whole pieces of cooked carrots and string beans as finger foods when baby can chew.
Fruits	*Fruit juice rich in vitamin C*—grapefruit juice or orange juice—not orangeade or orange drink. Start one at a time. Dilute juice with equal amounts of boiled and cooled water. Gradually leave out water.	*Fruit juice rich in vitamin C*—2 ounces undiluted. *Fruit*—start with one. Then add others: applesauce, ripe mashed banana, strained apricots, peaches, pears, prunes. You can prepare these fruits at home.	*Fruit juice rich in vitamin C*—baby takes up to 3 ounces undiluted. *Fruit*—add peeled, raw, ripe fruits such as apple slices, orange sections, or pear slices, as finger foods when baby can chew.	*Fruit juice rich in vitamin C* *Fruit*—all fruits as listed before.
Eggs and Meats		Start yolk of hard cooked egg about 5th month. White of egg will be added later. When baby takes egg well, start a strained meat by 5 to 6 months.	Yolk of hard cooked egg. Strained meat—beef, lamb, veal, chicken, liver, heart. Use liver often.	Egg yolk with some white, hard or soft cooked or scrambled. Finely ground meat without fat. Fish (one serving replaces egg or meat). At 8 to 12 months canned salmon or tuna may be given if oil is drained off.

Courtesy of Pennsylvania Department of Health.

school. Children of elementary school age have better dietary habits than adolescents.

Adolescence

Adolescence poses special problems. This period is characterized not only by profound physiological changes but also by an identity crisis in emotional development. The answer to the question, "Are adolescents well nourished?" is "No"; studies have shown that their food intakes are more variable and less adequate than those of any other group. Major nutritional problems among adolescents are overweight, obesity, dental caries, and iron-deficiency anemia. Adolescent obesity and overweight can be traced to overconsumption of high-caloric foods and underparticipation in active exercises. Teenagers are very sensitive to the comments and criticisms of their friends. Without fully understanding the relationship between good nutrition and good health, they will often discard good eating and health habits developed in earlier childhood. Pregnancy during adolescence poses another nutritionally-related problem with physical and psychological risks. Young pregnant girls, still experiencing their own growth process, are often in poor nutritional health and are vulnerable to anemia, toxemia, premature delivery, and prolonged labor. The *Nutrition News* of the Pennsylvania Department of Health (September 1972) cites the following factors as intensifiers of nutrition problems in adolescence: "growth, activity, lack of family commensality, peer acceptance, snacking, irregular meal patterns, physiological and psychological changes, misleading food advertisements, and lack of motivation." Adolescents need nutrition knowledge in spite of their lack of motivation and interest. Bizarre eating habits, which many of them assume, pose a serious threat for their future well-being.

Early and Middle Adult Years

As we reach adulthood in the course of growth and development, nutrition continues to hold a prominent position in health maintenance. It may be the major consideration from the early twenties through "middle age" in correcting or modifying some of the risk factors related to diabetes and heart disease—two serious threats in adult health. The nutritional-health problems that beset this age group are often an outgrowth of the life style which characterizes present-day society. Our way of life has changed markedly from that of the rugged, hardy pioneers. Even the most sedentary person in the frontier days led a more active life than do many busy persons of today. The affluence of twentieth century America has created an atmosphere where people tend to eat too much and exercise too little. These two factors have been pinpointed in the development of atherosclerotic coronary artery disease.

Another problem has been the growth of food cultism and food faddism—for example, the macrobiotic diet adapted from Zen Buddhist teachings; various crash diets for weight reduction such as the so-called Air Force Diet, the "Drinking Man's Diet," and the "Mayo Diet," and the current rage for vitamin E and organic foods. Problems have been created by widespread misuse and misapplication of these foods and diets. Such faddism is a byproduct of too much wealth and leisure and too little interest in serious learning and applying the basic facts of good nutrition. People look for, are impressed by, and foolishly spend their money on the newest or latest fad.

Paradoxically, in the midst of this affluence, many families exist who must try to maintain good nutrition as they struggle with poverty, near-poverty, or even with middle-income resources that are steadily eroded by continually spiraling food prices. Poverty has an adverse effect on nutritional status in all stages of the life cycle—mentioned earlier were pregnancy, infancy, and childhood as they are affected by undernutrition, often related to poverty.

Old Age

As we move into the final stage of the life cycle, we find that nutrition plays a most important role in health maintenance and disease prevention. The aged person is especially vulnerable with all of the biopsychosocial changes and adjustments he must face. (See page 159.) Often confronted with poverty and loneliness, he may eat poorly or not at all, and his problems are seriously compounded. However, as Figure 7-2 indicates, group dining programs may help to alleviate his problems.

NUTRITION SERVICES

Nutrition services are provided to the public, directly and indirectly, by various official and voluntary agencies, some of which are listed here:

OFFICIAL AGENCIES—EXAMPLES OF NUTRITION SERVICES

State and Local

Health departments—establishing and enforcing regulations for food sanitation; meat and milk inspection; local food processing standards; restaurant and food market inspections; foods and nutrition consultation and education.

Welfare departments—food subsidies for needy families; coordination of federal food stamp program; home economist services for family nutrition counseling, including budget planning.

Board of education—coordination of school lunch program; nutrition education.

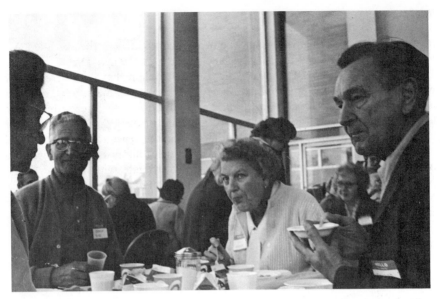

Figure 7-2 A group dining program at a senior citizens' center brings people together for socializing as well as for nutrition.

Agricultural Extension Service—home demonstration agents; nutrition education and consultation service using nutrition aides.

National

United States Department of Health, Education and Welfare—federal school lunch program; nutrition consultation, education, and research through the Maternal and Child Health Service and the National Institutes of Health; federal laws regulating standards of manufacturing purity and truthful labeling enforced by Food and Drug Administration.

United States Department of Agriculture—research in human nutrition; sale of surplus foodstuffs abroad; foods and nutrition consultation and education through extension services; food stamp program.

VOLUNTARY AGENCIES—EXAMPLES OF NUTRITION SERVICES

State and Local

Community health and welfare agencies—agencies: community nursing service, family service, Salvation Army; types of service: patient education; nutrition and family budget counseling; direct food contributions.

Church groups and other community groups—"meals on wheels"; food contributions.

Professional organizations—i.e., local chapters of the various national organizations (see list below).

National

National Academy of Sciences National Research Council—primarily research and consultation.

Professional organizations—e.g., American Academy of Pediatrics, American Dental Association, American Diabetes Association, American Dietetic Association, American Heart Association, American Home Economics Association, American Institute of Nutrition, American Medical Association Council of Foods and Nutrition, American Nurses' Association, American Public Health Association, National League for Nursing—research; education; consultation; resource; establishing standards.

Other—e.g., National Dairy Council (sponsored by industry)—research; resource; establishing standards.

In addition, many private firms (e.g. in the pharmaceutical and food industries) often publish nutritional health literature and specialized diets that are useful for patient teaching.

NATIONAL CONCERN WITH NUTRITION

The White House Conference on Food, Nutrition and Health, which was held in December, 1969, focused on the nutritional needs of our population with particular attention to the poor. The purpose of the Conference was twofold: (1) to advise the President, the Congress and the American people on the best methods of eliminating hunger and malnutrition, and (2) to develop a national nutrition policy. There were over 3000 participants from various professions, food industries, official and voluntary agencies, and community action groups. The Conference, in its final report, issued several hundred recommendations; one of these called for the Department of Health, Education, and Welfare to assume major responsibility for administration and coordination of all food and nutrition programs.

The Conference concluded that children at every stage of growth, from infancy through adolescence, must be considered to be at high risk because of their specific nutritional requirements for sound growth and development. The Maternal and Child Health Service of the Department of Health, Education, and Welfare is supporting national studies of the nutritional status of children. Preliminary findings of a study of preschool children indicate that "there are substantial proportions of preschool children who are at nutritional risk; e.g., considered to be anemic, to have iron deficiency and low levels of vitamin C in plasma. Low income children, particularly, show these deficiencies."[3] To provide nutritional services to these vulnerable groups, Maternal and Child Health and Crippled Children's Services grant-in-aid funds support personnel employed in state and local health agencies.[4]

Federally supported food programs—the Food Stamp Program, the Government Donated Foods Program, and the School Lunch Program—were also part of the Conference proceedings. There have been several major reforms to facilitate the purchase of food stamps by families in need. Additional funds have been allocated to improve the local administration and delivery of the Government Donated Foods Program. The School Lunch Program has received extra funds to provide free and reduced price lunches to 6.6 million needy children in the nation's schools, as well as funds for equipment and technical assistance.

Since the White House Conference there has been an increased interest in nutrition education for professional and community groups. Focusing on the need for nutrition education, the Senate Select Committee on Nutrition Needs opened hearings in the latter part of 1972. Senator Richard S. Schweiker of Pennsylvania, a member of the committee, called attention to the often-neglected problem of "middle class malnutrition." He declared that the hearings would "disprove the widespread belief that nutritional ignorance is limited to the poor . . . a moderate or upper income does not guarantee a nutritionally adequate diet." To educate the general public, films, filmstrips, TV spots and other commercial advertisements have been developed. The Expanded Nutrition Education Program, which employs nutrition aides to teach simple nutrition, food budgeting, purchasing, and preparation to needy families, has been increased in response to recommendations for individualized nutrition teaching.

The White House Conference stimulated nutrition activities at the state level; for example, individual states have established nutrition councils, held statewide conferences, and organized inter-agency task forces. They have emphasized the coordination of community efforts to make people aware of the importance of nutrition to health. They have expanded nutrition services, food assistance programs and community action nutrition programs.

INTERNATIONAL ORGANIZATIONS CONCERNED WITH NUTRITION

The Food and Agricultural Organization (FAO) of the United Nations was formed after the Second World War. It had as an immediate concern the provision of assistance to those who had suffered starvation, loss of means of food production, and other scars of warfare. As a long range goal, it seeks to expand the production and improve the distribution of food. It assists the 120 member states by an international intelligence service that gathers and distributes information; it acts in an advisory capacity; it provides technical assistance to nations that request help for such widely ranging problems as control of animal diseases, control of locusts, irrigation and drainage projects, and establishment of home economics programs in colleges. Other United Nations specialized agencies concerned with nutrition are the United Nations Children's Fund (UNICEF) and the World Health Organization (WHO).

The United States has sponsored international programs concerned with nutrition, including Agency for International Development (AID), an official agency, and CARE, a voluntary organization, which, through individual contributions, has helped those less fortunate.

REFERENCES

1. Bertrand Russell, "The Springs of Human Action," *Atlantic Monthly* (1952), as cited in George Seldes, *The Great Quotations* (New York: Pocket Books, 1967), p. 363.

2. Clinical Research Advances in Human Growth and Development, *How Children Grow* (Bethesda, Md.: National Institute of Health, June 1972), p. 26.

3. United States Department of Health, Education, and Welfare, *Maternal and Child Health Service Reports on Promoting the Health of Mothers and Children, 1970* (Washington, D.C.: Government Printing Office, 1971), p. 4.

4. A significant development in response to the nutritional needs of young children was the launching of a federally supported food program in 1974 for pregnant or lactating women, infants, and children up to four years of age (WIC). The WIC program, established through federal legislation, is supported through cash grants received by individual states from the United States Department of Agriculture. Under the terms of the WIC program, food vouchers are issued directly to participants, and they must be used for the purchase of specified essential foodstuffs.

ADDITIONAL READINGS

Benarde, Melvin A., and Norge W. Jerome, "Food Quality and the Consumer: A Decalog," in *American Journal of Public Health,* 62 (September 1972) 1199–1201.

Burton, Lloyd E., and Hugh H. Smith, *Public Health and Community Medicine.* Baltimore: Williams and Wilkins, 1970.

Christakis, George, ed., "Nutritional Assessment in Health Programs," in *American Journal of Public Health,* 63 (November 1973, supplement) 1–82.

Church, C. F., and H. N. Church, *Bowes and Church's Food Values of Portions Commonly Used.* 12th ed. Philadelphia: J.B. Lippincott Co., 1975.

Craig, D. C., "Guiding the Change Process in People," in *Journal of the American Dietetic Association.* 58(1) (January 1971) 22–25.

Egan, M. C., "Combating Malnutrition through Maternal and Child Health Programs," in *Children,* 16(2) (1969) 67.

Forbes, Allan L., "The Role of the Food and Drug Administration in the Nutritional Quality of Foods," in *American Journal of Public Health.* 62 (September 1972) 1207–9

"Guidelines for Developing Dietary Counseling Services in the Community," *Journal of the American Dietetic Association,* 55 (October 1969) 343–47.

Henderson, L.M., "Nutritional Problems Growing Out of New Patterns of Food Consumption," in *American Journal of Public Health,* 62 (September 1972) 1194–98.

Holtzman, Neil A., Allen G. Meek, and E. David Mellits, "Neonatal Screening for Phenylketonuria. IV. Factors Influencing the Occurrence of False Positives," in *American Journal of Public Health,* 64 (August 1974) 775–79.

Huenemann, Ruth L., "A Review of Teenage Nutrition in the United States," in *Health Services Reports,* 87 (November 1972) 823–29.

Jane, Diane E., Jean H. Hankin, Setsu Furuno, and Neal E. Winn, "Nutrition in Action for Young Transients in Hawaii," in *American Journal of Public Health,* 62 (September 1972) 1202–6.

Keller, M. D. and C. E. Smith, "Meals on Wheels, 1960," in *Geriatrics,* 16 (1961) 237,

Law, H.M., et al, "Sophomore High School Students' Attitudes Toward School Lunch," in *Journal of the American Dietetic Association,* 60(1) (January 1972) 38–41.

Leavell, Hugh R., and E. Gurney Clark, *Textbook of Preventive Medicine.* 3rd ed. New York: McGraw-Hill, 1965.

Lewin, K., "Forces Behind Food Habits and Methods of Change," in *The Problem of Changing Food Habits.* Washington, D.C.: National Academy of Sciences, National Research Council, 1943.

Lowenberg, M.E., et al., *Food and Man.* 2nd ed. New York: John Wiley and Sons, Inc., 1974.

Mann, George V., "Obesity, The Nutritional Spook," in *American Journal of Public Health,* 61 (August 1971) 1491–98.

Pennsylvania Department of Health, Division of Nutrition, *Nutrition News.* Harrisburg, Pa.: Department of Health, January–February 1971; July–August 1971; September 1972.

Robinson, Corinne H., *Normal and Therapeutic Nutrition.* 14th ed. New York: Macmillan Co., 1972.

Scholes, Robert T., and Kathryn T. Scholes, "The Health Survey for a Peasant Community," in *Journal of the American Dietetic Association,* 30 (June 1954) 1–24.

Scrimshaw, Nevin S., "Myths and Realities in International Health Planning," in *American Journal of Public Health,* 64 (August 1974) 792–98.

Spindler, E.B., and G. Asher, "Teenagers Tell Us About Their Nutrition," in *Journal of the American Dietetic Association,* 43 (1963) 228.

Watt, B. K., and A. L. Merrill, *Composition of Foods.* Agricultural Handbook No. 8, Agricultural Research Service, Washington, D. C., 1963.

Williams, Sue Rodwell, *Nutrition and Diet Therapy.* 2nd ed. St. Louis: C. V. Mosby Co., 1973.

Wilson, Patience, "Iron-Deficiency Anemia," in *American Journal of Nursing,* 72 (March 1972) 502–4.

Youland, Dorothy M., "New Dimensions for Public Health Nutrition: The Challenge of Chronic Disease and Aging," in *Health and the Community.* Alfred H. Katz and Jean Spencer Felton eds. New York: The Free Press, 1965.

Appendix
Sample Forms

COMMONWEALTH OF PENNSYLVANIA
DEPARTMENT OF HEALTH
NUTRITION

DIET RECORD – 24 HOUR RECALL

DATE

NAME		SEX	AGE	HEIGHT	WEIGHT	NURSE

SPECIAL CONDITION OR DISEASE

FOR INFORMATION ON HOW TO TAKE A DIET RECORD REFER TO "INSTRUCTION FOR USING AND EVALUATING DIET RECORDS".

MEAL	FOODS	AMOUNT	HOW PREPARED
DAY OF WEEK			
TIME			
WHERE EATEN			

BETWEEN-MEAL
FOODS:

DAY OF WEEK			
TIME			
WHERE EATEN			

BETWEEN-MEAL
FOODS:

DAY			
TIME			
WHERE EATEN			

BETWEEN-MEAL
FOODS:

SUMMARY OF INTAKE							
VEGETABLE-FRUIT GROUP			MILK, CHEESE GROUP	MEAT, EGG GROUP	ENRICHED BREADS CEREALS	OTHER FOODS	
VITAMIN C FOODS	DARK GREEN, DEEP-YELLOW	OTHER FRUITS, VEGETABLES				FATS	SWEETS AND EXTRAS
TOTAL INTAKE							

AMOUNTS RECOMMENDED. REFER TO EVALUATION TABLE

Figure 7-3

Source Figures 7–3 and 7–4 were reprinted with permission of the Nutrition Services of the Pennsylvania Department of Health.

VITAMIN, MINERAL OR OTHER SUPPLEMENTS USED

KIND _____ DOSAGE _____ ARE THEY PRESCRIBED BY A PHYSICIAN ☐ YES ☐ NO

ECONOMIC CONSIDERATIONS

_____

HOW OFTEN IS FOOD PURCHASED

☐ BI-WEEKLY ☐ WEEKLY ☐ DAILY

SHOPPING FACILITIES

☐ SUPERMARKET ☐ NEIGHBORHOOD STORE

☐ OTHER (SPECIFY)

STORAGE AND COOKING FACILITIES (DESCRIBE CONDITION AS GOOD OR POOR)

REFRIGERATOR _____ RANGE _____

FREEZER _____ OVEN _____

CUPBOARD _____ HOT PLATE _____

OTHER _____ OTHER _____

FOOD STAMPS OR OTHER GOVERNMENT FOOD PROGRAM

LIST FOODS THAT ARE HOME PRODUCED OR DONATED

FOOD DISLIKES	FOOD ALLERGIES

CULTURAL FACTORS INFLUENCING FOOD HABITS

OTHER COMMENTS: INCLUDE DIET PRESCRIPTION, DEGREE OF ACTIVITY, AND COMPLICATING FACTORS SUCH AS POOR APPETITE, CONSTIPATION, EMOTIONAL FACTORS, CHEWING AND SWALLOWING DIFFICULTIES, UNDERWEIGHT, OVERWEIGHT, ETC.

SUGGESTIONS MADE FOR IMPROVING FOOD SELECTION

PLANS FOR NUTRITION FOLLOW-UP

PENNSYLVANIA DEPARTMENT OF HEALTH, DIVISION OF NUTRITION

ure 7-3 (Continued)

105

HOW TO SUMMARIZE AND EVALUATE THE DIET RECORD

Under **SUMMARY OF INTAKE**, list each food with the quantity in the appropriate food group column. Include all foods that appear in the record of the 24-hour intake. For guidance in classifying the foods and determining the amounts that count as one serving, refer to the information below and to **A DAILY FOOD GUIDE** from the Pennsylvania Department of Health.

1. **VEGETABLES AND FRUITS** — Count as one serving: ½ cup or a portion as commonly used such as one orange, ½ grapefruit or one medium potato.

Vitamin C Foods — Count as one serving of this vitamin may be substituted for one serving of a good source. Some good sources are orange, grapefruit and their juices, cantaloupe, strawberries and broccoli. Some fair sources are tomato, tangerine and their juices, raw cabbage, potato cooked in the skin, spinach, honeydew and watermelon.

Dark-Green and Deep-Yellow — These include broccoli, beet greens, chard, collards, dandelion greens, spinach, watercress, kale, turnip greens, other dark green leaves, carrots, sweet potatoes, winter squash, pumpkin, apricots and cantaloupe.

Other Vegetables and Fruits — These include all vegetables and fruits not listed under Vitamin C Foods or Dark-Green and Deep-Yellow Vegetables and Fruits. One cup of vegetable soup may be counted as one serving of Other Vegetables.

2. **MILK** — Count 8 ounces (½ pint or 1 cup) as one serving of milk. On the basis of calcium content, count as equivalents for 1 cup (8 oz.) of milk: 1½ ounces cheddar-type cheese; 1½ cups cottage cheese; 1 pint (2 cups) ice cream; 1 cup ice milk, custard or cornstarch pudding; or 1½ cups soup made with milk.

3. **MEAT, FISH, POULTRY, EGGS, OR ALTERNATES** — Count as one serving: 2 to 3 ounces cooked lean meat, poultry or fish — all without bone; 2 frankfurters (10 per lb.); 2 eggs; 1 cup cooked dry beans, dry peas or lentils; 1½ cups split pea or bean soup; 4 tablespoons peanut butter; or ½ cup roasted peanuts, shelled.

On the basis of protein content, one ounce cooked lean meat, poultry or fish or ½ cup cottage cheese may be substituted for one egg.

4. **BREADS AND CEREALS** — **Whole grain or enriched** — Count as one serving: 1 slice bread; 1 roll; 1 hamburger or hot dog roll; ½ to ¾ cup cooked cornmeal, rice, macaroni, spaghetti or noodles. Breads and cereals that are not enriched are classified as Extras since they contribute much less iron and B-vitamins to the diet.

5. **FATS** — List foods such as butter, margarine, cream, cream cheese, oils, other cooking fats, bacon, salt pork, mayonnaise, French dressing, etc.

6. **SWEETS AND EXTRAS** — List candies, jellies, sirups, honey, cakes, cookies, pastries, crackers, unenriched breads and cereals, coffee, tea, soft drinks, cocoa or "cream" soups made with water, and alcoholic beverages. Also list under this group snack foods such as potato chips, popcorn and pretzels; and clear soups or broths with rice, noodles or barley.

TO EVALUATE THE DIET RECORD: Compare the intake of each food group with the quantity suggested in the table. Note the groups that appear to be inadequate or excessive in amounts.

FOOD GROUPS	ADULT	ADULT WITH TUBERCULOSIS	PREGNANT WOMAN	LACTATING WOMAN	PRE-SCHOOL CHILD 1-6 YEARS	SCHOOL AGE CHILD 6-12 YEARS	ADOLESCENT 12-14 YEARS	ADOLESCENT 14-18 YEARS
1. Fruits and Vegetables Vitamin C Foods	1 Serving	2 Servings	1 Serving	1 Serving	1 Serving	1 Serving	1 Serving	1 Serving - Girls 1½ Servings - Boys
Dark Green and Deep Yellow	1 Serving	1 Serving	1 Serving	1 to 2 Servings	1 Small Serving (4-5 Tbs. per serving)	1 Serving	1 Serving	1 Serving
Other Fruits and Vegetables	2 Servings	2 Servings	2 Servings	2 Servings	2 Small Servings (4-5 Tbs. per serving)	2 Servings	2 to 3 Servings	2 to 3 Servings
2. Milk Or equivalents as described above	2 cups (16 fl. oz.)	4 cups (32 fl. oz.)	3 to 5 cups (24 to 40 fl. oz.)	4 to 6 cups (32 to 48 fl. oz.)	2 to 3 cups (16 to 24 fl. oz.)	3 cups or more (24 fl. oz.)	4 cups (32 fl. oz.)	4 cups (32 fl. oz.)
3. Meat, Fish, Poultry Or equivalents as described above	2 Servings (Total of: 4 oz.-Women 6 oz.-Men)	2 Medium Servings (Total of: 5 to 6 oz.)	2 Medium Servings (Total of: 5 oz.)	2 Medium Servings (Total of: 6 oz.)	2 Small Servings (Total of: 1½ to 2 oz.)	2 Servings (Total of: 2 to 4 oz.)	2 Servings (Total of: 4 to 5 oz.)	2 Servings (Total of: 4 oz.-Girls 6 oz.-Boys)
Eggs	3 to 5 per week	1 per day	1 per day	1 per day	1 per day	1 per day	1 per day	1 per day
4. Breads and Cereals Whole Grain, Enriched or Restored	4 Servings	4 Servings	4 to 5 Servings	5 Servings	3 to 4 Servings (2-3 slices of bread ½ to ¾ cup cereal)	4 Servings	4 or more Servings	4 to 5 Servings or more

106

Figure 7-4

	Age (years)	Weight (kg)	Weight (lbs)	Height (cm)	Height (in)	Energy (kcal)[b]	Protein (g)	Vitamin A Activity (RE)[c]	Vitamin A (IU)	Vitamin D (IU)	Vitamin E Activity[e] (IU)	Ascorbic Acid (mg)	Folacin[f] (ug)	Niacin[g] (mg)	Riboflavin (B2) (mg)	Thiamin (B1) (mg)	Vitamin B6 (ug)	Vitamin B12 (ug)	Calcium (mg)	Phosphorus (mg)	Iodine (ug)	Iron (mg)	Magnesium (mg)	Zinc (mg)
Infants	0.0-0.5	6	14	60	24	kg x 117	kg x 2.2	420[d]	1,400	400	4	35	50	5	0.4	0.3	0.3	0.3	360	240	35	10	60	3
	0.5-1.0	9	20	71	28	kg x 108	kg x 2.0	400	2,000	400	5	35	50	8	0.6	0.5	0.4	0.3	540	400	45	15	70	5
Children	1-3	13	28	86	34	1300	23	400	2,000	400	7	40	100	9	0.8	0.7	0.6	1.0	800	800	60	15	150	10
	4-6	20	44	110	44	1800	30	500	2,500	400	9	40	200	12	1.1	0.9	0.9	1.5	800	800	80	10	200	10
	7-10	30	66	135	54	2400	36	700	3,300	400	10	40	300	16	1.2	1.2	1.2	2.0	800	800	110	10	250	10
Males	11-14	44	97	158	63	2800	44	1,000	5,000	400	12	45	400	18	1.5	1.4	1.6	3.0	1200	1200	130	18	350	15
	15-18	61	134	172	69	3000	54	1,000	5,000	400	15	45	400	20	1.8	1.5	2.0	3.0	1200	1200	150	18	400	15
	19-22	67	147	172	69	3000	54	1,000	5,000	400	15	45	400	20	1.8	1.5	2.0	3.0	800	800	140	10	350	15
	23-50	70	154	172	69	2700	56	1,000	5,000		15	45	400	18	1.6	1.4	2.0	3.0	800	800	130	10	350	15
	51+	70	154	172	69	2400	56	1,000	5,000		15	45	400	16	1.5	1.2	2.0	3.0	800	800	110	10	350	15
Females	11-14	44	97	155	62	2400	44	800	4,000	400	12	45	400	16	1.3	1.2	1.6	3.0	1200	1200	115	18	300	15
	15-18	54	119	162	65	2100	48	800	4,000	400	12	45	400	14	1.4	1.1	2.0	3.0	1200	1200	115	18	300	15
	19-22	58	128	162	65	2100	48	800	4,000	400	12	45	400	14	1.4	1.1	2.0	3.0	800	800	100	18	300	15
	23-50	58	128	162	65	2000	46	800	4,000		12	45	400	13	1.2	1.0	2.0	3.0	800	800	100	18	300	15
	51+	58	128	162	65	1800	46	800	4,000		12	45	400	12	1.1	1.0	2.0	3.0	800	800	80	10	300	15
Pregnant						+300	+30	1,000	5,000	400	15	60	800	+2	+0.3	+0.3	2.5	4.0	1200	1200	125	18[h]	450	20
Lactating						+500	+20	1,200	6,000	400	15	60	600	+4	+0.5	+0.3	2.5	4.0	1200	1200	150	18	450	25

[a] The allowances are intended to provide for individual variations among most normal persons as they live in the United States under usual environmental stresses. Diets should be based on a variety of common foods in order to provide other nutrients for which human requirements have been less well defined. See text for more detailed discussion of allowances and of nutrients not tabulated.

[b] Kilojoules (kJ) = 4.2 x kcal

[c] Retinol equivalents

[d] Assumed to be all as retinol in milk during the first six months of life. All subsequent intakes are assumed to be half as retinol and half as β-carotene when calculated from international units. As retinol equivalents, three fourths are as retinol and one fourth as β-carotene.

[e] Total vitamin E activity, estimated to be 80 percent as ∝-tocopherol and 20 percent other tocopherols.

[f] The folacin allowances refer to dietary sources as determined by Lactobacillus casei assay. Pure forms of folacin may be effective in doses less than one fourth of the recommended dietary allowances.

[g] Although allowances are expressed as niacin, it is recognized that on the average 1 mg of niacin is derived from each 60 mg of dietary tryptophan.

[h] This increased requirement cannot be met by ordinary diets; therefore, the use of supplemental iron is recommended.

Source Reprinted by permission. National Academy of Sciences, National Research Council, Food and Nutrition Board from Recommended Dietary Allowances, 8th ed., 1974, NAS publ. No. 2216.

Figure 7-5 Food and Nutrition Board, National Academy of Sciences-National Research Council Recommended Daily Dietary Allowances,[a] Revised 1974 (Designed for the maintenance of good nutrition of practically all healthy people in the U.S.A.)

Recommended Dietary Allowances
Revised 1974

─── SUMMARY ───

The 1974 Recommended Dietary Allowances (RDA), published by the Food and Nutrition Board, National Academy of Sciences—National Research Council, include several important changes as compared to the 1968 edition of the RDA. Of particular significance are two new introductory sections: general considerations regarding what the RDA are and appropriate uses of the RDA. The following changes should be noted:

(1) The age-weight-sex groupings are broadened, thus explaining some minor changes in the table for most nutrients.

(2) The energy allowances, although expressed in the table as kilocalories, may also be stated in joules—a conversion factor appears in a footnote to the table.

(3) It is recommended that dietary fat be reduced from the present level of consumption of 42 percent to 35 percent.

(4) The protein RDA is lowered from 0.9 to 0.8 g/kg body weight—a decrease from 65 g to 56 g for males, aged 23-50 years and 55 g to 46 g for females, 23-50 years of age.

(5) The term "retinol equivalents", in preference to International Units, is introduced for delineating vitamin A activity. During a period of transition allowances will be expressed both ways in the table.

(6) The vitamin E RDA is lowered significantly—50 percent for the adult male—thus the allowance is closer to the average vitamin E intake in the usual American diet.

(7) The ascorbic acid RDA is reduced 25 per cent for the adult male—from 60 mg to 45 mg.

(8) Niacin is no longer expressed as niacin equivalents, simply as niacin. However, a statement indicating that 60 mg of dietary tryptophan will provide approximately 1 mg of niacin is included in both the table and the text.

(9) The RDA for vitamin B_{12} is lowered appreciably for all age-sex groups.

(10) Although the calcium RDA is maintained at 800 mg for the adult, consideration is given to the positive correlation between protein intake and urinary calcium excretion. A high protein intake increases the need for calcium.

(11) The single addition to the table is the RDA for zinc—15 mg for adult males and females. Marginal deficiencies of this trace element may be evident in the U.S.

(12) The changes recommended during pregnancy include increases in the energy, protein, and iron allowances; decreases in the RDA for vitamins E and B_{12}; and the addition of a zinc RDA (20 mg). During lactation, the energy, vitamin E, and vitamin B_{12} RDA are reduced from the previous recommendations; ascorbic acid is increased; and an allowance of 25 mg zinc is added.

Figure 7-6

Source Reprinted through courtesy of the National Dairy Council. Information supplied as a public service of Dairy Council Inc.

108

UNIT III
CURRENT
HEALTH PROBLEMS
AND TRENDS

Chapter 8
Health Problems in the Community: Specific Diseases or Conditions

A health problem "becomes a public responsibility if or when it is of such character or extent as to be amenable to solution only through systematized social action. Its relative importance varies with the hazard to the population exposed. This hazard may be qualitative, in terms of disability or death; quantitative, in terms of proportion of population affected; it may be actual or potential."[1]

INTRODUCTION

A public health problem exists when the well-being of individuals or communities is threatened by conditions requiring organized community action. We can formulate a historical perspective of our society's health problems by examining current morbidity and mortality data and comparing them with similar data from some other point in time. For example, when we look at mortality data from the turn of the century we see that the three leading causes of death were communicable diseases—(1) influenza and pneumonia, (2) tuberculosis, and (3) gastroenteritis. For many years, communicable diseases were recognized as major public health problems and were the main target in organized public health programs. Today, the three leading causes of death are (1) heart disease, (2) cancer, and (3) stroke. These are chronic, degenerative processes, which reflect an increasing proportion of older age groups in our population. Chronic diseases, disabling conditions, and health needs of elderly people are now recognized as serious public health problems and are receiving greater emphasis in our health programs.

Contemporary public health problems are broader, more insidious, and less amenable to prevention, treatment, and control than those of an earlier era. Drug abuse, alcoholism, environmental pollution, mental illness, accidents, malnutrition—these are the targets of public health practice in the final quarter of the twentieth century. There are no immunizations against these conditions. They do not respond to the antibiotics and chemotherapy that have previously been so effective in curing disease and prolonging life. We are speaking about problems that urgently require that we find ways to help improve the quality as well as the longevity of life.

There are other problems and social forces that have a bearing on the health of the nation: poverty in the midst of abundance; racist feelings which have emerged; pollution of our mass media with crudeness, violence, and hard-core pornography; reexamination of traditional social roles and the place of the nuclear family in society; widespread experimentation with new life styles. Society seems to be in a constant state of flux; indeed, the only certainty in contemporary society is change, which is all-pervasive and never-ending. Modern man is forced to develop mechanisms to cope with this change at a whirling rate of speed for which he is not prepared.[2] Since World War II, there has been a breathtakingly rapid development of modern technology and automation. The appearance of automatic machines, which process information rather than energy, has ushered in what might aptly be termed the Second Industrial Revolution. Surely this has affected and will continue to affect community health as much as, if not more than, the original Industrial Revolution.[3]

Looking at current trends in public health, one recognizes that numerous conditions have helped bring about change. These conditions might be summarized as follows: (1) the population is growing and it has basic health needs that must be met; (2) people are living longer, increasing the needs characteristic of an aging population; (3) a greater concentration of population in urban areas has resulted in pollution of the air, water, and space, burdening city residents with an additional stress of "modern living"; (4) there is a movement in disease control from the acute, communicable diseases to the chronic, degenerative diseases with a concomitant need to emphasize prevention as well as treatment; (5) there is growing concern about the need for long-term care; (6) there is a tremendous increase in knowledge and technology used in the detection and treatment of disease; (7) improved communications systems utilizing computers, telephones, space satellites, television, radio and newspapers make it possible for more people to be aware of new types of services: people see the inequality between what they have and what they could have; (8) the public is becoming aware that good health care is a right rather than a privilege; and (9) there is a critical shortage of adequately trained public health personnel. As we review these factors, we see a wide gap between the "need" or demand for health services and the available resources to meet these needs and demands. This disparity makes it necessary to seek improvements in the delivery of health services.

In this chapter and the following one, we will discuss some of our present-day problems that require systematized community health action. We will present basic facts that should help you to understand the extent of the problems, their impact on our society, and the need to organize programs for prevention and control.

COMMUNICABLE DISEASES

General Information

Although great strides have been made in the control of many of these diseases, there is no cause for complacency; communicable disease still remains a problem in community health. Improved sanitation, specific protection through immunization, early case finding, treatment (particularly with antibiotics), follow-up, health education and health department surveillance have all had a part to play in organized communicable disease control. Some communicable diseases have been virtually eliminated from our country, for example, smallpox and poliomyelitis. Others, however, such as influenza and viral hepatitis, have eluded eradication. Other types of infections have emerged to pose special problems in the realm of communicable disease control, for example, nosocomial infections, particularly those caused by gram-negative organisms.

The United States has not had a case of smallpox since 1949. Towards the end of 1971, the Public Health Service recommended that routine smallpox vaccinations be discontinued. This historic decision was taken after careful study of evidence showing that while smallpox has been wiped out, there are an average of six to nine deaths and hundreds of complications related to smallpox vaccination each year. It is too early to evaluate the outcome of this action, but there is every indication of a need for continued, strict surveillance at all ports of entry from abroad. This was dramatically highlighted in 1972 by an outbreak of smallpox in Yugoslavia and West Germany, and in 1973 by reports of cases in England and Japan. In Yugoslavia, where there had been no known cases for forty years, a serious epidemic occurred, and it was ultimately brought under control through nationwide mass vaccination together with surveillance and international epidemiologic control efforts. Poliomyelitis has continued to decline since the widespread use of the safe and effective vaccines developed first by Dr. Jonas Salk for parenteral administration and then introduced in oral form by Dr. Albert Sabin. The number of cases dropped from 3,190 in 1960 to 5 in 1974.[4]

Influenza and viral hepatitis, on the other hand, are two diseases that take a serious toll (see Figure 8-1). In personal correspondence with the authors, Dr. Michael B. Gregg, Chief of the Viral Diseases Branch, Bureau of Epidemiology of the Center for Disease Control, stated that influenza is "a disease that causes tremendous morbidity and mortality when it occurs in epidemic fashion, a disease that so far is totally uncontrollable, and one that has an economic impact far greater than most communicable diseases that oc-

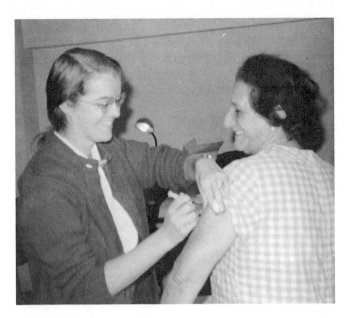

Figure 8-1 A nursing student giving an influenza vaccine injection to an elderly resident of a local public housing unit.

cur in the United States." He also points out that viral hepatitis, notably hepatitis-B, has been on the increase since 1966. Hepatitis has not been controlled by vaccines, and it ranks as a continuing and important health problem responsible for considerable morbidity and mortality.

Another area of deep concern is the emergence of new and insidious infections that are often hospital acquired. In addition to the gram-negative infections mentioned earlier, there are other problems. Modern medical intervention includes organ transplants, the use of poisonous substances to treat disease, and the employment of immunological suppressant therapies (for example, X-rays, anti-metabolites, and steroids). These measures, which are aimed at increasing the life span of people, alter the body defense mechanisms, thus predisposing patients to infections from organisms that would be resisted under normal conditions. This situation is causing great suffering and expense in the United States. There are few, if any, vaccines to combat these kinds of infections, which will be with us for many years to come as we keep people alive longer and longer.

Strict vigilance is a key element in communicable disease control. We speak of health workers developing a "high index of suspicion." For example, reported cases of chickenpox in adults should be investigated to rule out the possibility of smallpox. A history of miscarriages after the fourth month should be checked for the possibility of untreated syphilis. Adults with long-term, chronic, productive cough should be screened for the presence of tubercle bacilli.

114

Several critical factors have emerged which pose obstacles to the control of infectious disease:

(1) rapid growth of population and urbanization, which creates additional demands for safe water supply and sewage disposal systems;

(2) increasing mobility, which hastens the spread of disease nationally and internationally;

(3) declining levels of acquired immunity, which pose problems in diseases such as diphtheria where the immunity levels in adults may fall below the point of protection;

(4) excessive reliance on antibiotics and insecticides, many of which have become ineffective through increased resistance of biological agents and vectors;

(5) declining diagnostic acuity;

(6) lack of concern about reporting cases to health authorities; and

(7) individual carelessness regarding basic precautionary measures, such as scrupulous adherence to hand washing, cleansing, and sterilization procedures.

An important line of defense in the control of communicable disease is conscientiousness on the part of the nurse, physician, or other health worker in reporting these diseases to the appropriate health authority. Unfortunately, such morbidity reporting in the United States is relatively poor. Dr. Gregg, in his communication with the authors (see page 113) stated "perhaps only one out of ten or one out of twenty communicable disease cases gets into the reporting system." Therefore, all nurses, as professional practitioners and as concerned citizens, have a responsibility to become familiar with the list of notifiable diseases and the method of reporting in their state and local jurisdiction.

Each state has its own set of requirements and a list of reportable diseases. As reports come into the state health department, the data are tabulated and sent on to the National Center for Disease Control (United States Department of Health, Education, and Welfare) in Atlanta, Georgia. This center assumes responsibility for analyzing the data at the national level and issuing reports to the individual states and to the World Health Organization. (See pages 72 and 73.)

Figure 8-2 shows the list of reportable diseases for the Commonwealth of Pennsylvania.

Tuberculosis

The tuberculosis death rate has dramatically declined from 200 per 100,000 population in 1900 to less than 2 per 100,000 population in 1974.[5] Nevertheless, tuberculosis remains a serious public health problem because of the nature of the disease and its occurrence in the population. Recent figures show that among the reportable infectious diseases, tuberculosis ranks as the principal cause of death. The disease exists in almost every community, especially in lower socio-economic groups. Although most states and cities have reported

HB02.033 REV. 10/72 COMMONWEALTH OF PENNSYLVANIA
DEPARTMENT OF HEALTH
COMMUNICABLE DISEASE CONTROL

REPORTABLE DISEASES

The Advisory Health Board declares the following communicable diseases, unusual outbreaks of illness, non-communicable diseases and conditions to be reportable. (1)

Actinomycosis
Amebiasis (Amebic Dysentery)
* Anthrax
Brucellosis
Chancroid
Chickenpox —
  only if occurring in persons
  15 years of age and older
* Cholera
* Diarrhea of the Newborn
* Diphtheria, Cases and Carriers
Encephalitis
a. Primary
  (1) Arthropod-Borne Viral
  (2) Other Infections - identified by
    name of etiologic agent
b. Secondary, as a complication of
  other infections
* Food Poisoning
* a. Salmonellosis
* b. Staphylococcal Intoxication
* c. Clostridium Perfringens
* d. Botulism
German Measles (Rubella)
Conococcal Infection
a. Gonococcal Urethritis (Gonorrhea)
b. Gonococcal Vulvovaginitis of Children
c. Ophthalmia Neonatorum, Gonococcal
d. Gonococcal conjunctivitis
Granuloma Inguinale
Hepatitis, viral
a. Infectious (Acute Catarrhal Jaundice)
b. Serum (Homologous Serum Jaundice)
Histoplasmosis
Lead Poisoning, Childhood
a. Cases - blood lead level of 80 micro-
  grams% or higher
b. Suspected - blood lead level of 40
  micrograms% to 79 micrograms%
Leptospirosis (Weil's Disease)
Lymphocytic Choriomeningitis
Lymphogranuloma Venereum

Malaria
Measles (Rubeola)
Meningococcal Infection
a. Meningitis
b. Meningococcemia
Mononucleosis, Infections
Mumps
Ophthalmia Neonatorum, Gonococcal
Pertussis (Whooping Cough)
* Plague
Poliomyelitis
a. Paralytic
b. Non-Paralytic
* Psittacosis
"Q" Fever
* Rabies
* Relapsing Fever, Louse-Borne
Rickettsialpox
Rocky Mountain Spotted Fever
Rubella (German Measles)
Rubeola (Measles)
Salmonellosis, Cases, Carriers or
  Asymptomatic Infections
Shigellosis (Bacillary Dysentery)
* Smallpox
Streptococcal Disease, Hemolytic
a. Streptococcal Sore Throat with Rash
b. Streptococcal Sore Throat without Rash
c. Puerperal Infections
d. Erysipelas
Syphilis, All Stages
Tetanus
Toxoplasmosis
Trachoma
Trichinosis
Tuberculosis, All Forms
Tularemia
Typhoid Fever, Cases, Carriers or
  Asymptomatic Infections
Typhus Fever, Endemic, Flea-Borne
* Typhus Fever, Epidemic, Louse-Borne
* Yellow Fever

For these diseases, telephone your report to the local health authority immediately.

UNUSUAL OR ILL-DEFINED DISEASES, ILLNESSES OR OUTBREAKS — The occurrence of any unusual disease or group expression of illness which may be of public concern whether or not it is known to be of a communicable nature should be reported to the local health officer of the municipality in which it occurs; in areas which have no local health officer, reports should be made to the representative of the Secretary of Health (Regional Medical Director). Included among such diseases or illnesses are: fevers of unknown origin, unusual incidence of respiratory illness such as pneumonia or influenza and the infections due to adenoviruses, Coxsackie viruses and ECHO viruses; epidemic gastroenteritis (non-bacterial), epidemic keratoconjunctivitis, and pleurodynia. Individual cases of diseases of public concern are: aseptic meningitis, cat scratch fever, complications of smallpox vaccination, cryptococcosis, herpangina, listeriosis and varicella pneumonia.

ANIMAL BITE OR OTHER TRAUMA — Any bite or injury resulting in laceration or puncture of the skin and inflicted by an animal susceptible to rabies shall be reported to the local health authority.

(1) Rules and Regulations, Commonwealth of Pennsylvania, Department of Health, Chapter 3, Article 355, Regulations for Communicable and Non-communicable Diseases, Section 2, Reportable Diseases, Paragraphs A, B and C. See also Section 3, Paragraphs A, B, C and D.

Figure 8-2

Source Courtesy of the Pennsylvania Department of Health.

reductions in the incidence and prevalence of tuberculosis in recent years, there are a few areas where comparatively little progress has been made. During the three-year period between 1971 and 1974, new cases of active disease were reported in nearly 2,700 counties. Even though the number of cases and case rates continues to drop, there is no state in which tuberculosis has been eradicated.[6]

Tuberculosis infection rates as measured by tuberculin testing offer a sensitive index to the number of active cases in a population. It is estimated that approximately 15 million persons (7 percent of the total population) are presently infected with tubercle bacilli. A breakdown by age is shown in Figure 8-3. However, the active stage of the disease develops in only a small number. The 1974 total of 30,122 new active cases represents a rate of 14.2 per 100,000 population.[7] Distribution of new active cases by age, sex, and race has remained relatively unchanged in the last few years. The rate among non-whites in this group is four times that of the white population; the rate for the male population twice the female rate. Since the introduction of preventive therapy and chemotherapy, tuberculosis has been going down steadily among five-to fourteen-year-olds and young adolescents. The reduction of new cases in adults has not kept pace: Case rates for persons forty five years or older

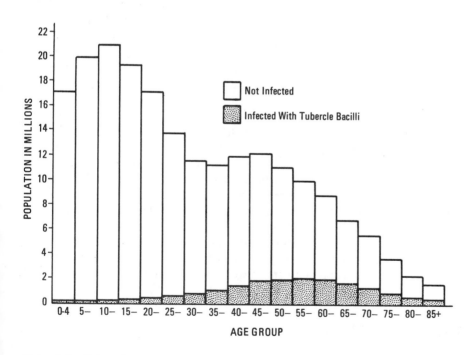

Figure 8-3   Tuberculosis infection by age group, United States population.

Source   U.S. Department of Health, Education, and Welfare, Center for Disease Control, Tuberculosis Programs 1973, Tuberculosis Program Reports, December 1974.

have been slow in dropping. Tuberculosis is found to be most prevalent in males of all races over fifty years of age.[8]

Although tuberculosis is decreasing as an endemic disease, intermittent outbreaks or small epidemics may result when active, infectious cases go unrecognized. Once a case of tuberculosis is identified, intensive public health measures are indicated. These measures include early recognition and prompt treatment with antituberculosis drugs along with careful investigation of contacts to detect the source case and other suspects.[9] One of these drugs, isoniazid, may be used as preventive treatment for persons with tuberculosis infection which has not progressed to disease and those at high risk of infection. In persons who have never been infected, active immunization against tuberculosis may be produced by the vaccine of Calmette and Guerin (BCG). Although the use of BCG vaccine for tuberculosis prevention has never gained universal acceptance in the United States, it has been used extensively and successfully in the Scandinavian countries, Japan, the Soviet Union, Yugoslavia, and other countries.

Around the turn of the century, specialized hospitals, or sanatoria, were developed, where patients with tuberculosis could be isolated for treatment, which extended over long periods of time. A real breakthrough in treatment came by mid-century with the discovery of the antibiotic streptomycin and the synthetic chemicals isoniazid (INH) and para-aminosalicylic acid (PAS), which were effective in arresting the disease and preventing its spread. Their effectiveness was readily demonstrated with a resulting decrease in the need for isolation of tuberculosis patients in sanatoria. Today, we know that patients with infectious tuberculosis under appropriate therapy can be rendered virtually noninfectious within a short time, usually two to three weeks. There has been a marked trend away from treatment in specialized hospitals or sanatoria to treatment in general hospitals, as well as in the home.

In the forefront of the battle against tuberculosis has been the American Lung Association (formerly the National Tuberculosis and Respiratory Disease Association) an organization supported by private contributions, essentially from the sale of Christmas seals. Originally established for the control of tuberculosis, it now supports research, education, treatment, and control of other respiratory diseases including chronic bronchitis, emphysema, pneumoconiosis, histoplasmosis, and lung cancer. The organization sponsors community chest X-ray screening and tuberculin testing programs, and helps in the campaign against air pollution and smoking. Through a network of individual state and local chapters, it works with local communities to provide services in tuberculosis and respiratory disease control.

Syphilis and Gonorrhea (Venereal Diseases)

While other venereal diseases (chancroid, granuloma inguinale, and lymphogranuloma venereum) pose problems individually for those whom they strike, they do not present the same overall public health problem as the two major venereal diseases, syphilis and gonorrhea. These two diseases have wreaked havoc with the lives of millions of people for centuries and have caused an immeasurable waste of human resources.

From the end of World War I until the mid-fifties, venereal disease control had received national attention, with interest peaking in the late thirties and forties. However, with the advent of penicillin and a subsequent decline in the incidence of venereal disease, support for control programs was withdrawn, so that by the late fifties, many venereal disease control activities had been seriously curtailed. Since 1957, reported cases of infectious syphilis increased, reaching a peak in 1965, with a leveling-off until 1970. At that time, the trend changed to an upward direction until 1974, when a slight decrease was noted. With regard to the incidence of gonorrhea: Since 1958 it has increased with no sign of leveling off, and it has been a matter of grave concern in community health, as indicated in Figure 8–4.

Figure 8-4 shows the reported cases per 100,000 population, but does not reveal the whole picture, for there is considerable underreporting of venereal disease. Estimates vary, but the Public Health Service points out that in 1974 there were at least 81,000 new cases of infectious syphilis although only 24,728 were reported; and 2,700,000 cases of gonorrhea, although only 874,161 were reported.[10] Of the reported cases, analysis reveals the highest incidence of gonorrhea and primary and secondary syphilis occurring in the twenty- through twenty-four-year-old age group, as shown in Table 8–1. Though venereal diseases spare no one group or individual, reported cases are higher in urban areas and are more common in the male than in the female. Venereal diseases (gonorrhea and syphilis) are the leading communicable diseases in the United States with gonorrhea far outstripping all others. (See Figure 8–5.)

In venereal disease control, constant alertness and a high index of

Table 8-1   Gonorrhea and Primary and Secondary Syphilis—Morbidity and Age-Specific Rates per 100,000 Population by Age Groups of Reported Cases (United States, Calendar Year 1974)

Age Group	Gonorrhea		Primary and Secondary Syphilis	
	Number of Reported Cases	Rate per 100,000 Population	Number of Reported Cases	Rate per 100,000 Population
0-14	11,510	21.1	270	0.5
15-19	248,757	1216.5	3,992	19.5
20-24	354,150	1984.0	7,296	40.9
25-29	165,048	1041.2	5,498	34.7
30-39	89,729	365.6	5,477	22.3
40-49	21,610	93.5	2,057	8.9
50 +	8,139	15.3	795	1.5
TOTAL	898,943	428.7	25,385	12.1

Source   Department of Health, Education, and Welfare, Public Health Service, Center for Disease Control, Venereal Disease Control Division, 1975.

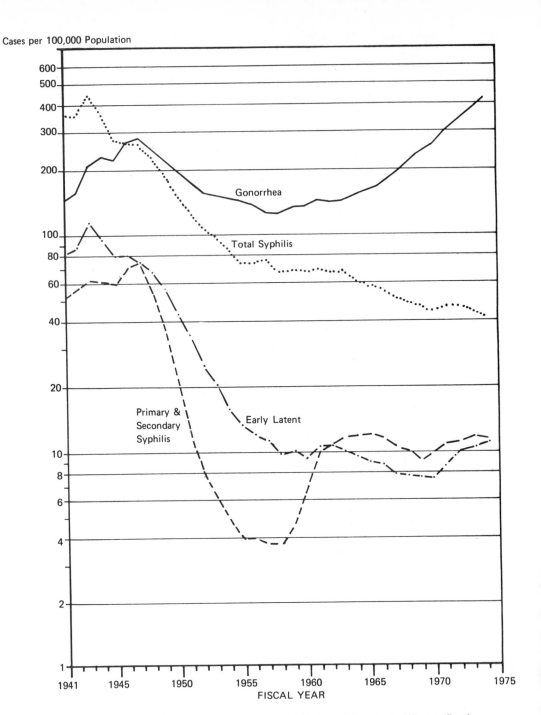

Cases per 100,000 Population

Gonorrhea

Total Syphilis

Primary &
Secondary
Syphilis

Early Latent

FISCAL YEAR

Figure 8-4 Reported cases of syphilis and gonorrhea per 100,000 population, United States, fiscal years 1941-1974.

Source Department of Health, Education, and Welfare, Public Health Service, Center for Disease Control, Venereal Disease Control Division, 1975.

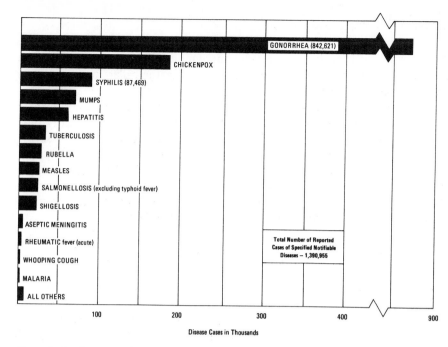

GONORRHEA (842,621)

CHICKENPOX

SYPHILIS (87,469)

MUMPS

HEPATITIS

TUBERCULOSIS

RUBELLA

MEASLES

SALMONELLOSIS (excluding typhoid fever)

SHIGELLOSIS

ASEPTIC MENINGITIS

RHEUMATIC fever (acute)

WHOOPING COUGH

MALARIA

ALL OTHERS

Total Number of Reported
Cases of Specified Notifiable
Diseases — 1,390,955

100   200   300   400   900

Disease Cases in Thousands

Figure 8-5   Communicable diseases—number of reported cases, United States, calendar year 1973.

Source   Department of Health, Education, and Welfare, Public Health Service Center for Disease Control, Venereal Disease Control Division, 1975.

suspicion are essential. Syphilis has been called "the great imitator," and gonorrhea may often go unnoticed. Every case of congenital syphilis must be regarded as a public health failure. One of the problems that has emerged in gonorrhea control is the development of strains of the organism resistant to penicillin and other antibiotics. Another problem is the asymptomatic female carrier who is a reservoir of infection. Venereal disease control involves case finding, early diagnosis (including history, examination, and laboratory studies), prompt treatment, contact investigation, patient education, and follow-up.

By 1975 all states had laws permitting minors to give their own consent for the diagnosis and treatment of venereal disease. Throughout the country, innovative approaches to venereal disease control have been attempted in order to reach the vulnerable population under eighteen years of age. For example, Philadelphia's "Operation Venus" program has met with considerable success, since its inception in 1972. Under this program, an information source has been established for young people who think they might have contracted venereal disease and need help. The telephone number has been widely publicized and is listed in the telephone directory. A central telephone is manned by youth volunteers who provide information to troubled callers.

Anyone who calls for help may remain anonymous. The volunteers have been trained to handle difficult questions and to direct the callers to appropriate diagnostic and treatment facilities.

Active in the dissemination of information on venereal disease control is the American Social Health Association. With headquarters in New York, it is a voluntary health organization financed through individual contributions. It supports legislative efforts, provides educational materials, and attempts to promote venereal disease control and sex education activities at the national level. The Planned Parenthood Federation of America and the Sex Information and Education Council of the United States (SIECUS) also promote educational programs in efforts to control venereal disease.

DEGENERATIVE AND DISABLING DISEASES, INJURIES, OR CONDITIONS

Chronic Illness

Chronic disease has been termed America's number one health problem. The National Health Survey has estimated that more than 94 million Americans, nearly 50 percent of the population, have one or more chronic conditions. Of these, 22 million are limited to some extent in their activity; 6.3 million have some limitation of mobility. Limitation of activity refers not only to the person's major activity (his ability to work, keep house, or engage in school or preschool activities) but also to his other activities, such as participation in recreational, civic, or church activities. Limitation of mobility refers to the ability to move about freely. The major causes of activity and mobility limitation are heart conditions and arthritis. Other conditions that cause limitation of activity or mobility are impairments of the back, spine, lower extremities and hips, as well as visual impairments, mental and nervous conditions, complete or partial paralysis, and hypertension.[11]

Chronic health problems may strike at any age, but they increase sharply with advancing age. The lives of millions of older Americans are affected daily by illnesses or impairments. Indeed, chronic diseases might aptly be termed "companions of the aged."[12] The figures are striking: 85 percent of those sixty-five and over living outside institutions (15 million people) have at least one chronic condition, and about half of these individuals suffer some limitation of activity because of chronic conditions. Heart disease, hypertension, diabetes, and arthritis occur more frequently with advancing age (45 years and over), and all four are more common among women than among men (in this age group). The leading causes of activity limitation or prevention of activities in older people are heart conditions and arthritis.

Effective chronic disease control is hampered by the fact that the health care delivery system is crisis oriented. The public's attitudes and the structure of the health care delivery system hinder efforts at prevention and early detection on a broad scale. Yet, it is prevention, early detection, and treatment that must be at the core of all efforts aimed at chronic disease control if disability is to be avoided or minimized. Early treatment could postpone or prevent the development of the life-threatening stage or the disability associated with a particular disease. Follow-up care could help to maintain achieved stability.

Nursing can make a most valuable contribution at all levels of prevention in the field of chronic disease control. At the primary prevention level, nurses have organized and directed screening programs for hypertension, diabetes, uterine cancer, and other conditions (Figures 8-6 and 8-7). Examples of nursing practice at the secondary and tertiary levels of prevention would include measures such as administering specific medications in the treatment of illness, moving and positioning patients to prevent complications, assisting with passive and active exercises to prevent limitation of disability, and continued health supervision for rehabilitation. We find nurses involved at all levels of prevention through health teaching with individuals, families, and groups in the community.

Individual members of society must assume a great deal of personal responsibility if chronic illness is to be prevented or reduced to a minimum.

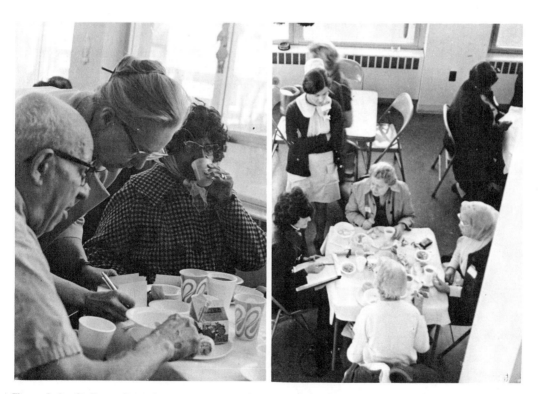

Figure 8-6   Staff members of a community nursing agency, assisted by nursing students and community volunteers, conduct a diabetes screening program for elderly residents of a public housing unit.

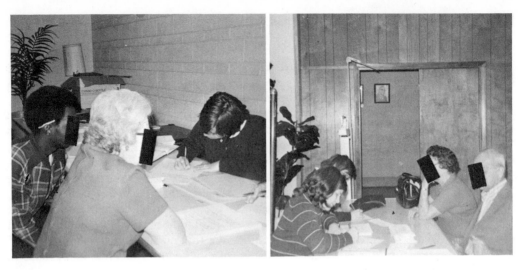

Figure 8-7 A volunteer nurses' group, assisted by nursing students, conducts a hypertension screening program in the community.

They must learn to appreciate the value of prevention through positive health promotion, health maintenance, and screening. Indeed, health screening should be a routine practice before the development of obvious disease symptoms. The growing public acceptance of Pap smears, mammography, and chest X-rays points the way. With increasing education, the public should be getting more information about chronic disease and the importance of prevention.

There are many voluntary health organizations, such as the American Heart Association, American Cancer Society, and United Cerebral Palsy, involved in dissemination of information to the public about chronic disease. These organizations are supported largely through private contributions. Through their network of state and local chapters, they assist communities in some or all of the following ways: supporting research efforts; educating the public; supplying professional educational materials; promoting health screening programs; maintaining diagnostic and treatment facilities; providing supplies and equipment for patients; lobbying in legislative bodies for appropriate laws.

Mental Health Problems

Mental Illness Mental and emotional problems have reached epidemic proportions in the United States. According to a report from the National Association for Mental Health, at least one person in ten (a total of 20 million people), will be afflicted during their lifetime with some form of mental or emotional illness that may require professional help. This report also points out that 1.4 million persons affected are children under eighteen years of age, and of those only about one-half are receiving some form of treatment. The loss to the individual and community is staggering when measured in terms of human misery, family disruption, cost of care, and the economic waste from mental and physical disability. Emotional factors play an important role in many physical illnesses; the report cited above indicates that more than fifty percent of all medical and surgical problems are complicated by an emotional crises.[13]

Mental illness is a public health problem that has been aggravated by the prejudices and attitudes of the community. Historically, the mentally ill person has been viewed as one who poses a threat and must be shut away from the mainstream of society, stripped of his rights and privileges. Such persons were often cruelly bound and shackled behind iron bars. Humanitarian efforts to improve the care of the mentally ill were in evidence nearly two centuries ago with the famous "unchaining of the insane" by Dr. Philippe Pinel, as illustrated by Figure 8–8. In recent years enlightened legislation has had the effect of protecting individual rights of patients, and has helped to reduce the use of compulsory hospitalization. Compulsory hospitalization is limited to emergency situations where there is evidence that a person has attempted to harm himself or others. The emphasis today has shifted from involuntary confinement in an "insane asylum" to the patient's voluntary acceptance of treatment in the most appropriate setting, whether it is the hospital, the community mental health center, or his own home.

Major advances within the last decade, such as the use of psychotropic drugs, group and individual therapy, and better diagnostic and screening methods, have contributed to the reduction of lengthy in-hospital treatment and encouraged the patient's early return home. With the focus of care shifting to the community, it is possible, through careful intervention, to prevent hospitalization or to limit the inpatient days to the acute phase of the psychotic episode. Thus, though numbers of admissions to mental hospitals are on the increase, the average length of stay has been shortened.

Federal legislation has been instrumental in supporting early discharge. In 1963 Congress passed the Community Mental Health Act for construction of mental health centers and provision of basic mental health services. Subsequent amendments in 1968 and 1970 broadened the services to include special programs for drug abuse and alcoholism. Regionalization of the services for population groups of 75,000 to 200,000 people, later termed "catchment areas," formed the "base service units" that helped make a range of services readily accessible to a target population. To be eligible for federal support these centers must provide five essential services—inpatient care, outpatient care, partial hospitalization, emergency service and consultation, and education.

Some dramatic changes have resulted from the development of community mental health units. For example, the population in state mental hospitals was reduced from 550,000 in 1955 to 338,000 in 1970. Furthermore,

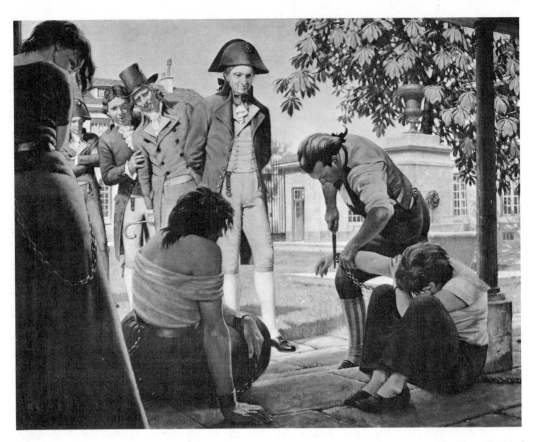

Figure 8-8 In the 1790s the French physician Philippe Pinel demanded humane treatment for the patients of the large Parisian insane asylums. A pioneer in improving conditions for the mentally ill, he ordered their chains and fetters removed and insisted upon kindness, understanding, and rational therapy in their treatment. His success with these methods paved the way for modern psychiatry.

Source A History of Medicine in Pictures, a pamphlet accompanying photographs presented by Parke, Davis. ©1960 by Parke, Davis and Company.

the expansion and increased use of outpatient facilities as an alternative to in-hospital care may help prevent the dismantling effect of long-term confinement. The fear and prejudice that constitute the chief barriers to the patient's return to the community can be dealt with early through group and family therapy at the community centers. In community mental health programs, every effort should be made to effect a coordinated community approach for the alleviation of mental health problems. The utilization of existing community health resources and the inclusion of the community health nurse as a member of the mental health team are two major factors that can help to broaden the service.

As a key person on the mental health team, the nurse is in a strategic position to identify problems that disrupt family life. Her broad knowledge of the community and its resources, her easy entree into the home, and her ability to communicate with families as a whole are part of her special expertise. She offers encouragement and support to families as they begin to develop new and more rewarding efforts of coping with problems that affect daily living. In several communities throughout the country where the nurse-therapist role has been recognized (Dothan, Alabama; LaGrange, Georgia; and Columbus, Georgia),[14] the public health nurse has served as the primary care professional in the mental health treatment centers.

A moving force for the improvement of mental health services is the National Association for Mental Health, a voluntary organization made up of lay and professional persons. Through its state and local chapters, it is involved in research, education, and legislative action for the prevention and treatment of mental illness. Its official symbol is the Mental Health Bell (Figure 8-9), which was cast in 1953 from chains and handcuffs formerly used to bind mental patients.

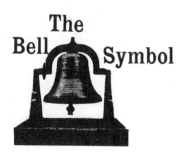

"Cast from shackles which bound them, this bell shall ring out hope for the mentally ill and victory over mental illness"

Figure 8-9

Source   Reproduced courtesy of the National Association for Mental Health, Inc.

Mental Retardation   There are an estimated six million mentally retarded persons in the United States. The number varies depending on the particular definition employed to identify the condition. Epidemiologic information indicates a higher incidence of mental retardation among males than females. There is an increased incidence among low-income groups where mothers and children receive inadequate medical care. The etiology of mental retardation in approximately 25 percent of the cases identified is unknown. Known biological causes of the condition include heredity, infection, nutritional deficiencies during pregnancy, injuries, and "prematurity."[15]

Mental retardation ranges from mild to severe. Some conditions of retardation, for example, Down's syndrome, may be recognizable at birth. However, certain physical features that have come to be regarded as identifying characteristics of retardation, for example, small head size, small anatomical build and features, and slanted eyes, are not sufficient evidence for diagnosis. The impaired ability to learn, inadequately developed intelligence, and the failure to adapt to the demands of society are additional factors to be considered before the final diagnosis is made.

The degrees of mental retardation are based on measured assessment of learning abilities, as seen in Table 8-2.

Today, the emphasis is on community based treatment and education for the retarded person, avoiding long-term institutionalization. Many communities now have respite care centers where the retarded person can be cared for on a short-term basis whenever necessary. Community diagnostic centers, special education classes, day care centers, sheltered workshops, occupational training centers, and recreational programs are some of the specialized services organized to help retarded persons reach their maximum ability. Enlightened legislation in some states has made it possible for even the severely retarded to achieve some potential through public education programs. For example, in Pennsylvania, retarded children have been given the right to free public education on the basis of a federal court ruling in a case brought by the Pennsylvania Association for Retarded Children. West Virginia has enacted legislation requiring special education for children with developmental handicaps.

Prevention of mental retardation consists of genetic counseling for couples who have a history of metabolic disease, or contemplate pregnancy after age thirty-five. Early and comprehensive prenatal care, avoidance of unnecessary drugs during pregnancy, prevention of infection, family planning, and early detection of inborn errors of metabolism in the newborn infant offer new hope for the prevention and eventual eradication of mental retardation.

Many citizens volunteer their time in behalf of retarded persons. Working quietly behind the scenes they have formed several voluntary organizations, such as the National Association for Retarded Children (NARC). This group, through its 1300 local member units, promotes and supports research, provides parent counseling, stimulates legislative action, and gives interested citizens an opportunity to serve others.

Drug Abuse

Drug abuse has infiltrated all levels of society and poses a serious threat to the well-being of our people. The problem is increasing despite concentrated ef-

Table 8-2   Developmental Characteristics of the Mentally Retarded

Degrees of Mental Retardation	Pre-School Age 0-5 Maturation and Development	School Age 6-20 Training and Education	Adult 21 and Over Social and Vocational Adequacy
Mild I.Q. 52-67	Can develop social and communication skills; minimal retardation in sensorimotor areas; often not distinguished from normal until later age.	Can learn academic skills up to approximately sixth grade level by late teens. Can be guided toward social conformity. "Educable."	Can usually achieve social and vocational skills adequate to minimum self-support but may need guidance and assistance when under unusual social or economic stress.
Moderate I.Q. 36-51	Can talk or learn to communicate; poor social awareness; fair motor development; profits from training in self-help; can be managed with moderate supervision.	Can profit from training in social and occupational skills; unlikely to progress beyond second grade level in academic subjects; may learn to travel alone in familiar places.	May achieve self-maintenance in unskilled or semi-skilled work under sheltered conditions; needs supervision and guidance when under mild social or economic stress.
Severe I.Q. 20-35	Poor motor development; speech is minimal; generally unable to profit from training in self-help; little or no communication skills.	Can talk or learn to communicate; can be trained in elemental health habits; profits from systematic habit training.	May contribute partially to self-maintenance under complete supervision; can develop self-protection skills to a minimal useful level in controlled environment.
Profound I.Q. less than 20	Gross retardation; minimal capacity for functioning in sensorimotor areas; needs nursing care.	Some motor development present; may respond to minimal or limited training in self-help.	Some motor and speech development; may achieve very limited self-care; needs nursing care.

Source   United States Department of Health, Education, and Welfare, Secretary's Committee on Mental Retardation, The Problem of Mental Retardation, 1969.

forts to halt its spread. Many therapeutic drugs—once hailed as a boon to relieve pain and illness—are now often employed illegally to alter one's state of consciousness and create euphoria as an alternative to facing life's frustrations. Precise statistics on drug abuse are difficult to gather; even if they were readily obtainable, numbers alone could not measure the real costs to society and to the individual victims. Drug abuse is a human problem—the human price is paid in lives wasted and talents lost, and in the social by-products of crime, disintegration of communities, and despair.

The Drug Enforcement Administration has classified drugs with substantial abuse potential into four major groups according to their pharmacological properties as follows: [16]

Narcotics are primarily opium derivatives and synthetic opiates and are utilized in medical treatment for their analgesic effects. The fact that these drugs produce euphoria and are addictive gives them a high abuse potential. Examples: morphine, opium, codeine, and demerol. (Heroin is also included in this group; however, it is not utilized in medical treatment.)

Depressants are primarily barbiturates, tranquilizers, and bromides and are utilized medically for their sedative and sleep-producing qualities. Abuse of these drugs produces acute intoxication similar to that of alcohol. Examples: seconal, valium, and chloral-hydrate.

Stimulants are primarily amphetamines and cocaine; amphetamines are prescribed for weight reduction, cocaine is used as a topical anesthetic. They are abused because of the high level of excitation they cause. Examples: dexedrine, "speed," cocaine, and methamphetamine.

Hallucinogens. Although chemically dissimilar, most hallucinogens produce some degree of sensory distortion; there are few medical uses except under experimental conditions. Examples: LSD, mescaline, PCP, and cannabis.

Narcotic addiction is only one part of the total drug problem. Non-narcotic substances mentioned above are greatly overused. There is legitimate access to depressants and stimulants, which are often prescribed for therapeutic purposes. The extent of the abuse of non-narcotic drugs can only be grossly measured. Inferences as to the size of the problem can be drawn from production figures of leading drug companies. It is estimated that nearly half of all the barbiturates and amphetamines produced in this country annually are diverted to the illegal market.[17] "The availability of the drug combined with the existence of a personality disorder" are two major factors, leading ultimately to drug dependence (see Alcoholism, p. 133).[18] Studies have failed to identify a specific personality involved in drug dependence. Users of narcotics and other dangerous drugs often develop a high level of resistance to their effects. This increasing tolerance leads to dependence and the need for larger dosages to maintain the achieved state of euphoria.[19]

Among the narcotic drugs, heroin ranks first both in popularity and in long-range addiction. The total number of heroin users in the United States is not known and can only be estimated from two basic sources, as follows:

(1) treatment centers where heroin users voluntarily come for help;
(2) law enforcement agencies which apprehend heroin users on criminal charges.[20]

Young people between the ages of fifteen and twenty-five are thought to be the most vulnerable group. Surveys of students in elementary schools indicate that heroin abuse may be found among children as young as eleven.[21]

There is some evidence to indicate a changing pattern in the spread of heroin throughout the United States. Reports from major United States cities suggest 1968 to 1970 as a peak period for heroin use, with a subsequent decline.[22] However, one study points out that heroin use continues to peak, but that this peak usage has shifted from larger cities to smaller communities.[23] Estimates vary, but according to statistics compiled by federal authorities, the number of heroin addicts may have decreased from an estimated 273,000 in 1971 to approximately 250,000 in 1973; however, in 1974 the number went up to 310,000.[24] Guarded optimism was expressed over the fact that for a brief period between 1971 and 1973 there was a substantial decrease in the availability of heroin at the "street" or retail level.[25] A very important event which affected the supply of the drug was Turkey's temporary ban on the production of opium (from which heroin is derived) after the harvest of 1972. However, the ban was lifted in 1974, and there are real indications that Turkey may once again become a major supplier, along with Mexico and the so-called "Golden Triangle" between Burma, Laos, and Thailand.

Although drug detoxification and rehabilitation are aimed at all forms of drug addiction, heroin has been given priority, because it is the most difficult drug problem to treat. Several approaches have been used in the treatment of heroin addiction, all of which have had some measure of success, as follows:

The British System[26]   The basic premise of the British approach is the belief that drug addiction is a medical problem and should be treated by a physician. The person addicted to heroin or morphine may present himself voluntarily at an outpatient clinic for treatment. These clinics are also rehabilitation centers where every effort is made to help the addict understand his problem and voluntarily undergo withdrawal. The emphasis is on persuasion, without coercion. If the addict does not choose to withdraw, he is encouraged to substitute methadone for heroin in his maintenance program. If, however, he does not accept either withdrawal or methadone maintenance, he can be given a maintenance dose of the narcotic drug to which he is addicted—prescribed and administered by a physician at the specialized treatment center.

The Methadone Maintenance Program[27]   This method was first introduced in 1964 by Dr. Vincent Dole and Dr. Marie Nyswander. The treatment consists of gradually decreasing the patient's intake of heroin until he is completely detoxified and then administering increasing doses of methadone. A synthetic chemical, methadone is said to block the euphoric effects of heroin, thus breaking the dependency of the patient on the drug. Maintenance on methadone is for life.

Long Term Institutionalization[28]   The federal government hospitals at Fort Worth, Texas, and Lexington, Kentucky, before they were closed in 1973, had used the long-term treatment approach. The patient was completely withdrawn from heroin over a two-week period. After the patient completed physical withdrawal, he entered a rehabilitation program. This program was tailored to his individual needs as determined by a complete physical and psychological evaluation. He was then given vocational or other educational training according to his potential. The average length of stay was about three and one-half years; the average cost per year was approximately $30,000. The combined cost of both federal facilities was estimated at $50 million per year.

The Therapeutic Community[29]   This is an in-residence program using the group therapy approach. The principle behind the therapeutic community is that the addict treats himself, the assumption being that his drug dependency is only a symptom of a deeper emotional problem. He may enter the residence voluntarily, but he continues with the program only if he leads a nonaddictive life. He must be gainfully employed, helping to keep the center financially self-sufficient while he develops ego strength and deals with his problems. Representative of this type of treatment center is Synanon in California, founded in 1958 and based on the Alcoholics Anonymous principle (see Alcoholism, p. 134). Here the length of stay averages three to five years. Other examples of the therapeutic community are Gaudenzia House (Philadelphia), Daytop Village and Phoenix Houses (New York), and Gateway Houses (Chicago).

The methods within the established professional care system, some of which we have just outlined, are unable to meet the present demands for treatment. The growing public disenchantment with formal treatment programs has stimulated the emergence of a wide variety of "self-help" groups organized by ex-addicts or those people in local communities who feel committed to helping ex-addicts remain free of drugs. Dumont, who has studied the counterculture organizations engaged in helping those suffering from the horrors of drug abuse, describes the reward and punishment system that encourages upward mobility among the clients.[30] Loosely structured and relatively flexible in their approach, these groups are nevertheless committed to the type of therapy that extends individual ego strength through the collective sharing of the discomfort of withdrawal and the struggle for a life free from drugs.

Intensive efforts have been made to prevent drug abuse. Legislation aimed at importation control, mandatory treatment programs, imprisonment of drug users and vendors has failed to substantially reduce the drug problem in the United States. Organized crime perpetuates illicit drug traffic. However, the federal government has taken major steps to try to stop the illegal flow of heroin and opium from other countries. Activities and programs in drug abuse education, training, treatment, rehabilitation, and research are conducted at the federal level by numerous agencies.

Individual communities must take greater responsibility for the eradication of the drug problem. Communities should develop and expand recreational programs for youth, and parents must become involved in these programs. And, most important, adults must set examples for the youth by eliminating their own dependence on alcohol and other drugs. From the growing body of literature on drug abuse, we begin to realize that the solution to this devastating problem remains elusive. "No man is an island"—each one of us is a part of the problem and therefore must become a part of the solution. Unless society can find ways to improve the quality of life for all people and instill a meaningful value system in our youth, the drug problem will remain a part of our culture for a long time.

Alcoholism

Alcoholism ranks as one of the major drug abuse problems that plague the nation's health. The National Council on Alcoholism estimates that 80 million Americans drink alcohol in one form or another. Some drinkers experience no serious effects, others (one out of every sixteen persons) are "problem drinkers." Five million lose control under the influence of alcohol and are considered "chronic alcoholics." Problem drinking has infiltrated every level of society. The alcoholic puts unnecessary strain on our social institutions—the family, church, police, and courts. Problem drinking is often a contributing factor in many criminal acts such as assault and battery, auto theft, and non-support. Alcoholism and alcohol abuse are a special threat on our highways. One out of every fifty drivers is drunk, and alcohol is involved in about 25 to 50 percent of all fatal traffic accidents. Moreover, the alcoholic occupies one out of every seven beds in our mental institutions and one out of every six beds in our veterans' hospitals. Sixty percent of men in prisons are there because of crimes committed while under the influence of alcohol. Although alcohol kills and maims more persons than drug overdose, alcoholism as a cause of death is seriously under-reported.[31] The figures for 1974 show cirrhosis of the liver to be one of the ten leading causes of death.[32]

There is a widespread attitude that the alcoholic is not a sick person but is morally weak. Nothing could be further from the truth. Despite the myriad of theories that have been offered to explain the cause of alcoholism, it is an illness whose etiology is still obscure. Heavy drinking does not always produce an alcoholic. Some psychologists and psychiatrists hold that the alcoholic is an insecure, self-centered, immature individual. Biochemists offer the theory that in certain individuals alcohol causes a metabolic disturbance, a condition which reduces the level of tolerance and produces pathological intoxication. A combination of the psychological traits and biochemical effects has produced another theory similar to that of drug addiction, that is "the availability of the drug combined with the existence of a personality disorder."[33]

Alcoholism is a condition that can be controlled but not cured. The alcoholic should be given the same consideration as the victim of other chronic conditions such as diabetes, heart disease, and cancer. Only then will the victim of this disease be removed from the degraded and disinherited ranks of society. More than a decade ago, the American Medical Association and the American Bar Association issued a joint statement recognizing alcoholism as an illness and one of the nation's major health problems. Both organizations declared that the alcoholic was entitled to the same rights and privileges in law and medical treatment as granted to the victims of other disease conditions.

The most successful treatment so far has been the approach used by Alcoholics Anonymous (AA), a voluntary organization of recovered alcoholics. Founded in 1935, it now has chapters in major cities and many small communities across the United States. The program operates on the principle that one admits to being an alcoholic and is motivated to conquer his drinking problem. Alcoholism is incurable, but can be controlled through total abstinence from alcoholic beverages. The alcoholic sets his goals a day at a time, recognizing that under circumstances that produce extreme stress he may be tempted to reach for a drink. To avoid this temptation, he uses the network set up by his local AA chapter, whereby he can call a "helping hand" (a recovered alcoholic) who will try to dissuade him from taking that drink.

The alcoholic needs all the support he can get from family and friends to "stay on the wagon." Alanon and Alateens are subsidiary branches of Alcoholics Anonymous whose members are spouses and children of alcoholics. These two organizations work closely with AA to help wives, husbands, children, and other relatives of the victim gain insight into the alcoholic problem. In many communities, meetings of Alanon and Alateen are held concomitantly with Alcoholics Anonymous meetings. When there is a mutual understanding of the alcoholic's problem by family and friends, the home environment may become more conducive to his rehabilitation, thus increasing the alcoholic's chances for a complete recovery.

The key to the control and prevention of alcoholism is education. In American society where drinking is socially acceptable, almost everyone is threatened with the disease. Educational programs, counseling and guidance services, parent-teacher groups, and neighborhood organizations can be tremendous assets in controlling social drinking before its participants become victims of alcoholism. To be effective, a public education program about alcoholism and alcohol abuse must present accurate, scientifically sound information. Resource material should be readily available for those who wish it. Alcoholism Information Centers are found in many cities and towns across the country. They may be located in churches, industrial organizations, or health and welfare agencies. These resource centers provide programs and furnish speakers for interested groups. They may supply books, leaflets, films, and research material on alcoholism.

The *Twelve Steps* program of Alcoholics Anonymous is really a reeducation process for the alcoholic. The success of the program depends on the alcoholic's desire for sobriety. The organization recognizes that many victims of alcoholism must "hit bottom" before they will seek help. Attention should be directed toward helping the families of alcoholics. Every effort should be made to support them throughout those trying days before their sick member is ready to recognize his problem and accept treatment.

THE TWELVE STEPS OF ALCOHOLICS ANONYMOUS

(1) We admitted we were powerless over alcohol, that our lives had become unmanageable.

(2) Came to believe that a power greater than ourselves could restore us to sanity.

(3) Made a decision to turn our will and our lives over to the care of God as we understand Him.

(4) Made a searching and fearless moral inventory of ourselves.

(5) Admitted to God, to ourselves and to another human being the exact nature of our wrongs.

(6) Were entirely ready to have God remove all these defects of character.

(7) Humbly asked Him to remove our shortcomings.

(8) Made a list of persons we had harmed and became willing to make amends to them all.

(9) Made direct amends to such people whenever possible except when to do so would injure them or others.

(10) Continued to take personal inventory and when we were wrong, promptly admitted it.

(11) Sought through prayer and meditation to improve our conscious contact with God as we understand Him, praying only for knowledge of His will for us and the power to carry that out.

(12) Having had a spiritual awakening as the result of these steps, we tried to carry this message to alcoholics and practice these principles in all our affairs.

Accidents

The National Safety Council in its 1975 preliminary condensed edition of *Accident Facts* points out that accidents are the fourth leading cause of death for all age groups and the number one cause for all persons between the ages of one and thirty-eight. The report lists the principal classes of accidents and the number of deaths as shown in Table 8–3.

Motor vehicles are involved in nearly one-half of all fatal accidents. The automobile, originally created to serve man, becomes a deadly weapon in the hands of a careless driver. Attitude, personality, and life-adjustment are important factors in safe driving.[35] Anxiety, tension, heavy drinking, drug abuse, and driving at an excessive rate of speed have been identified as specific causative factors in many fatal and non-fatal accidents.[36] The National Safety Council pointed out that the 1974 figures for motor vehicle fatalities represented a 17 percent decrease from 1973. Can it be that the nationwide reduc-

Table 8-3 Accident Fatality Toll—United States, 1974

Class of Accident	Number of Deaths
All accidents	105,500
Motor vehicle	46,200
Public non-motor-vehicle	24,500
Home	25,000
Work	13,500

Note: Motor vehicle totals include some deaths already included in the Work and Home totals. This duplication amounts to about 3,700.

Source Accident Facts, 1975 Preliminary Condensed Edition. Chicago: National Safety Council, February, 1975.

tion of the speed limit, imposed at the onset of the "energy crisis," had a salutory effect on this serious problem?

In the home setting, falls, fires, and burns account for over one-half of the accident fatalities. Especially vulnerable are those persons over seventy-five years of age. Work-related accidents are a matter of great concern to industry and the community, although there has been a slight downward trend in fatalities over the last two decades. Public non-motor-vehicle accidents include falls, transportation accidents (rail, air, water, and other), fires, drowning, suffocation, poisoning, and firearms, and account for 23 percent of the fatal accidents.

Loss of life, tragic as it is, is only part of the total human loss from accidents. See Table 8-4 below showing disabling injuries that result from accidents:

Table 8-4 Accident Disability Toll—United States, 1974

Class of Accident	Number of Disabling Injuries
All accidents	11,000,000
Motor vehicle	1,800,000
Public non-motor-vehicle	2,900,000
Home	4,000,000
Work	2,400,000

Note: Duplication of motor vehicle with other classes numbers 100,000.

Source Accident Facts, 1975 Preliminary Condensed Edition. Chicago: National Safety Council, February, 1975.

Each one of these numbers stands for a victim who has endured pain, loss of potential, economic deprivation, and in some cases permanent disability.

These overwhelming conditions cost the American public $43.3 billion in 1974. Included in this figure are $13.0 billion in loss of wages, $5.5 billion in medical expenses, $8.2 billion in administrative and claim settlement costs, $6.7 billion in property damage from motor vehicle accidents, $3.1 billion in property loss from fires, and $6.8 billion for the "indirect" costs of work accidents. Marked public apathy to the problem persists in spite of the staggering cost in terms of death, disability, and economic waste. The same type of citizen involvement that helped to conquer poliomyelitis and to control cancer, heart disease, and mental illness must be employed to lower the accident rate.

One of the major goals of nursing care is accident prevention. In formulating a plan of care, the nurse will observe and assess the condition of the individual patient and other family members—can they see well? do they move about without difficulty? do they remember to turn off the burners on the stove? She will also observe and evaluate the environmental factors—are there slippery throw-rugs in the halls? are there loose objects lying on the floor? are electrical outlets protected? are poisonous detergents and cleaning fluids out of reach of small children? Health teaching for accident prevention is a most important nursing function whether in the home or in hospitals, nursing homes, other health care institutions, schools, industry, or any setting. The nurse has a professional obligation to be knowledgeable about and involved with the legislative processes responsible for establishing and enforcing safety codes and regulations.

Education for prevention is the keystone to building a program for the control of the accidental death and injury problem. Educators, industrialists, public health officials, and all citizens have a major responsibility in accident prevention. Strict adherence to safety codes in industry and building construction, continued surveillance of marketed products, and greater individual concern for human life are several ways in which accidents might be prevented.

Safety on highways is everyone's concern. The increase in the number of automobiles has intensified the motor vehicle accident problem. The National Safety Council, a nongovernmental public service organization, has worked diligently to provide leadership in the safety movement. This agency is responsible for instituting special seminars in defensive driving for all operators of motor vehicles. They support driver education in public schools by providing speakers, films, and literature. They are engaged in ongoing education and research for the safety of the nation.

REFERENCES

1. Harry S. Mustard and Ernest L. Stebbins, *An Introduction to Public Health* 4th ed. (New York: Macmillan,© 1959), p. 15-16.

2. Alvin Toffler, *Future Shock* (New York: Random House, 1970), p. 2.

3. Anatol Rapoport, "Foreword" in Walter Buckley, *Modern Systems Research for the Behavioral Scientist* (Chicago: Aldine Publishing Co., 1968), p. XIII-XXII.

4. Center for Disease Control, *Morbidity and Mortality, Weekly Report,* for week ending December 28, 1974.

5. Center for Disease Control, *Tuberculosis Statistics: States and Cities* (July 1975), Table 1.

6. U.S. Department of Health, Education, and Welfare, *Tuberculosis Programs 1973, Tuberculosis Program Reports* (Atlanta, Georgia: Center for Disease Control, December, 1974), pp. 1 and 8.

7. Center for Disease Control, *Tuberculosis Statistics,* Table 1.

8. U.S. Department of Health, Education, and Welfare, *Tuberculosis Programs 1973,* p. 6.

9. James F. Jekel, "Communicable Disease Control and Public Policy in the 1970s—Hot War, Cold War or Peaceful Coexistence?" *American Journal of Public Health,* 62 (December 1972) 1578-85.

10. U.S. Department of Health, Education, and Welfare, *VD Fact Sheet 1974* (Atlanta, Georgia: Center for Disease Control, edition 31, #75-8195).

11. U.S. Department of Health, Education, and Welfare, National Center for Health Statistics, *Chronic Conditions and Limitations of Activity and Mobility,* Series 10, No. 61, (January 1971), p. 1.

12. U.S. Department of Health, Education, and Welfare, National Center for Health Statistics, *Health in the Later Years of Life* (October 1971) p. 17.

13. National Association for Mental Health, *Facts About Mental Illness,* 1971-72 (pamphlet).

14. Leonard T. Maholick, "A Delivery System for Local Mental Health Services," *American Journal of Public Health,* 62 (March 1972) 364-70.

15. U.S. Department of Health, Education, and Welfare, Secretary's Committee on Mental Retardation, *The Problem of Mental Retardation* (Washington, D.C.: Government Printing Office, 1969).

16. *Statistical Briefing Book. Statistics Updated through December 1974.* U.S. Department of Justice, Drug Enforcement Administration (Washington, D.C.: Government Printing Office), p. 1.

17. National Institute of Mental Health, *Recent Research on Narcotics, LSD, Marihuana, and Other Dangerous Drugs* (Washington, D.C.: Government Printing Office, October, 1969), p. 2.

18. Morton J. Rodman and Dorothy W. Smith, *Pharmacology and Drug Therapy in Nursing* (Philadelphia: J.B. Lippincott Co., 1968,) p. 44.

19. Ibid.

20. Mark H. Greene, "An Epidemiologic Assessment of Heroin Use," *American Journal of Public Health,* 64 (December 1974) 1–10, Supplement.

21. Kit G. Johnson, John H. Donnelly, Robert Scheble, Richard L. Wine, and Morris Weitman, "Survey of Adolescent Drug Use I—Sex and Grade Distribution," *American Journal of Public Health,* 61 (December 1971) 2418-32.

22. Mark H. Greene, "An Epidemiologic Assessment."

23. Leon G. Hunt, "Recent Spread of Heroin Use in the United States," *American Journal of Public Health,* 64 (December 1974) 16-23, Supplement.

24. *Statistical Briefing Book,* page 61.

25. Ibid, page 3.

26. National Clearinghouse for Drug Abuse Information, "The British Narcotics System," *Report Series,* 13:1 (Washington, D.C.: Government Printing Office, April, 1973), pp. 1–12.

27. V.P. Dole and Marie E. Nyswander, "Rehabilitation of Heroin Addicts after Blockade with Methadone." *New York Journal of Medicine,* 66 (August 1966) 2011-17.

28. S.B. Sells, "Rehabilitating the Heroin Addict," *Report of the Institute on New Developments in the Rehabilitation of the Narcotic Addict, Fort Worth, Texas, February, 1966* (Washington, D.C.: Government Printing Office, 1966).

29. Jerome H. Jaffe, "Whatever Turns You Off," *Psychology Today,* 3 (12), (May 1970): 43–44, 60–62.

30. M.P. Dumont, "Drug Problems and Their Treatment," in G. Caplan, ed. *American Handbook of Psychiatry. Vol. II.* (New York: Basic Books, 1973).

31. William O. Penrose, "Counseling the Alcoholic—A New Source of Help," *Pennsylvania's Health,* 33 (Spring 1972) 2-10.

32. Monthly Vital Statistics Report, *Annual Summary for the United States, 1974, Births, Deaths, Marriages, and Divorces* (Rockville, Maryland: National Center for Health Statistics. May 30, 1975), p. 3.

33. Morton J. Rodman and Dorothy W. Smith, *Pharmacology and Drug Therapy in Nursing* (Philadelphia: J.B. Lippincott Co., 1968), p. 44.

34. Abstracted from *Patient Information Booklet* (Alcoholic Rehabilitation Unit, Haverford State Hospital, Haverford, Pa.).

35. National Safety Council, *Accident Facts, 1973 Preliminary Condensed Edition* (February 1973).

36. *Accident Facts,* 1972 edition (Chicago: National Safety Council, 1972) pp. 52-53.

ADDITIONAL READINGS

Brockington, C. Fraser, *World Health.* Boston: Little, Brown and Company, 1968.

Burton, Lloyd E., and Hugh H. Smith, *Public Health and Community Medicine.* Baltimore: Williams & Wilkins, 1970.

Cornely, Paul B., "The Hidden Enemies of Health and the American Public Health Association," in *American Journal of Public Health,* 61 (January 1971) 7-18.

Hanlon, John J. *Public Health: Administration and Practice.* 6th ed. St. Louis: C.V. Mosby Co., 1974.

Leavell, Hugh R., and E. Gurney Clark. *Preventive Medicine for the Doctor in His Community.* 3rd ed. New York: Blakiston McGraw-Hill, 1965.

Sartwell, Philip E., ed. *Maxcy-Rosenau Preventive Medicine and Public Health.* 10th ed. New York: Appleton-Century-Crofts, 1973.

Wilner, Daniel M., Rosabelle Price Walkley, and Lenor S. Goerke, *Introduction to Public Health.* New York: Macmillan Co., 1973.

Communicable Disease

General Information

Benenson, Abram S., ed. *Control of Communicable Diseases in Man.* 12th ed. New York: American Public Health Association, 1975.

Francis, Byron John. "Current Concepts in Immunization." in *American Journal of Nursing,* 73 (April 1973) 646-49.

Garner, Julia S., and Allen B. Kaiser. "How Often Is Isolation Needed?" in *American Journal of Nursing,* 72 (April 1972) 733-37.

Gregg, Michael B., "Communicable Disease Trends in the U.S.," in *American Journal of Nursing,* 68 (January 1968) 88–93.

Johnston, Dorothy F., *Essentials of Communicable Disease with Nursing Principles.* St. Louis: C.V. Mosby Co., 1968.

Keusch, Gerald, "Bacterial Diarrheas," in *American Journal of Nursing,* 73 (June 1973) 1028-32.

Lane, J., et al., "Smallpox and Smallpox Vaccination Policy," in *Annual Review of Medicine,* 22 (1971) 251–72.

Lentz, Josephine, "The Nurse's Role in Extending Infection Control to the Community," in *Nursing Clinics of North America,* 5 (March 1970) 165-73.

Morrison, Shirley T., and Carolyn R. Arnold, *Landow and Sider's Communicable Diseases.* 9th ed. Philadelphia: F.A. Davis, 1969.

Morrison, Shirley and Carolyn R. Arnold, "Patients with Common Communicable Diseases—Preventive Measures, Treatment, and Rehabilitation," in *Nursing Clinics of North America,* 5 (March 1970) 143-55.

Taylor, Andrew, "Botulism and Its Control," in *American Journal of Nursing,* 73 (August 1973) 1380-82.

Tuberculosis

Atkinson, Mary Louise, and Frances R. Ogasawara, "The New TB Evaluation Indexes," in *Bulletin of the National Tuberculosis and Respiratory Disease Association* (November 1972) pp. 14–16.

Barham, Virginia, "Changing the Attitudes of Hospital Nurses," in *Nursing Outlook,* 19 (August 1971) 538–40.

———, "How I Wanted to be Treated," in *Nursing Outlook,* 19 (January 1971) 48–49.

Brooks, Wanda, "Replacing Ritual with Reason in Tuberculosis," in *American Journal of Nursing,* 69 (November 1969). 2410–11.

Diagnostic Standards and Classification of Tuberculosis. New York: American Lung Association, 1974 (with the supplement *The Tuberculin Skin Test*).

Edwards, Phyllis G., "Is Tuberculosis Still a Problem?" in *Health Services Reports,* 88 (June-July 1973) 483–85.

Kelly, Hugh, "Patient Population and Treatment Choices," in *Nursing Outlook,* 19 (August 1971) 541-42.

Murphy, Patricia, "Satellite Clinics for Tuberculosis Care," in *Nursing Outlook,* 20 (March 1972) 186–87.

Mushlin, I., and H.R. Nayer, "Big City Approach to Tuberculosis Control," in *American Journal of Nursing,* 71 (December 1971) 2342-45.

Nursing Care in Tuberculosis—A Programmed Course of Instruction. New York: National League for Nursing, 1970 (also *Patient Care in Tuberculosis,* 2nd ed., 1973).

Ogasawara, Frances R., and Mary Louise Atkinson, "New Guidelines on TB Infection Control," in *American Lung Association Bulletin* (September 1974), pp.11–14.

Tizes, Reuben, Christopher Hayden, and Carol W. Tizes, "The Source of Notification in Tuberculosis," in *American Journal of Public Health,* 64 (August 1974) 809–11.

Weg, John C., "Tuberculosis and the Generation Gap," in *American Journal of Nursing,* 71 (March 1971) 495–500.

Syphilis and Gonorrhea (Venereal Diseases)

Atwater, John B., "Adapting the Venereal Disease Clinic to Today's Problem," in *American Journal of Public Health,* 64 (May 1974) 433-37.

Blount, Joseph H., "A New Approach for Gonorrhea Epidemiology," in *American Journal of Public Health,* 62 (May 1972) 710-12.

Brown, Mary Agnes, "Adolescents and VD," in *Nursing Outlook,* 21 (February 1973) 99–103.

Brown, William J., "Acquired Syphilis—Drugs and Blood Tests," in *American Journal of Nursing,* 71 (April 1971) 713–15.

Caldwell, Joseph G., "Congenital Syphilis: A Nonvenereal Disease," in *American Journal of Nursing,* 71 (September 1971) 1768-72.

Ennis, Michael J., "Week of VD Awareness in Erie County, New York, 1972," in *Health Services Reports,* 88 (May 1973) 463-68.

Lenz, Philomene E., "Women, the Unwitting Carriers of Gonorrhea," in *American Journal of Nursing,* 71 (April 1971) 716-19.

Mathews, Rosemary, "TLC with the Penicillin," in *American Journal of Nursing,* 71 (April 1971) 720-23.

Rosebury, T., *Morals and Microbes: The Strange Story of Venereal Disease.* New York: Viking Press, 1971.

Schwartz, William F., "Communities Strike Back," in *American Journal of Nursing,* 71 (April 1971) 724.

Taylor, Jody, and Robert W. Gonring, "Venereal Disease Campaign in Colorado—A Model for Community Action," in *Health Services Reports,* 89 (January–February 1974) 47–52.

Degenerative and Disabling Diseases, Injuries, or Conditions

Chronic Illness

American Public Health Association, *Control of Chronic Diseases in Man.* New York: American Public Health Association, 1966.

Christensen, Kathryn A., and Marylou Kiley, "The Public Health Nurse and the Long-Term Neurologic Patient," in *Nursing Clinics of North America,* 4 (June 1969) 275-83.

Commission on Chronic Illness, *Chronic Illness in the United States.* Cambridge: Harvard University Press (Commonwealth Fund), 1957.

Lilienfeld, Abraham, and Alice J. Gifford, eds. *Chronic Diseases and Public Health.* Baltimore: Johns Hopkins Press, 1966.

McIntyre, H. Mildred, and Carol L. Betson, "Unified Approach to Heart Disease: Inter-Society Commission for Heart Disease Resources," in *American Journal of Nursing,* 71 (December 1971) 2369-74.

Wang, Mamie Kwoh, "A Health Maintenance Service for Chronically Ill Patients," in *American Journal of Public Health,* 60 (April 1970) 713-21.

Mental Health Problems

Mental Illness

Caplan, G., *Principles of Preventive Psychiatry.* New York: Basic Books, 1964.

"Community Mental Health Nursing," in *American Journal of Nursing,* 70 (May 1970) 1019-21.

Cowen, E., E. Gardner, and M. Zax, eds. *Emergent Approaches to Mental Health Problems.* New York: Appleton-Century-Crofts, 1967.

Duran, Fernando A., and Gerald D. Errion, "Perpetuation of Chronicity in Mental Illness," in *American Journal of Nursing,* 70 (August 1970) 1707-09.

Goldman, Elaine, ed. *Community Mental Health Nursing.* New York: Appleton-Century-Crofts, 1972.

Hankoff, L.D., L.G. Bernard, and J. Omura, "Visiting Nurse Consultant in a Community Psychiatry Program," in *Journal of Psychiatric Nursing,* 5(3) (1967) 217-32.

Keyes, Joan, and Charles Hofling, *Basic Psychiatric Concepts.* Philadelphia: J.B. Lippincott, 1974.

Klerman, Gerald L. "The Therapeutic Future of Mind-Altering Drugs," in *Nursing Digest,* 1 (October 1973) 73-79.

Mouw, Mildred L., and Clarence H. Haylett, "Mental Health Consultation in a Public Health Nursing Service," in *American Journal of Nursing,* 67 (1967) 1447-50.

Rosenzweig, Simon, "Compulsory Hospitalization of the Mentally Ill," in *American Journal of Public Health,* 61 (January 1971) 121-26.

Mental Retardation

Curran, William J., "Rights for the Retarded," in *American Journal of Public Health,* 62 (February 1972) 264-65.

Haynes, Una, *A Developmental Approach to Casefinding.* Washington, D.C.: Government Printing Office, 1967. (Children's Bureau Publication, No. 449-1967).

Mandelbaum, Arthur, "The Group Process in Helping Parents of Retarded Children," in *Children,* 14 (1967) 227-32.

Nichtern, Sol, *Helping the Retarded Child.* New York: Grosset and Dunlap, 1974.

Piaget, J., *Psychology of Intelligence.* Translated by Malcolm Piercy and D.E. Berlyne. London: Routlege and Kegon Ltd., 1950.

President's Committee on Mental Retardation, Third Report, *MR 69: Toward Progress—The Story of a Decade.* Washington, D.C.: Government Printing Office, 1969.

Drug Abuse

Advisory Committee on Drug Dependence, *The Rehabilitation of Drug Addicts. Report of the Advisory Committee on Drug Dependence.* London: Her Majesty's Stationery Office, 1968.

Charalampous, K.D., "Drug Culture in the Seventies," in *American Journal of Public Health,* 61 (June 1971) 1225-28.

Distasio, Carol, and Marcia Nawrot, "Methaqualone," in *American Journal of Nursing,* 73 (November 1973) 1922–25.

Duvall, H. J., B.Z. Locke, and Leon Brill, "Follow-up Study of Narcotic Drug Addicts, Five Years After Hospitalization," in *Public Health Reports,* 78 (March 1963) 185-93.

Fink, Max, Alfred M. Freedman, Arthur M. Zaks, and Richard B. Resnick, "Narcotic Antagonists: Another Approach to Addiction Therapy," in *American Journal of Nursing,* 71 (July 1971) 1359-63.

Fisher, Gary, and Irma Stantz, "An Ecosystems Approach to the Study of Dangerous Drug Use and Abuse with Special Reference to the Marijuana Issue," in *American Journal of Public Health,* 62 (October 1972) 1407-14.

Foreman, Nancy J., and Joyce Zerwekh, "Drug Crisis Intervention," in *American Journal of Nursing,* 71 (September 1971) 1736-41.

Garvey, B., "The Kilburn Square Drug Abuse Center," in *British Journal of Addiction,* 64(3) (1970) 383-94.

Greene, Mark H., and Robert L. Dupont, eds., "The Epidemiology of Drug Abuse," in *American Journal of Public Health,* 64 (December 1974) 1-56, Supplement.

Hughes, P.H., G.A. Crawford, and N.W. Barker, "Developing an Epidemiologic Field Team for Drug Dependence," in *Archives of General Psychiatry,* 24 (May 1971) 389-94.

———, Noel W. Barker, Gaila Crawford, and Jerome H. Jaffe, "The Natural History of a Heroin Epidemic," in *American Journal of Public Health,* 62 (July 1972) 995-1001.

Kromberg, Carol J., and Judith Betz Proctor, "Methadone Maintenance: Evolution of a Drug Program," in *American Journal of Nursing,* 70 (December 1970) 2575-77.

Levengood, Robert, Paul Lowinger, and Kenneth Schoof, "Heroin Addiction in the Suburbs—An Epidemiologic Study," in *American Journal of Public Health,* 63 (March 1973) 209-14.

Levin, Gilbert, Gary Hirsch, and Edward Roberts, "Narcotics and the Community: A System Stimulation," in *American Journal of Public Health,* 62 (June 1972) 868-73.

Lipp, Martin R., Samuel G. Benson, and Patricia S. Allen, "Marijuana Use by Nurses and Nursing Students," in *American Journal of Nursing,* 71 (December 1971) 2339-46.

Louria, Donald, "A Critique of Some Current Approaches to the Problem of Drug Abuse," in *American Journal of Public Health,* 65 (June 1975) 581-83.

Lucas, Warren C., Stanley E. Grupp, and Raymond L. Schmitt, "Single and Multiple Drug Opiate Users: Addicts or Nonaddicts?' in *HSMHA Health Reports,* 87 (February 1972) 185-92.

Maidlow, Spencer T., and Howard Berman, "The Economics of Heroin Treatment," in *American Journal of Public Health,* 62 (October 1972) 1397-1406.

McKee, Michael, "Drug Abuse Knowledge and Attitudes in 'Middle America' ", in *American Journal of Public Health,* 65 (June 1975) 584–91.

Morgan, Arthur James, and Judith Wilson Moreno, "Attitudes Toward Addiction," in *American Journal of Nursing,* 73 (March 1973) 497-501.

National Commission on Marihuana and Drug Abuse (Shafer Report), *Drug Use in America: Problem in Perspective.* Washington, D.C.: Government Printing Office, March, 1973.

National Institute for Drug Programs, Center for Human Services, *Bibliography on Drug Abuse: Prevention, Treatment, Research.* Washington: Human Service Press, 1973.

Nelson, Karin, "The Nurse in a Methadone Maintenance Program," in *American Journal of Nursing,* 73 (May 1973) 870-74.

Nelson, Scott H., Barak Wolff, and Paul B. Batalden, "Manpower Training as an Alternative to Disadvantaged Adolescent Drug Misuse," in *American Journal of Public Health,* 65 (June 1975) 599-603.

Pearson, Barbara, "Methadone Maintenance in Heroin Addiction," in *American Journal of Nursing,* 73 (December 1970) 2571-74.

Russaw, Ethel, "Nursing in a Detoxification Unit," in *American Journal of Nursing,* 70 (August 1970) 1720-23.

Singer, Ann, "Mothering Practices and Heroin Addiction," in *American Journal of Nursing,* 74 (January 1974) 77–82.

Winek, C.L., *All You Wanted to Know About Drug Abuse, But Were Afraid to Ask.* New York: Marcel Dekker, 1973.

Yablonsky, L., *Synanon: The Tunnel Back.* Baltimore: Penguin Books, 1967.

Alcoholism

Chafetz, Morris E., "New Federal Legislation on Alcoholism—Opportunities and Problems," in *American Journal of Public Health,* 63 (March 1973) 206-08.

Cornwell, Georgia, "Factors in Interpersonal and Family Relationships and Alcoholism," in *Journal of Psychiatric Nursing and Mental Health Services,* 6 (1968) 274-78.

Fitzig, C., "Nursing in an Alcoholic Program," in *American Journal of Nursing,* 66 (October 1966) 2218-21.

Fox, Ruth, "A Multidisciplinary Approach to the Treatment of Alcoholism," in *American Journal of Psychiatry,* 123 (January 1967) 769-78.

Gelperin, Abraham, and Eve Arlin Gelperin, "The Inebriate in the Emergency Room," in *American Journal of Nursing,* 70 (July 1970) 1494-97.

Gillespie, Cecilia, "Nurses Help Combat Alcoholism," in *American Journal of Nursing,* 69 (September, 1969) 1938–41.

Hecht, Murray, "Children of Alcoholics are Children at Risk," in *American Journal of Nursing,* 73 (October 1973) 1764–67.

Holder, Harold D., and Jerome Hallan, "Systems Approach to Planning Alcoholism Programs in North Carolina," in *American Journal of Public Health,* 62 (October 1972) 1415-21.

Jellinek, E.M., "Phases in the Drinking History of Alcoholics," in *Quarterly Journal of Studies on Alcohol,* 7 (1946) 1–88.

Mueller, John F., "Treatment for the Alcoholic: Cursing or Nursing?" in *American Journal of Nursing,* 74 (February 1974) 245-47.

Accidents

Brenner, B., "Alcoholism and Fatal Accidents," in *Quarterly Journal of Studies on Alcohol,* 28 (1967) 517–28.

Eelkema, Robert C., James Brosseau, Robert Koshnick, and Charles McGee, "A Statistical Study on the Relationship between Mental Illness and Traffic Accidents—A Pilot Study," in *American Journal of Public Health,* 60 (March 1970) 459-69.

O'Neill, Brian, and Richard S. Eiswirth, "Screening Drivers for Alcohol—An Application of Bayes' Formula," in *American Journal of Public Health,* 62 (November 1972) 1468-71.

Public Health Service, Division of Emergency Health Service, *Accidental Death and Disability: The Neglected Disease of Modern Society.* Washington, D.G.: Government Printing Office, 1970 (Public Health Service Publication 1071-A-13).

Schaplowsky, A.F., "Community Injury Control—A Management Approach," in *American Journal of Public Health,* 63 (March 1973) 252-54.

Chapter 9
Health Problems
of Special Population Groups
in the Community

*"Health problems cannot be separated from the world's social ills.
Neither can they be dealt with effectively by means of disease-oriented
measures."* [1]

INTRODUCTION

In the preceding chapter we described several specific diseases and conditions
that are considered to be public health problems. In this chapter we will discuss
health problems in relation to special population groups at risk. Two of these
groups, mothers and children, have been given priority in organized health
programs (Maternal and Child Health) from the earliest days of the public
health movement (see page 12). The well-being of other vulnerable segments of
the population has also been a matter of special concern in public health;
however, only recently has there been substantial public response to the needs
of some of these groups, namely, the elderly, certain minority groups, and the
poor. Before we begin to discuss these groups and their health needs, we will
present selected demographic data used in describing a population. For example, what is the size and the composition of our population? What is the birth
rate, the marriage rate, the divorce rate, the death rate?

Certainly the situation in the United States today is quite different from
what it was a generation ago, or even a decade ago. We are living in a
technologically complex and highly industrialized society with a population
that continues to change, in size and composition. According to the 1970 census, the total population of the United States was about 204,000,000, i.e., an
increase of 13.3 percent over the 1960 total. (By the end of 1974, the
population of the United States rose to nearly 213,000,000,[2] exceeded only by

145

China, India and the Soviet Union.) With regard to the population's composition, the 1970 census showed an increase in urban concentrations, with declines in many central city areas offset by a heavy rise in suburban populations. Farm populations dropped from fifteen million to ten million. The composition by age has also changed with an absolute and relative increase of older people. Since 1900 the number of persons age sixty-five and over has grown much faster than the rest of the population; according to the 1970 census, nearly 10 percent of the population is sixty-five years of age or over.

While the population has continued to increase in numbers, the growth rate has diminished: By the early 1970s the annual rate of growth was about 1 percent. This rate is influenced by the number of births, the birth rate, and the fertility rate, all of which declined in spite of an increase in the number of women of childbearing age. By 1973, with 3,136,965 live births (fewer than any since 1945), the birth and fertility rates declined to record low levels: Birth rate—14.9 per 1000 population; fertility rate—69.3 births per 1000 women fifteen through forty-four years of age.[3]

The fertility rate, which reflects the extent of childbearing, is an important barometer for observing population trends. In reviewing the fertility rate over the past few decades, we find that the previous low was recorded during the economic depression period of 1933-39. The close of that decade marked the end of a long-term decline in fertility in the United States. Beginning in the early 1940s there was an increase in births that grew to massive proportions after World War II and reached its peak in 1957.[4] Subsequently, a downward trend in fertility set in, which, since 1970, has offset the rate of population growth. No expert has been willing to predict how long this decrease in fertility will continue without interruption. As far as numbers of births are concerned, we must assume that they can go up again and, indeed, there was a slight rise in 1974 (to 15 per 1000 population, with an increase of 30,000 births).[5] Since the fertility rate in 1974 continued to decline, this rise in births would reflect the fact that the large numbers of children born in the late 1950s and early 1960s were entering the childbearing age.

Marriages in the United States declined both in number and rate in 1974, thus interrupting the continuous upward trend of the previous fifteen years. With 2,223,000 marriages (10.5 per 1000 population), there were 60,000 less than in 1973.[6] Some observers regard this as the beginning of a downward trend resulting from the precarious economic situation as well as changing mores.[7] The number and rate of divorces and annulments increased for the twelfth consecutive year. Provisional reports indicate that 970,000 divorces were granted, giving a rate of 4.6 per 1000 population, almost twice the rate for 1964.[8]

With regard to mortality, the crude death rate has remained relatively unchanged for more than two decades. The data for 1974 show 9.1 deaths per 1000 population; this represents a 5 percent decrease from 1950, which showed 9.6. Perhaps a better measure of mortality than the crude death rate is the expectation of life at birth—the average number of years an infant can be expected to live if the age-specific death rates observed during the year of his birth were to continue unchanged during his lifetime. The estimated expectation of life at birth in 1974 was 72.0 years for the total population, the highest life expectancy ever attained in the United States.[9] Based on the respective annual age-specific death rates, the expectation of life at birth for the years 1965 through 1974 may be seen in Table 9-1.

Table 9-1   Life Expectancy 1965-1974, United States

Year	Life Expectancy	Year	Life Expectancy
1974 (est.)	72.0	1969	70.4
1973	71.3	1968	70.2
1972	71.1	1967	70.5
1971	71.1	1966	70.1
1970	70.9	1965	70.2

Source   United States Department of Health, Education and Welfare, National Center for Health Statistics Annual Summary for the United States, 1974, Births, Deaths, Marriages, and Divorces, May 1975, p. 8.

HEALTH OF MOTHERS AND CHILDREN

Maternal and child health encompasses the physical, mental, and social well-being of childbearing women and their offspring. Emphasis is placed on promotion of health and prevention of death, disease, and defects. Traditionally mothers and children have been regarded as the most vulnerable members of society. From earliest times, they have constituted a special risk group in terms of human survival. The level of a society's advancement from "survival of the fittest" to adequate health protection of all its members is often reflected in the kinds of services provided to mothers and children.

Mortality rates for children and for childbearing women are very sensitive indexes to the health of a population. When a large number of children die at an early age, you may assume that any or all of the following conditions exist: inadequate sanitation, lack of food, poor weaning and feeding practices, and a high prevalence of infectious diseases. Maternal and child health programs attempt to identify and correct these factors.

In 1973 it was estimated that 470 women died from "complications of pregnancy, childbirth, and the puerperium."[10] This placed the maternal mortality rate at 15.2 per 100,000 live births, the lowest rate ever recorded. Provisional data for 1974 place the maternal mortality rate at a new high of 20.8, indicating an interruption of the long-term downward trend in maternal mortality since 1950. (See Table 9-2.)

The infant mortality rate in 1974, based on the estimate of 52,400 infant deaths, was 16.5 per 1000 live births.[11] This was the lowest annual rate ever recorded in the United States. Both the neonatal (under twenty-eight days) and the postneonatal (twenty-eight days to eleven months) mortality rates declined in 1974. See Table 9-3.

Table 9-2   Maternal Mortality Rates per 100,000 live births 1950 and 1960-74, United States

Year	Rate	Year	Rate
1974 (est.)...................	20.8	1966.......................	29.1
1973.......................	15.2	1965.......................	31.6
1972.......................	18.8	1964.......................	33.3
1971.......................	18.8	1963.......................	35.8
1970.......................	21.5	1962.......................	35.2
1969.......................	22.2	1961.......................	36.9
1968.......................	24.5	1960.......................	37.1
1967.......................	28.0	1950.......................	83.3

Source   United States Department of Health, Education, and Welfare, National Center for Health Statistics, Annual Summary for the United States, 1974. Births, Deaths, Marriages, and Divorces. May 1975, p. 5.

Table 9-3   Infant Mortality Rates per 1000 live births 1950 and 1960-74, United States

Year	Under 1 year	Under 28 days	28 days to 11 months
1974 (est.)	16.5	12.1	4.4
1973...............................	17.7	13.0	4.8
1972...............................	18.5	13.6	4.8
1971...............................	19.1	14.2	4.9
1970...............................	20.0	15.1	4.9
1969...............................	20.9	15.6	5.3
1968...............................	21.8	16.1	5.7
1967...............................	22.4	16.5	5.9
1966...............................	23.7	17.2	6.5
1965...............................	24.7	17.7	7.0
1964...............................	24.8	17.9	6.9
1963...............................	25.2	18.2	7.0
1962...............................	25.3	18.3	7.0
1961...............................	25.3	18.4	6.9
1960...............................	26.0	18.7	7.3
1950...............................	29.2	20.5	8.7

Source   United States Department of Health, Education and Welfare, National Center for Health Statistics Annual Summary for the United States, 1974. Births, Deaths, Marriages, and Divorces. May, 1975, p. 4.

Many factors contribute to mortality and morbidity in maternal and child health. When we speak of the threats to the life and health of mothers and children, we include all those conditions that adversely affect the well-being of childbearing women and their offspring. All the factors that pose threats to the health of mothers affect the course of a baby's development. The life style and health of the mother have a marked influence on the well-being of her offspring, especially before and just after birth. One study points out that the "fate of the mother, of the fetus before birth, and the infant after birth are part of an inseparable whole and . . . any effort toward bettering the condition of one will be reflected in the condition of the other."[12]

What, then, are these factors which pose special risks? Tables 9-4 and 9-5 outline some, but by no means all, of the threats to the life and health of mothers and infants.

Table 9-4   Some Factors Which Interfere with the Course of Normal Pregnancy and Delivery ("High-Risk Mothers")

Socioeconomic and Demographic Factors	Problems of Previous Pregnancies	Chronic Systemic or Metabolic Disorders	Systemic Infections
Age of mother: under 16 or over 35	Death of previous live birth	Diabetes	Tuberculosis
Parity: those undergoing first or fifth or more pregnancy	Previous fetal death	Heart disease	Syphilis
Education of mother: eight years or less	Too frequent pregnancies, e.g., previous delivery within a year	Hypertension	Rubella
	Repeated abortions	Renal disease	Other viral diseases
Illegitimacy	Previous Caesarean section	Hyper- or hypo-thyroidism	
Inadequate prenatal care	RH incompatibility	Anemia	
Poverty, substandard housing, and nutritional deprivation	Toxemia	**Complications at Time of Labor and Delivery**	
Migrant family status	Multiple pregnancy		
Other environmental factors, e.g., X-ray irradiation, occupational hazards, pollution	**Genetic Risks**	Rupture of the uterus	
Mental-Emotional Problems	History of children born with: congenital abnormalities or inborn errors of metabolism	Placenta previa, premature separation, abruptio placentae	
Drug abuse		Difficult or prolonged labor	
Alcoholism		Uterine inertia	
Smoking		Cephalo-pelvic disproportion	
History of mental illness		Premature labor	
Mental retardation		Abnormal presentation	

In addition to the risk factors for mothers and infants cited in Tables 9–4 and 9–5, we can identify many other problems that pose threats to the life and health of young children, for example, child abuse, accidents and accidental poisoning, phenylketonuria, sickle cell anemia, cystic fibrosis, lead poisoning, mental retardation. Over and above these high risk factors there are other adverse conditions created by the inadequacies of our health care delivery system (see Chapter 11). According to one report, "one-third or more of the resident births in our large cities are to women who are dependent upon community agencies for their medical care."[13] This demand for services has placed a heavy burden on public facilities, which are chronically understaffed and overcrowded. Inadequate and inaccessible facilities and the long hours spent waiting for impersonal care have actively discouraged mothers and children

Table 9-5   Some Factors Which Interfere with Normal Fetal, Neonatal, and Infant Development ("High-Risk Babies")

Factors Related to Maternal Health

All the factors which pose threats to the health of mothers affect the course of a baby's development. Thus, for example, we might expect to find "high-risk babies" born to mothers who:

(a) were poorly nourished or anemic;

(b) had not received adequate prenatal care;

(c) smoked or used drugs unwisely;

(d) were over 35 years of age;

(e) suffered a viral disease, such as rubella, during pregnancy;

(f) were under 16 years of age, were unwed and had little formal education;

(g) had numerous previous births or miscarriages;

(h) or were subject to any of the risk factors cited in Table 9-4.

Factors Related to the Newborn

"Prematurity"

The greatest hazards to infant survival are physical underdevelopment and immaturity at time of birth. "Premature" is the term used to describe those newborn infants who are not fully developed because of curtailed gestation, low birth weight, or both. The "premature" baby is a high-risk baby. In the United States, the risk of death in the first year of life among infants who weigh 2500 grams or less at birth is 17 times the risk among infants weighing 2501 grams or more. Infants of low birth weight are subject not only to greater risk of death, but also to higher morbidity, particularly from those conditions affecting the central nervous system. Evidence points to a greater prevalence of cerebral palsy, epilepsy, mental retardation, congenital anomalies, etc., among infants of low birth weight and/or curtailed gestation than among normal full-term infants.*

We can size up the problem of infants at risk by looking at numbers and rates of "premature" births. In the United States, for example, reliable estimates indicate that annually more than one quarter of a million infants of low birth weight are born alive. In addition, there has been an overall rise in the "prematurity" rate: the proportion of low birth weight infants to the number of live births increased from 7.5% in 1950 to 8.2% in 1967. In analyzing these figures, we find that the rate among white infants remained relatively stable (around 7%). However, the rate among those classified as "other" (i.e., Black, American Indian, Chinese, Japanese, Hawaiian, Aleuts, and Eskimo) increased markedly from 10.2% to 13.6%.**

Other Factors Related to the Newborn

Low Apgar score	Failure to thrive
Prolonged hospital stay	Poor progress in hospital
Congenital malformations	Poor home environment
Other physical or mental handicaps	Sudden infant death syndrome

---

*National Center for Health Statistics, Trends in "Prematurity" United States: 1950-67 (Washington, D.C.: Government Printing Office, January 1972), p. 2.

**Ibid., p. 41.

from obtaining preventive health services. Indeed, it is not surprising that many expectant mothers from low-income families have given birth with little or no prenatal care.

Public programs designed to alter some of the conditions posing threats to the life and health of mothers and children operate under local, state, and federal auspices. Basically, each state has its own organization for maternal and child health. However, this pattern is not static, and undoubtedly will be affected by current demands for regional and comprehensive health care planning. Among the states and within each state there is great variation in the amount and kind of MCH services available to the population. At the local level, qualified public health departments include MCH programs through which services are provided directly or indirectly. In the following discussion, we will cite examples of maternal and child health programs and services.

State Maternal and Child Health Services

The creation of maternal and child health services at the state level was assisted by the federal government originally through the Sheppard-Towner Act of 1921. Further development, improvement, and extension of MCH programs were stimulated by Title V of the Social Security Act of 1935, with the subsequent passage of the Maternal and Child Health and Mental Retardation Planning Amendments, 1963, and the Child Health Amendments, 1967. MCH services are aimed at preventing disability and illness, protecting the period around pregnancy, and identifying hazards to health as early as possible. These services include maternity clinics, family planning, in-hospital maternity care, expectant parents' classes, well-child conferences, inpatient care for premature infants, dental care, health screening (for anemia, vision, developmental, tuberculin, hearing, dental, and other problems), immunization programs (for rubella, diphtheria, mumps, poliomyelitis, pertussis, tetanus, and measles), and nursing service to mothers and children.

State Crippled Children's Services

With the Social Security Act of 1935, the federal government began to provide annual grants to the states to help them extend and improve "services to crippled children and children suffering from conditions that lead to crippling. These services were to include case-finding programs, diagnostic services, medical and surgical care, hospitalization, and aftercare for crippled children."[14] Before that time, there was no nationally organized program to help children and adults with crippling conditions. The Maternal and Child Health and Mental Retardation Planning Amendments of 1963 identified mental retardation as a national health problem, and charged state crippled children's programs to become concerned with and to provide services for retarded children. The Child Health Amendments of 1967 required state crippled children's programs to extend the coverage of their state programs and to become involved with screening and case-finding programs for the identification of disabling conditions.[15]

There has been a steady increase in the numbers of children using services available under the crippled children's program since its inception. Within the last few decades, the number of children using the crippled children's program has more than doubled. In 1950 there were 214,405 children served; by 1972 the number had exceeded 500,000.[16] However, these figures represent only a small part of the total need. Though no one knows just how many children there are with handicapping conditions, the U.S. Department of Health, Education, and Welfare has pointed out that "the number of children with orthopedic handicaps alone is estimated to be well over a million . . . hundreds of thousands of children have cerebral palsy, and over a million may have epilepsy. Vision, hearing, and speech disorders affect millions of children. About 2½ million children are mentally retarded to some degree."[17]

More than three decades ago when the program was first instituted, poliomyelitis with its after effects contributed heavily to the case load. In recent years there has been a marked decline in the number of new cases related to the residual effects of poliomyelitis. Diseases of the nervous system and sense organs, and diseases of the bones and organs of movement each accounted for about one-fourth of all conditions noted in children served in 1970. Congenital malformations accounted for one-fifth of all conditions.[18]

There are numerous voluntary, nonprofit community organizations that provide services for crippled children, such as the National Foundation, the National Easter Seal Society for Crippled Children and Adults, the American Heart Association, the United Cerebral Palsy Associations, Inc., the National Cystic Fibrosis Research Foundation, the National Association for Retarded Children, and the National Hemophilia Foundation. Many have branches in the states and local communities so that the public and private agencies can work together effectively in behalf of handicapped children.

Maternity and Infant Care Projects

The threats to the life and health of mothers and children were the prime target of the 1963 Maternal and Child Health and Mental Retardation Planning Amendments to the Social Security Act (Section 508, Title V of the Social Security Act). Under this section, grants were authorized for the establishment of Maternity and Infant Care (MIC) Projects "to help reduce the incidence of mental retardation and other handicapping conditions caused by complications associated with childbearing and to help reduce infant and maternal mortality by providing necessary health care to high-risk mothers and their infants."[19]

Within ten years after the first MIC project was funded in 1964, fifty-six programs were operating in thirty-four states, the District of Columbia, and Puerto Rico. Each was established to serve a locality showing much higher infant and maternal mortality rates than the nation as a whole. While the majority of the projects were located in cities of 100,000 and more, they were also established in smaller cities and rural areas. The MIC projects have served

as catalysts, helping communities to mobilize their health resources for improved care to mothers and children. Reports indicate that they have made
progress in the whole area of maternity care, and have helped to bring about a
reduction in infant mortality.

Projects for Intensive Care of Infants

One of the provisions of Title V of the Social Security Act was the
authorization of grants for projects "to provide necessary health care to
infants during their first year of life when they have conditions or are in
circumstances which increase the hazards to their health, in order to help
reduce the incidence of mental retardation and other handicapping conditions
caused by complications associated with childbearing."[20] Special programs
for premature infants were initiated in the 1940s. Emphasis was placed on
highly skilled nursing care. Since the 1960s these special premature nurseries
have undergone a transition and become intensive care units for high-risk
newborn infants. Special equipment, laboratory services, and increased
medical and nursing care have made these special units another force in this
country's efforts to reduce the infant death rate. Eight such units were
receiving direct federal support until mid-1974, when an amendment to Title V
charged each state with the responsibility for a program of projects covering
the services previously available through special MCH project grants. To help
the states discharge this responsibility, the amount of direct formula grants
authorized to the states was increased by the federal government.[21]

Comprehensive Care for Preschool and School Age Children

Children and Youth Projects were developed to extend the concept of family
centered health care beyond the first year of life. Grants for comprehensive
programs to meet the medical, dental, physical, and emotional needs of
children and youth were authorized under Title V of the Social Security Act.
These projects were aimed at the areas with high concentrations of low-income
families.

From late 1968 to the beginning of 1972 the number of persons being
served at C and Y projects increased from 254,000 to 475,000. The percentage
of all program registrants hospitalized had decreased from 1.5 to 0.7 in that
same period. Other benefits growing out of the C and Y projects have been (1)
increased community involvement, (2) increased attention to particular area
needs through consumer participation on policy boards, and (3) increased job
opportunities for area residents because of added services and the need for
personnel.[22]

The C and Y projects concentrate on the preschool group and maintain
close working relationships with other federal and state programs within the

communities they serve. Other programs, such as neighborhood health centers, MIC projects, community mental health centers, and family planning projects, work on a cooperative basis with C and Y programs to coordinate comprehensive health care for families.

Dental Health Projects

Over the years interest has grown in the dental health of children as a public health concern. In the early 1960s, despite the increase in fluoridated water supplies, the incidence of dental cavities continued to rise each year. Estimates show that by age fifteen, the average child has eleven teeth that are either decayed, missing, or filled. About half the children under fifteen in the nation have never been to a dentist.[23]

In 1971 special project grants became available under Title V of the Social Security Act "to promote the dental health of children and youth of school and preschool age, particularly in areas with concentrations of low-income families."[24] By 1974, nineteen dental health projects were in operation.[25] Under this program dental care is provided through a variety of approaches, emphasizing prevention and continuing dental supervision. These special projects augment the dental care available through the states' Maternal and Child Health and Crippled Children's Programs and the Children and Youth and Maternity and Infant Care Projects. In addition to these projects, there are regulations under Medicaid (Title XIX of the Social Security Act) that require dental screening and care for children (see Early and Periodic Screening, Diagnosis, and Treatment Programs, page 155).

Family Planning Services

Studies have shown that family planning is a leading factor in the reduction of the infant mortality rate in the United States. Every child coming into this world has the natural right to be born well to healthy parents. "Children by choice and not by chance" is the theme of the Planned Parenthood movement. Parents have the right and the responsibility to decide how many children they want, and how often they want to have them. Until very recently many families living in poverty have had little or no access to family planning services.

Family planning is defined as the "voluntary planning and action by individuals to have the number of children they want, when and if they want them."[26] Family planning involves fertility regulation, which has been defined as "medical and nonmedical techniques that enable individuals to engage in voluntary planning and action to have the number of children they want, when and if they want them."[27] These techniques include contraception, infertility diagnosis and treatment, abortion, and sterilization.[28] Family planning services are those services that provide the means to enable individuals to meet their family planning objectives. These services may be found in a variety of settings: in special family planning clinics, as an integral part of maternity and infant care projects, in hospital and outpatient departments, and elsewhere. Services include outreach, follow-up, and education.

Since the mid-1960s, family planning programs have advanced rapidly in the United States, moving toward the desired goal of assuring that services are available to all women. A significant factor in the expansion of family planning services has been a change in the attitude on the part of the public toward birth control information. State laws that prohibited the dissemination of contraceptive information and family planning services have been rejected as unconstitutional by the United States Supreme Court. Such information, when requested, may not be withheld from anyone, regardless of age or marital status.

In the public sector, support for family planning programs has come from both official and voluntary sources. The federal government has provided support with project grants through the Economic Opportunity Act, the Social Security Act, and the Family Planning Services Act. Title V of the Social Security Act specifies that "not less than 6 percent of the annual appropriation for formula grants to the states for maternal and child health services, the Maternity and Infant Care Projects, and research grants shall be used for family planning services." Additional project grants, administered by the National Center for Family Planning Services, became available through Title X of the Public Health Service Act, often referred to as the Family Planning Services and Population Research Act of 1970.

The major voluntary agency that supports family planning programs is the Planned Parenthood Federation of America. This organization can trace its origins to the era preceding the first world war and to the tireless efforts of Margaret Sanger. In the early years of the present century, Ms. Sanger, as a nurse working in the community, had been deeply moved by the sad plight of women in poverty who had no means to prevent unwanted pregnancies. Undaunted by the hostility from a large segment of her contemporary society, she pressed on in her mission to help these women who needed and would have welcomed a respite from uninterrupted childbearing. More than half a century has passed since those early days, and the Planned Parenthood movement, which she had inspired, has expanded its programs in many directions.

Early and Periodic Screening, Diagnosis, and Treatment Programs (EPSDT)

In response to public criticism of Title XIX programs' emphasis on treatment rather than prevention, Congress amended this portion of the Social Security Act in 1972. Under the new amendment, federal regulations were issued that would require participating states to begin to establish and maintain a program of early and periodic screening, diagnosis, and treatment for all eligible individuals under twenty-one years of age. These regulations signaled an official recognition by the federal government of the tremendous need for primary prevention and health maintenance programs, and the potential saving in human lives through a positive approach to health care. This amendment requires the development and implementation of new approaches to the delivery of health care. The new methods must be consolidated into a patient-centered health care delivery system—accessible, acceptable, and available to all who are eligible.

The EPSDT program has five phases, as follows:[29]

Phase I—Outreach and Case Finding   Phase I includes all casework services necessary to find, identify, inform, and assist eligible persons to utilize the program. Under federal regulations, county assistance offices are required to actively seek out and identify eligible children and bring them into the screening process. Recipients of welfare and all other residents must be made aware of the existence of the program, its benefits, its purpose, and the application procedures.

Phase II—Screening Administration   Phase II includes coordination of existing resources, development of new resources as required, and the establishment of a network of qualified screening units within given geographical areas to serve the eligible population. Continuing review, evaluation, and monitoring of services provided by screening units and the revision of procedures is handled under Phase II.

Phase III—Testing   Phase III includes the direct provision of screening and evaluation services. The following basic screening services are to be offered by participating testing facilities: an unclothed physical examination, developmental appraisal, growth measurements, anemia screening, lead poisoning screening, tuberculosis testing, vision and hearing testing, dental screening, evaluation of nutritional status.

Phase IV—Compilation and Reporting of Results   Phase IV includes the forwarding of test results for processing, compilation of findings, and the translation of these findings into a health profile for each individual screened.

Phase V—Follow-through and Treatment   Phase V includes follow-up measures to insure provision of indicated treatment services to eligible persons and continued monitoring for services provided.

School Health Programs

The health of school age children has long been recognized as a matter of public concern—back at the turn of the present century we saw the beginnings of school health and school nursing (see p. 12). These earliest programs were essentially limited to preventing the spread of communicable diseases. The need to broaden the scope of attention on the health of school children was dramatized during the first world war. At that time, the American people were greatly dismayed to learn that over one-third of its young men were turned down for military service because of health defects, many of which might have been prevented or corrected. Interest in school health continued to grow: In 1918 the Commission on the Reorganization of Secondary Education named health as a major educational goal.[30] Today, although primary responsibility for the health of their children rests with the parents, school health programs exist in virtually every community. Their basic goals are health education, health promotion, prevention of illness, case finding, and correction of defects.

The organization and administration of school health services is generally a local function with authority delegated by the state government. School health programs may be administered in one of the following ways: (1) through the local Board of Education, as a specialized program with a specially assigned staff of school nurses and school physicians; (2) through the Department of Public Health, as part of the generalized health program under the direction of the regular staff; or (3) through a combination of the resources of the Board of Education and the Department of Public Health. Sometimes school districts contract with voluntary agencies for school nursing services. However it may be organized and administered, the school health program will include basic services such as health teaching, periodic health examinations of students and teachers, immunizations, first aid, follow-up remedial procedures, supervision of environmental sanitation and safety, health counseling and health supervision, and nutrition education. The nurse, who is a key member of the school health team, is involved in all of these activities through planning, coordinating, acting as a resource person, providing direct service, and serving as a liaison with community agencies.

HEALTH OF THE ELDERLY

"Grow old along with me! The best is yet to be, The last of life, for which the first was made . . . "[31] For whom did the poet intend these lines? Undoubtedly for one who is aging gracefully, blessed with good health, in full command of his physical and mental endowments, surrounded by loving family and friends, and in reasonably comfortable circumstances. A friend of ours from Europe speaks of her father, a retired general, who, now in his early nineties, is busy writing his memoirs, but manages to find time for a daily swim in the river near his home. He has a colleague nearing ninety who, after gaining international renown as an epidemiologist and medical historian, has recently embarked on a new career as a lexicographer and has nearly completed a manuscript for a bilingual dictionary. We can point to other examples closer to home: One of our colleagues, an energetic septuagenarian in good health, is a registered nurse who maintains an active interest in the profession through membership in the ANA, participation in continuing education programs, and occasional private duty practice; her older sister, a busy, alert octogenarian, matriarch, and "elder statesman" of a large and widespread family, is always ready at a moment's notice to come and help whenever and wherever she is needed. Are these exceptional people? If so, then what about the thousands upon thousands of those aged persons for whom "the best" has already been, and who must face an uncertain future in days and years of idleness, illness, immobility, instability, and/or isolation?

Throughout the civilized world, we are witnessing an increased popular concern for the health needs of the elderly. This is particularly evident in those industrialized and developing countries where the numbers of old people continue to grow. According to United Nations estimates, the world population of older persons (sixty-five years of age and over) is now about 200 million, a number that is expected to double by the end of the century.[32] In the United States, which has over 20 million elderly, this segment of the population has been characterized as the "fastest growing minority."[33] How do we measure the health of this group? How do we go about meeting their needs? To begin with, what do we mean by aging and the aging population? Who are the elderly? On the basis of epidemiologic studies, and through common usage and custom, the age of sixty-five has arbitrarily been chosen as the designated starting point of the aging population. To help us arrive at a common level of understanding about pertinent concepts related to the health of the aging population, we have listed the following definitions:[34]

(1) *Aged*—a concept that fixes the individual at a point in time, usually age 65. This arbitrary age is used, not because of an actual change that takes place in the individual, but because it has become the usual age of "retirement" in our society.

(2) *Aging*—a term used to describe the processes of biological, psychological, and sociological change from one point of time to another.

    (a) *Chronological aging*—the use of a birth date in defining an individual's age and, by implication, his appropriate social roles and functions.

    (b) *Biological aging*—a term that describes the changes in biological processes with the passage of time, and the variations of degree and consequence of these changes from one individual to another.

    (c) *Psychological aging*—those changes and degrees of change in sensory function and perception, memory, learning, intelligence—as well as in the dynamics of personality.

    (d) *Sociological aging*—the changing roles, functions and status—as these are defined by the various social institutions, including family, economic, government, recreational, church, educational, and medical.

(3) *Geriatric*—referring to the medical treatment of old age and its diseases.

(4) *Gerontology*—the study of aging processes—from the Greek "geron," old man—originating in the biological sciences and expanding more recently into the social and behavioral sciences.

(5). *Senescence*—a state of growing old; physical aging.

(6) *Senility*—a traditional term for degenerative change in old people, including illness and weakness, especially mental.

We look upon aging as something more than a chronological entity or a biological phenomenon. We can point to no single process that determines aging. The question "When is a person old?" cannot be answered unless we know something about the individual and his total being. All old people are not alike, and it is a mistake to characterize or stereotype them according to any fixed ideas we may have. Certainly, heredity is of utmost importance as an influence in the aging process. Psychological factors and social role are also essential determinants. An Olympic swimmer may be old in his twenties; a professional ball player may be old in his thirties. But a history professor may only be approaching his prime at fifty. And there are the hill folk in the remote and mountainous regions of the Caucasus, the Andes, and the Karakorams who are young at eighty! [35]

What, then, are the changes associated with aging? When you begin to look at the changes that occur in an aging individual, you will find that it may often be difficult to determine which ones are due to "normal aging" and which ones to pathology.

> Changes that come with age include alterations in the structure of cells, in their numbers, in the substances surrounding them, in the blood and the' vessels that supply tissues and organs, in the organ systems and the regulating endocrinal and nervous systems they depend on, and in the system of systems—the whole organism. The organism's interaction with its environment, including social interactions, also must be considered for repercussion on its physical and psychological state. [36]

Some processes may show little or no significant change with age; others may change during the fifth or sixth decade and stabilize. Still others may remain essentially unchanged until relatively late in life and then slowly decline. All of the body systems may be affected. Some of the body changes associated with aging are displayed in Table 9-6.

If we recognize these changes, we can help the elderly person understand them; we can use them as a basis for identifying the needs of the elderly. For example, with a lessening of visual acuity, older people may have a tendency to fall; therefore we must be alert to the need for accident prevention. Or, with stiffening of joints and changes in bone structure, elderly persons may need assistance in ambulation. Physical needs such as these must be viewed along with emotional and social needs. For example, let us consider nutritional needs of the elderly, over and above those dictated by changes in digestive processes or metabolism. Old people who live alone often have little motivation to prepare adequate food. Or they may experience loss of appetite from anxiety and internal tensions. On the other hand, they may indulge in compulsive

Table 9-6 Body Changes in Aging

Body system	Some of the changes in "normal aging"
Skin and subcutaneous tissues	The skin becomes lax, inelastic, dry, and wrinkled; there is graying or whitening with progressive loss or thinning of hair; old people sweat less than younger ones.
Musculo-skeletal system	Changes in appearance and limitations in mobility occur with the stooped posture, stiffened joints and porous bone structure characteristic of advancing age.
Nervous system	Reflexes are slower with a concomitant decrease of responses to various stimuli; there may be tremors, with alterations in facial expression and mental reactions.
Special senses	The senses—hearing, sight, taste, smell, touch, balance—become less sharp with age.
Cardiovascular system	There is a decline in cardiac output at rest; there is a progressive increase in peripheral resistance to the flow of blood, and a tendency for increased systolic blood pressure.
Respiratory system	The following components of the respiratory system may show age-related impairments: ventilation (breathing), diffusion (exchange of oxygen and carbon dioxide between lungs and blood), and pulmonary circulation.
Gastro-intestinal tract	The stomach shows a reduction in gastric motility, with an increased tendency towards achlorohydria (loss of digestive acid) and a reduction in gastric volume; there is diminished peristalsis, which may be responsible for the constipation that is common in old people; hemorrhoids may develop.
Urinary tract	Filtration rate in the kidney and renal blood flow are diminished; polyuria (excessive urination) and nocturia (nighttime urination) are common.
Reproductive organs	With advancing years, the capacity for reproduction ebbs—earlier in the female than in the male; however, sexual needs and desires do not undergo an abrupt change, and sexual activity may continue long after reproductive powers have diminished.
Endocrine system	Structural changes occur in the endocrine glands, which indicates there may be a central endocrine deficit.
Hemopoietic system	There appears to be a diminished leucocytic response to infection; responses of the lymphoid system appear to diminish with age.
Nutrition and Metabolism	Digestive processes slow down, and food habits change.

Source United States Department of Health, Education, and Welfare, Working with Older People. Vol. 1: The Practitioner and the Elderly (Washington, D.C.: Government Printing Office, PHS Pub: 1459, March 1971), pp. 12-21.

eating to compensate for emotional isolation, loneliness, and other stress. Such problems require nursing intervention through health teaching, supervision, and follow-up.

The changes that accompany aging do not necessarily impair the efficiency of the body or lead to disease or death. They may bring about modification in the individual's power of adaptation and his ability to function well under strain. Health must be viewed in terms of function, and older people should be regarded as normal people who may or may not become ill. Nevertheless, chronic illness is one of the major problems for our aging citizens, as was pointed out in Chapter 8. National Health Survey findings show that compared with the population as a whole, older people do tend to have more hospital stays (for longer periods of time), more physician visits, more days of disability, and they spend more on drugs.

A common misconception among many people is that a high percentage of the elderly are institutionalized. The fact is that over 95 percent of older Americans live outside of institutions. However, many of them live alone, in relative isolation, with no close family ties. They are cut off from the mainstream of a society that adulates youth. Thus, even though over 80 percent of the elderly have no limitation of mobility, they need encouragement to remain active, alert, and independent. "Aging can be either good or bad, depending on what the aged person and his society do with it."[37]

When institutionalization cannot be avoided, an elderly person and/or his family may be faced with a serious problem—to find, within their financial limitations, a suitable long-term care facility, most probably some type of nursing home. In its Master Facility Inventory, the Public Health Service National Center for Health Statistics defines nursing homes as "establishments with three beds or more which provide nursing or personal care to the aged, infirm, or chronically ill."[38] In the 1971 survey of facilities, there were 22,004 nursing homes in the United States caring for 1,075,000 persons. These homes have been classified according to the primary type of service offered—nursing care homes, personal care homes with nursing, personal care homes without nursing, and domiciliary care homes. There are three types of nursing homes according to ownership—proprietary, nonprofit (church and other), and government (state or local and federal). Most of the nursing homes (78 percent) are proprietary; 16 percent are nonprofit, and 6 percent are government operated.

The emphasis today is on maintaining the elderly person in his own surroundings, and to avoid institutionalization insofar as possible. The nurse can make a unique contribution to the care of the elderly in their own home setting by acting as patient advocate and by providing primary health care service with emphasis on health maintenance. Across the nation, nursing has responded to the needs of the elderly in a variety of ways. Some of these activities have been documented in the hearings held by the United States Subcommittee on Health of the Elderly in the summer of 1973. These hearings were held to explore barriers to health care for older Americans. For example, many nursing agencies have established health center services in senior citizens' housing units and apartment buildings as well as in area schools and churches. These services include health screening clinics for diabetes, blood pressure, glaucoma, tuberculosis, hearing, emphysema, and other problems;

information and referral to physicians as needed; classes in nutrition, therapeutic exercise, and personal safety; immunization clinics; podiatric care; counseling in problems of daily living; sick care and personal services. Other activities organized or sponsored by nursing agencies include meals-on-wheels, group dining programs, mobile health units, friendly visitor services, telephone reassurance program, and thrift shops and other fund raising projects to support senior citizen centers.

At the national level, the federal government has made attempts to respond to the health needs of the elderly in their home setting. Provisions under the Medicare and Medicaid programs were intended to remove financial barriers to medical care for our senior citizens. Designed as they are around medical functions, neither of these programs was intended to meet overall health needs. Although they do provide for home health services, their reimbursement policies exclude many elderly people who are in need of supportive and maintenance services. They provide no mechanisms for health promotion, health maintenance, or prevention. The Older Americans Act of 1965 with its subsequent amendments was designed to help communities develop programs offering home health services for the aging. Title III . . . authorizes projects to increase the capability of the elderly to maintain independent living. Many of the projects contain explicit home health components and many others have health-related aspects. Besides visiting nurses and home health aid services for the home-bound elderly, services include homemaker, immunization, screening programs, health education, accident prevention techniques, home repairs, and delivered meals. . . . Under title IV . . . research and demonstration projects have been conducted to test alternatives to institutionalization for the elderly [39]

HEALTH OF MINORITY GROUPS AND THE POOR

The 1960s witnessed two major developments in the United States—the Civil Rights Movement and the War on Poverty—which directly or indirectly had an effect on the health and welfare of many citizens. Both of these movements focused national attention on the problems of minority groups and the poor. We view these groups jointly in our discussion, because poverty and class or racial inequality often go hand-in-hand as causally related factors in illness or disability.

What do we mean by minority groups? Strictly speaking, a minority group is any group—racial, ethnic, religious, occupational, national—making up less than a numerical majority of a population. Throughout history, minority groups have existed in virtually every country, and have often been victims of persecution, discrimination, or ostracism. The United States was populated by immigrant minority groups, many of whom had fled from hostile surroundings to seek a better life for themselves and their children in a new land.

The history of the United States in the last 100 years may be viewed in terms of "the history of successive minority groups attempting to move up in American society, and the reaction of the older established groups in opposing them."[40] As succeeding waves of immigrants arrived, they found, all too often, that older, established groups of settlers looked down on them as foreigners, newcomers, "greenhorns." It was not unusual for them to be excluded from the more attractive residential neighborhoods and better jobs. They lived in grinding poverty in the worst kinds of slum dwellings or "company houses," and received starvation wages for the most menial labor. Many arrived here worn out and in a poor state of health. Health care was often inadequate, and largely dependent upon a relatively few dedicated, fearless, and/or philanthropic individuals (Figures 9–1 and 9–2). The Scandinavians, Germans, Irish, Italians, Slavs, Greeks, Armenians, and Jews are but a few of the many groups over the last century whose descendants have reaped the benefits of those early years of hardships. Today, when the children and grandchildren of these immigrant peoples recount the deprivations and strivings of their forbears, they do so from the vantage point of a relatively secure place in the mainstream of American society.

In the process of its settlement, this country saw its own indigenous population—the American Indians—reduced to a minority status (the total population of Indians in the last census was under 800,000). Today, they and other minority groups—Blacks, Mexican-Americans, Puerto Ricans—are seeking equal participation in a society they feel has attempted to exclude them. In the last few years we have seen a concerted effort to stir up interest and concern for these groups in their struggle for upward mobility. A disproportionate number of people in these groups live in poverty—for example, Bureau of Census figures show that 33 percent of all Blacks were classified as poor; among the whites, 10 percent were considered to be living at the poverty level. Or to put it another way, Blacks constitute about 11 percent of the total population (22.5 million) but about 30 percent of the population living in poverty.

What is poverty and who are the poor? "Poverty is a relative term that reflects a judgment made on the basis of standards prevailing in the community."[41] While standards may change in time and place, the poor are those "who, by the prevailing standards, are found to be deficient in means of subsistence and privileges of life."[42] By certain objective criteria, we can point to some degree of progress over the last few years. For example, the number of persons in families below the federally defined low-income or poverty level dropped from 40 million in 1960 to 25.5 million in 1971.[43] However, the situation is aggravated by the fact that, in spite of this progress, harsh poverty continues to exist in the midst of great affluence.

We often hear about the culture of poverty, a term which has come to have real meaning for nurses who work in the community. As a nurse —especially if you have grown up in a middle- or upper-class milieu—you may experience a kind of "culture shock" when you are first exposed to the

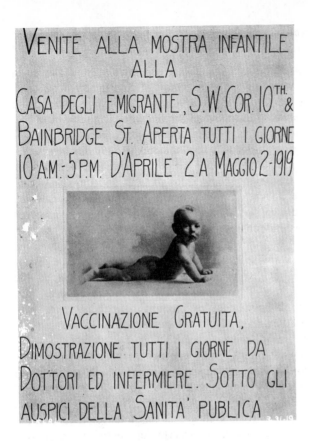

Figure 9-1 A baby health exhibit in an immigrant neighborhood, 1919. <u>Translation:</u> ''Come and bring your baby for a checkup at the Immigrants' Center, S.W. Corner, 10th and Bainbridge; open every day 10 AM–5 PM, April 2–May 2, 1919. Free vaccination. Demonstration every day by the doctor and the nurse. Under the auspices of the Department of Public Health.''

Source From the Philadelphia Department of Public Health.

sights and sounds and smells of poverty. This culture shock may be just as profound as one you might encounter when you come in contact with an alien culture in a foreign land. Be prepared for this because the attitudes and values by which you are influenced will affect the way you relate to your patients and their families. Your focus, of course, will be on the health problems that you identify. From the standpoint of poverty, the picture is clear. In every aspect of health and every state of illness or disabling conditions, the poor are at a disadvantage—they have more illness and more serious illness than their more affluent neighbors. Elsewhere in the book we refer to some of the indices—for example, the infant mortality rate, tuberculosis case rate, inaccessibility of

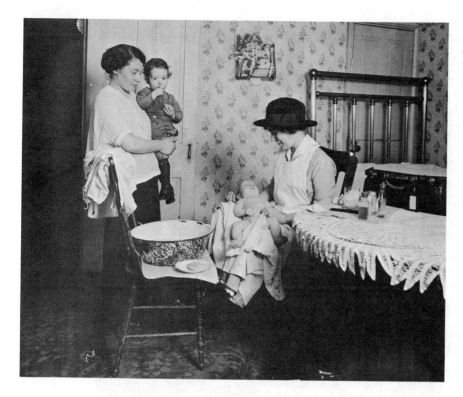

Figure 9-2 A public health nurse visits an immigrant family for maternal and child health care, circa 1915.

Source Courtesy of the Visiting Nurse Society of Philadelphia.

health care—that reflect the health risks to which minority groups and the poor are exposed. In concluding this section, we would like to present two specific conditions that have gained wide attention in recent years as hazards to which the Blacks and the poor are vulnerable—namely, sickle cell disease and lead poisoning.

Sickle Cell Anemia

First described as a clinical entity in 1910, sickle cell disease has only recently become a matter of national concern. Sickle cell anemia is found predominantly, although not exclusively, among Blacks. Estimates vary, but it is believed that the incidence of the primary disease is about one in every 400 Black Americans. About 10 percent, or 2.5 million Blacks, carry the sickle cell trait, although they are not afflicted with the disease.[44]

Sickle cell anemia, a chronic blood disease characterized by the presence of sickle or crescent shaped blood cells (see Figure 9–4), can be diagnosed

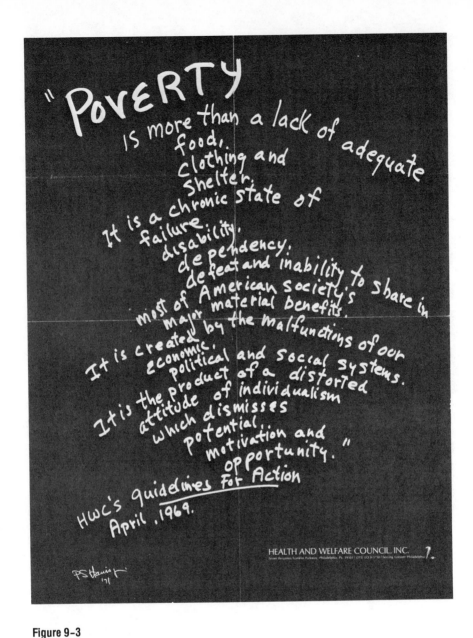

Figure 9-3

Source Reproduced with permission of the Health and Welfare Council, Inc., a United Fund agency.

readily through a simple blood test. The course is both predictable and tragic. While sickle cell anemia develops at the time of conception, signs and symptoms may not appear until the infant is stricken with an upper respiratory infection or tonsillitis, which may be accompanied by severe debilitation. The disease takes a heavy toll with a high death rate in the early years. Those in-

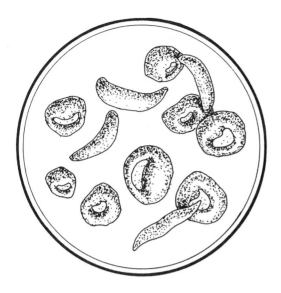

Figure 9-4 Sickle or crescent-shaped cells in Sickle Cell
Anemia, as viewed under the microscope.

fants who survive are vulnerable to additional enervating attacks, which may
impede their total development.

One of the major difficulties in the control of this disease stems from the
fact that is is genetically transmitted. Persons who unknowingly carry the
sickling trait may bear children with sickle cell anemia. See Figure 9-5 for the
genetic pattern of occurrence.

Public recognition of the genetic transmission of sickle cell anemia is
essential for the development of an effective control program. Control efforts
must be directed toward increased research in the cause and treatment of the
disease, and the education, screening, and counseling of the carriers of the
sickle cell trait. Simple and inexpensive screening tests have been devised to
identify those who have the disease or carry the trait.

Control programs must be based upon voluntary cooperation of the individuals involved. The attainment of better methods of control, diagnosis,
and treatment of sickle cell anemia deserves the highest priority. National concern for this problem culminated with the passage in 1972 of the National
Sickle Cell Anemia Control Act, authorizing funds for research, screening,
genetic counseling, and educational programs. The Sickle Cell Anemia Foundation, a nonprofit organization which receives voluntary support from well-
known athletes, entertainers, and other public figures, particularly among the
Black community, has given impetus to the promotion of control programs.

Lead Poisoning

The ingestion of paint and plaster by young children in the oral exploratory
phase of development (ages one to three) is responsible for 200 deaths in the

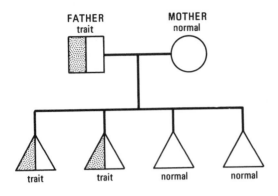

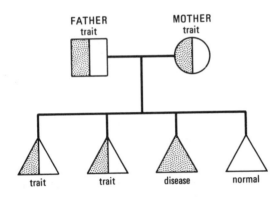

Figure 9-5   Sickle Cell Disease—genetic pattern of occurrence: If one parent carries the sickle cell trait, there is a 50 percent chance his children will have the trait. If both parents carry it, there is a 25 percent chance of having a child with the disease.

Source   Carl Pochedly, "Sickle Cell Anemia: Recognition and Management," **American Journal of Nursing**, 71:1948-51, October 1971. Copyright October 1971, The American Journal of Nursing Company. Reprinted from **American Journal of Nursing.**

United States each year. It is estimated that at least 250,000 children in the country develop lead poisoning from chewing and swallowing the peeling particles of paint and plaster from the window sills and walls of their dwellings.[45]

Childhood lead poisoning is significantly related to pica.[46] As many as 70 to 90 percent of the victims have a history of an abnormal appetite for nonedible substances. Environmental factors associated with the disease include overcrowded conditions, where large numbers of children are left unsupervised, and dilapidated housing with flaking paint and chipping plaster. Lead ingestion can result in lead encephalopathy—a condition that frequently

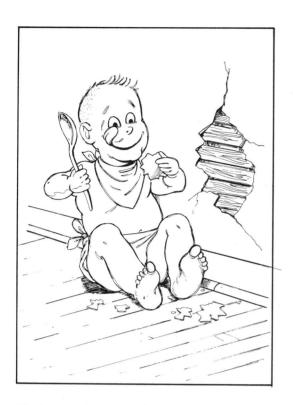

Figure 9-6

leads to convulsions and death. Children who survive may be left with long-term disabling effects such as blindness, learning defects, behavior disorders, kidney damage, and other handicaps.

Early detection of lead poisoning is difficult because of the insidious nature of this disease. The destructive process begins almost immediately. However, in most cases, the first clinical manifestations—anorexia, vague abdominal pain, nausea, vomiting—do not appear before three to six months of steady lead ingestion. These symptoms are often treated palliatively without further investigation. The relationship of these symptoms with the underlying cause may be overlooked if the health care worker is not attuned to the importance of taking a complete history. If pica is suspected, blood and urine testing for lead levels is mandatory. When dangerous lead levels are detected in a child, the treatment is directed toward reducing the lead concentration in the body through detoxification. Antidotal treatment of lead poisoning is accomplished through the use of a chelating agent such as calcium disodium edetate, but this treatment often fails to stop the corrosive action of lead on the brain tissue. Of utmost importance is the necessity to alter the environment. The child must be removed from the lead infested surroundings.

Lead poisoning prevention and control programs need a specific plan of action, which should include the following:

(1) education of professional health workers and the general public to increase their awareness of the problem;

(2) effective legislation aimed at improving housing and regulating the use of lead-based paint (an HEW regulation defines lead-based paint as paint containing more than 1 percent of lead by weight and prohibits the use of such paint in federally-approved housing);

(3) case finding, which incorporates the screening of vulnerable children;

(4) home visits to high-risk families;

(5) further research into causes and treatment of pica;

(6) provision of prompt service in blood level determinations by local health departments; and

(7) establishment and maintenance of a case registry.

A most important factor in a control program is individualized health teaching and follow-up for the prevention of reexposure. Since the families who comprise a high-risk population usually have a slim chance of moving to new surroundings, public health nurses and other health workers must seek ways to eliminate the existing hazards. For example, instructing a family to cover damaged paint and plaster with protective material is one simple means of prevention.

In 1971, the problem of lead poisoning was given national recognition through a series of Congressional hearings and the issuance of the Surgeon General's Policy Statement on Medical Aspects of Childhood Lead Poisoning emphasizing early detection and prevention. In that same year, the President signed the first federal law to help prevent lead poisoning in children.

HEALTH OF THE WORKING POPULATION

Occupational Health

Alice Hamilton is a name that stands out in the history of the development of occupational health programs in this country. Early in the present century, Dr. Hamilton stimulated interest in occupational disease by showing the correlation between illness in workers and their exposure to toxic materials in industry. Although she was greeted by apathy on the part of many of her physician colleagues, she persisted in her work. At first, the progress was slow, but gradually the occupational health movement began to grow. A major step forward was the adoption of Workmen's Compensation laws by most of the states in the decade before the first world war and the immediate postwar period. These laws were instrumental in directing public attention to the need for occupational health programs.

The earliest industrial health programs were limited to the treatment of injuries and diseases occurring to production workers while on the job. However, in time, it became apparent that absenteeism from work was a serious problem which interfered with productivity and that the underlying causes for most of this absenteeism were related to nonoccupational illness and accidents. It also became clear that prevention was more economical than treatment. Eventually, programs were broadened to include all workers, with emphasis on the positive aspects of health. In today's context, occupational health is concerned with the maintenance of health as well as prevention and treatment of diseases and accidental injuries in the working population.

Another milestone was reached toward improving the health of the working population with the passage of the Occupational Safety and Health Act of 1970—called a landmark in health legislation. This law, designed to "assure safe and healthful working conditions," is not so much a culmination as it is a beginning. It reaches out to more than 4 million business establishments and 55 million employees. (See Figure 9-7.) Under this law, the federal government is responsible for issuing and enforcing occupational safety and health standards. The law provides for effective sanctions where violations occur.

Occupational hazards linked to certain types of employment may be classified according to their causally related factors. We can identify occupational diseases which result from exposure to:

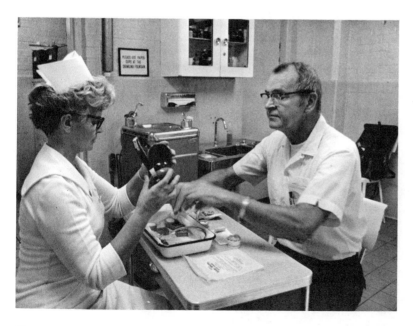

Figure 9-7 Occupational health nurse fitting a worker with a hearing protection device.

Source Courtesy of Scott Paper Company, Chester, Pennsylvania.

chemical substances—such as dusts, gases, or vapors;
the physical state of the environment—such as temperature, radiant energy, or noise;
mechanical factors—such as pressure, physical strain, and movement; and
infectious agents—such as bacteria, viruses, and fungi.

Hazards the worker brings with him to his job, which may be generated outside of his occupational setting, include pathophysiological and psychosocial problems such as high blood pressure, metabolic disorders, alcoholism, drug abuse, poor nutrition, and emotional crises. Specific programs of prevention must include environmental control, personal and individual health teaching, as well as initial health screening of job applicants and periodic examinations of the workers (Figure 9-8). Nursing is involved throughout every phase of the program—in planning, screening, follow-up, health counseling and teaching, establishing environmental safety measures, maintaining records, providing emergency care (Figure 9-9).

Migrant Workers

One large segment of the labor force, outside the mainstream of workers covered by occupational health programs, are the migrant laborers. "They

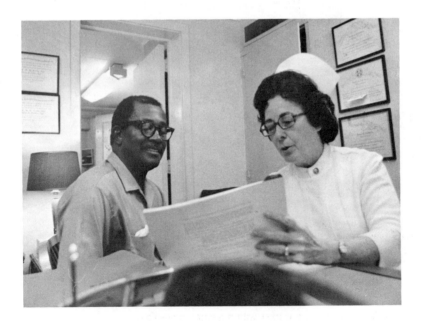

Figure 9-8   Occupational health nurse in a counseling session with a worker.

Source   Courtesy of Scott Paper Company, Chester, Pennsylvania.

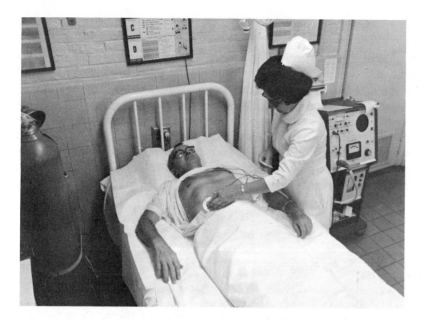

Figure 9-9 An occupational health nurse in an emergency care situation: She is applying electrodes to a worker with chest discomfort. A cardiac monitor will send the printout to a Heart Station at a local hospital, and the nurse will receive a physician's orders for emergency treatment within minutes.

Source Courtesy of Scott Paper Company, Chester, Pennsylvania.

come with the crop and go with the harvest.'' Thus are they described in the Public Health Service film, *The Forgotten Families,* which depicts their plight and their search for health care. These forgotten people, a million of them, earn their livelihood as agricultural workers on the move. We depend heavily upon them and their labor for our daily market supply of fresh fruits and vegetables, so essential to good nutrition.

Living from day to day, in crowded makeshift shelters, these families face dire hardships, drudgery, and frequent crisis situations. Their children are often two to three years behind in school. Rejected by the communities where they must make their temporary homes, they are welcome only for the labor they can perform. In many instances, they are not regarded as part of the community and are thus excluded from desperately needed health, welfare, education, and recreation services. As soon as the work season is over, the community is eager to see them go.

To help meet the health needs of migrant farm workers and their families, Congress passed the Migrant Health Act in 1962, authorizing grants for family health clinics and for other health services. Subsequent amendments in 1965, 1968, and 1970 continued and extended the migrant health program. About one hundred projects were funded in thirty-one states, the District of Columbia, and Puerto Rico. At least three of these were under the direction of nurses. The primary mission of the migrant health program is the development

173

of high quality, comprehensive, accessible health care services in rural areas for migrant and seasonal farm workers and their families.

By the mid-1970s there were substantial reductions in federal funding, and the burden of responsibility for these migrant health projects shifted to the states. Health problems among migrant workers and their families continue to exist and will not be resolved until each and every community involved displays genuine concern and assumes more responsibility for comprehensive health measures. Unfortunately, all too often, interest is aroused only after the occurrence of an emergency that threatens the entire community.

REFERENCES

1. Martha Rogers, *An Introduction to the Theoretical Basis of Nursing* (Philadelphia: F.A. Davis, 1970), p. 134.

2. As cited in *Current Population Reports,* Series P-25, #538, December 1974.

3. Monthly Vital Statistics Report, Provisional Statistics, *Annual Summary for the United States, 1974. Births, Deaths, Marriages, and Divorces* (Rockville, Maryland: National Center for Health Statistics; U.S. Department of Health, Education, and Welfare; May 30, 1975), p. 1.

4. National Center for Health Statistics, *Natality Statistics Analysis 1965-1967* (Washington, D.C.: Government Printing Office, May 1970), p. 1.

5. Monthly Vital Statistics Report, Provisional Statistics, *Annual Summary 1974,* p. 1.

6. Ibid., p. 8.

7. *The Evening Bulletin* (Philadelphia, January 6, 1975).

8. Monthly Vital Statistics Report, Provisional Statistics, *Annual Summary 1974*, p. 10.

9. Ibid., p. 8.

10. Monthly Vital Statistics Report, *Annual Summary for the United States, 1973. Births, Deaths, Marriages, and Divorces* (Rockville, Maryland: National Center for Health Statistics, U.S. Department of Health, Education, and Welfare, June 27, 1974), p. 4.

11. Monthly Vital Statistics Report, *Provisional Statistics, Annual Summary 1974,* p.4.

12. E. L. Potter and W. Jack, "Symposium on Obstetrics and Gynecology: Responsibility of Obstetrician in Perinatal Mortality," *Surgical Clinics of North America,* 33 (1953) 141-52.

13. Florence Haselkorn (ed.), *Mothers-at-Risk* (Washington, D.C.: Government Printing Office, 1968), p. 16.

14. Conference Proceedings, *The Role of Maternal and Child Health and Crippled Children's Programs in Evolving Systems of Health Care* (Ann Arbor, Michigan: The University of Michigan Medical Center, March 23-25, 1970), p. 60.

15. Ibid., p. 60.

16. U.S. Department of Health, Education, and Welfare, *Maternal and Child Health Service Reports on: Promoting the Health of Mothers and Children FY 1973* (Washington, D.C.: Government Printing Office, 1973), p. 26.

17. U.S. Department of Health, Education, and Welfare, *Services for Crippled Children* (Washington, D.C.: Government Printing Office, 1972, pamphlet).

18. U.S. Department of Health, Education, and Welfare, *Maternal and Child Health Service Reports on: Promoting the Health of Mothers and Children FY 1971* (Washington, D.C.: Government Printing Office, 1971), p. 16.

19. U.S. Department of Health, Education, and Welfare, *Maternal and Child Health Service Reports 1973,* p. 29.

20. U.S. Department of Health, Education, and Welfare, *Maternal and Child Health Service Reports on: Promoting the Health of Mothers and Children FY 1972* (Washington, D.C.: Government Printing Office, 1972), p. 35.

21. U.S. Department of Health, Education, and Welfare, *Projects for Intensive Infant Care* (Washington, D.C.: Government Printing Office, 1974), p. 2.

22. U.S. Department of Health, Education, and Welfare, *Maternal and Child Health Service Reports 1971,* p. 20.

23. U.S. Department of Health, Education, and Welfare, *Dental Health Projects for Children* (Washington, D.C.: Government Printing Office, June 1974), p. 1.

24. U.S. Department of Health, Education, and Welfare, *Maternal and Child Health Service Reports 1972,* p. 40.

25. U.S. Department of Health, Education, and Welfare, *Dental Health Projects,* p. 1.

26. National Family Planning Forum's Committee on Terminology, "A Glossary of Family Planning Terminology," *Family Planning Digest,* 2 (November 1973) 8-12.

27. Ibid.

28. Ibid.

29. Department of Public Welfare, "Medical Assistance: Early and Periodic Screening and Diagnosis of Persons under 21," *Pennsylvania Bulletin,* 3 (February 10, 1973) 296-303.

30. C. L. Anderson, *School Health Practice,* 5th ed. (St. Louis: C.V. Mosby, 1972), p. 18.

31. From Robert Browning's poem "Rabbi Ben Ezra."

32. Ethel Shanas, "Health Status of Older People: Cross-National Implications," *American Journal of Public Health,* 64 (March 1974) 261-64.

33. Herman B. Brotman, "The Fastest Growing Minority: The Aging," *American Journal of Public Health,* 64 (March 1974) 249-52.

34. U.S. Department of Health, Education, and Welfare, *Working with Older People. Volume I. The Practitioner and the Elderly* (Washington, D.C.: Government Printing Office [PHS Pub. 1459], March 1971), glossary in introduction

35. Alexander Leaf, "Every Day Is a Gift when You Are over 100," *National Geographic,* 143 (January 1973) 92-119.

36. U.S. Department of Health, Education, and Welfare, *Working with Older People, Vol. II. Biological, Psychological and Sociological Aspects of Aging* (Washington D.C.: Government Printing Office [PHS Pub. 1459], April 1970), pp. 2-3.

37. June S. Rothberg, "Nursing Assessment of the Aged Person," from *Papers Presented at the Third A. Daniel Rubenstein Lectureship in Gerontology* (Boston College, 1968), p. 3.

38. U.S. Department of Health, Education, and Welfare, *Inpatient Health Facilities as Reported from the 1971 MFI Survey* (Rockville, Maryland: National Center for Health Statistics, March, 1974), p. 1.

39. *Barriers to Health Care for Older Americans.* Hearings before the Subcommittee on Health of the Elderly of the Special Committee on Aging, United States Senate, Part 6, July 12, 1973, p. 579.

40. Bonnie Bullough and Vern L. Bullough, *Poverty, Ethnic Identity, and Health Care* (New York: Appleton-Century-Crofts,© 1972), p. 19. Reprinted by permission of Prentice-Hall, Inc., Englewood Cliffs, N.J.

41. John Kosa, "The Nature of Poverty" in John Kosa, Aaron Antonovsky, and Irving Kenneth Zola, *Poverty and Health: A Sociological Analysis* (Cambridge: Harvard University Press, 1969), p. 2.

42. Ibid. p. 2.

43. As of April 30, 1975, an American family of four in an urban area is considered "poor" by government standards if annual family income is $5050 or less in the continental United States, $5810 in Hawaii, or $6310 in Alaska. For farm families, the standard is somewhat lower—$4300, $4940 or $5360, respectively. *News Release,* Office of Information, U.S. Department of Labor, Washington, D.C., May 7, 1975.

44. Carl Pochedly, "Sickle Cell Anemia: Recognition and Management," *American Journal of Nursing,* 71 (October 1971) 1948-51.

45. A. Jane Reed, "Lead Poisoning: Silent Epidemic and Social Crime," *American Journal of Nursing,* 72 (December 1972) 2181-84.

46. H. Jacobziner and H.W. Raybin, "The Epidemiology of Lead Poisoning," *New York Journal of Medicine,* 64 (May 1964) 1233-35.

47. U.S. Department of Health, Education, and Welfare, Health Services and Mental Health Administration, *A Directory of Migrant Health Projects Supported under the Migrant Health Act* (May 1972), passim.

ADDITIONAL READINGS

Health of Mothers and Children

Bean, Margaret, "The Nurse-Midwife at Work," in *American Journal of Nursing,* 71 (May 1971) 949–52.

Bergman, Abraham B., "Sudden Infant Death," in *Nursing Outlook,* 72 (December 1972) 775–77.

Bozian, Marguerite W., "Nursing Care of the Infant in the Community," in *Nursing Clinics of North America,* 6 (March 1971) 93–101.

Bryan, Doris S., *School Nursing in Transition.* St. Louis: C. V. Mosby Co., 1973.

Chase, Helen C., ed., "A Study of Risks, Medical Care, and Infant Mortality," in *American Journal of Public Health,* 63 (September 1973) supplement 1–56.

Cohn, Helen D., and E. James Lieberman, "Family Planning and Health," in *American Journal of Public Health,* 64 (March 1974) 225–29.

Davis, Lucille, and Helen Grace, "Anticipatory Counseling of Unwed Pregnant Adolescents," in *Nursing Clinics of North America,* 6 (December 1971) 581–90.

Dickens, Helen, Emily Mudd, Celso-Ramon Garcia, Karen Tomar, and David Wright, "One Hundred Pregnant Adolescents, Treatment Approaches in a University Hospital," in *American Journal of Public Health,* 63 (September 1973) 794–800.

Eisner, Victor, *Dimensions of School Health.* Springfield, Ill.: Charles C. Thomas, 1974.

Fiedler, Dolores E., Dorothea M. Lang, and Judy M. Carlson, "Pathology in the 'Healthy' Female Teenager," in *American Journal of Public Health,* 63 (November 1973) 962-65.

Fischman, Susan H., "Change Strategies and Their Application to Family Planning Programs," in *American Journal of Nursing,* 73 (October 1973) 1771–74.

Fitzpatrick, Elise, Sharon Reeder, and Luigi Mastroianni, *Maternity Nursing.* Philadelphia: J.B. Lippincott, 1971.

Florentine, Helen G., *The Preparation and Role of Nurses in School Health Programs.* New York: National League for Nursing, 1962.

Greenberg, Eleanor M., "Standing Orders for the School Nurse," in *Nursing 75,* (February 1975) 62–63.

Grimm, Linda M., "Maternity Continuity Clinic," in *American Journal of Nursing,* 73 (October 1973) 1723–25.

Guttmacher, Alan F., "Commentary: Family Planning Need and the Future of the Family Planning Program," in *Family Planning Perspectives,* 5 (Summer 1973) 175-76.

Hanlon, John Joseph, and Elizabeth McHose, *Design for Health; School and Community.* Philadelphia: Lea & Febiger 1971.

Harris, David, Donna O'Hare, Jean Pakter, and Frieda G. Nelson, "Legal Abortion 1970-1971—The New York Experience," *American Journal of Public Health,* 63 (May 1973) 409-18.

Hubbard, Charles William, *Family Planning Education; Parenthood and Social Disease Control.* St. Louis: C. V. Mosby Co., 1973.

Humes, Charles, "Who Should Administer School Nursing Services?" in *American Journal of Public Health,* 65 (April 1975) 394–96.

Igoe, Judith Bellaire, "The School Nurse Practitioner," in *Nursing Outlook,* 23 (June 1975) 381–84.

Jekel, James F., Jean T. Harrison, D. R. E. Bancroft, Natalie C. Tyler, and Lorraine V. Klerman, "A Comparison of the Health of Index and Subsequent Babies Born to School Age Mothers," in *American Journal of Public Health,* 65 (April 1975) 370-83.

Kauffman, Margaret C., and Anne Cunningham. "Epidemiologic Analysis of Outcomes in Maternal and Infant Health in Evaluating Effectiveness of Three Patient Care Teams," in *American Journal of Public Health,* 60 (September 1970) 1712-25.

Knowles, John H., "The Health System and the Supreme Court Decision—An Affirmative Response," in *Family Planning Perspectives,* 5 (Spring 1973) 113–16.

Lewis, Robert, Mark Charles, and K.M. Patwary, "Relationships between Birthweight and Selected Social, Environmental, and Medical Care Factors," in *American Journal of Public Health,* 62 (November 1973) 973-81.

Maxwell, Jane E., "Home Care for the Retarded Child," in *Nursing Outlook,* 19 (February 1971) 112–14.

Miller, C. Arden, "Health Care of Children and Youth in America," in *American Journal of Public Health,* 65 (April 1975) 353–58.

Morris, Naomi, J. Richard Udry, and Charles L. Chase, "Shifting Age-Parity Distribution of Births and the Decrease in Infant Mortality," in *American Journal of Public Health,* 65 (April 1975) 359-62.

O'Brien, Margaret, Margery Manly, and Margaret C. Heagarty, "Expanding the Public Health Nurse's Role in Child Care," in *Nursing Outlook,* 23 (June 1975) 369-73.

Oppel, Wallace and Sanford Wolf, "Liberalized Abortion and Birth Rates Changes in Baltimore," in *American Journal of Public Health,* 63 (May 1973) 405–8.

Pavenstedt, Eleanor, "An Intervention Program for Infants from High Risk Homes," in *American Journal of Public Health,* 63 (May 1973) 393–95.

Rubin, Reva, "Maternity Care in Our Society," in *Nursing Outlook,* 11 (July 1963) 519–22.

Schiffer, Clara G., and Eleanor P. Hunt, *Illness among Children. Washington, D.C.:* Government Printing Office, 1963.

Schmidt, William M., "Public Health Then and Now: The Development of Health Services for Mothers and Children in the United States," in *American Journal of Public Health,* 63 (May 1973) 419-27.

Sells, Clifford, and Eleanor May, "Scoliosis Screening in Public Schools," in *American Journal of Nursing,* 74 (January 1974) 60–62.

Stoeffler, Victor R. Reuben Mayer, and Donald C. Smith, "Lessons To Be Learned from New Child Health Programs—Where Do We Go from Here?" in *American Journal of Public Health,* 62 (November 1972) 1444–47.

Wallace, Helen M., Hyman Goldstein, Edwin M. Gold, and Ira W. Gabrielson, "A Survey of Health Status and Needs of Urban Mothers and Children," in *HSMHA Health Reports,* 86 (September 1971) 829-38.

Wallace, Helen M., Hyman Goldstein, and Allan C. Oglesby, "The Health and Medical Care of Children Under Title 19 (Medicaid)," in *American Journal of Public Health,* 64 (May 1974) 501-6.

Weinberger, Caspar W., "Population and Family Planning," in *Family Planning Perspectives,* 6 (Summer 1974) 170–72.

Williams, Cicely D., and Derrick B. Jelliffe, *Mother and Child Health—Delivering the Services.* London: Oxford University Press, 1972.

Health of the Elderly

American Nurses Association Committee on Standards for Geriatric Nursing Practice, "Standards for Geriatric Nursing Practice," in *American Journal of Nursing,* 70 (September 1970) 1894–97.

Anderson, Edna, and Avery A. Andrew, "Senior Citizens Health Conferences," in *Nursing Outlook,* 21 (September 1973) 580–82.

Birchenall, Joan, and Mary Eileen Streight, *Care of the Older Adult.* Philadelphia: J.B. Lippincott, 1973.

Brody, Stanley J., "Evolving Health Delivery Systems and Older People," in *American Journal of Public Health,* 64 (March 1974) 245-48.

Butler, Robert N., and Myrna I. Lewis, *Aging and Mental Health. Positive Psychosocial Approaches.* St. Louis: C.V. Mosby Co., 1973.

Curtin, Sharon R., *Nobody Ever Died of Old Age.* Boston: Little, Brown and Company, 1972.

DeBeauvoir, Simone, "Old Age: End Product of a Faulty System," in *Saturday Review* (April 8, 1972). 39-45.

"Exercises for the Elderly," in *American Journal of Nursing,* 72 (August 1972) 1401.

George, Janet A., "Teaching the Young about the Old," in *Nursing Outlook,* 20 (June 1972) 405-7.

Hammerman, Jerome, "Health Services: Their Success and Failure in Reaching Older Adults," in *American Journal of Public Health,* 64 (March 1974) 253–56.

Kazmierczak, Frances, Dorothy H. Moser, and Mary A. Russo, "Communication Problems Encountered When Caring for the Elderly Individual," in *Journal of Gerontological Nursing,* 1 (March, April 1975) 21-27.

Kinoy, Susan K., "Home Health Services for the Elderly," in *Nursing Outlook,* 17 (September 1969) 59-62.

Lawton, M. Powell, "Social Ecology and The Health of Older People," in *American Journal of Public Health,* 64 (March 1974) 257-60.

Long, Janet M., ed., *Caring for and Caring about Elderly People.* Philadelphia: J.B. Lippincott Co., 1974.

Ornstein, Sheldon, "Objective—A National Policy on Aging," in *American Journal of Nursing,* 71 (May 1971) 960-63.

Proceedings of the 1971 White House Conference on Aging, *Toward A National Policy on Aging.* Washington, D.C.: Government Printing Office, 1973.

Robison, Sandy, "Home Visits to the Elderly," in *American Journal of Nursing,* 74 (May 1974) 908-9.

Rodstein, Manuel, "Health Problems of the Aged," in *R.N.,* 35 (August 1972) 39-43.

Stone, Virginia, "Give the Older Person Time," in *American Journal of Nursing,* 69 (October 1969) 2124-27.

U.S. Department of Health, Education, and Welfare, *Health in the Later Years of Life.* Washington, D.C.: Government Printing Office, October 1971.

U.S. Department of Health, Education, and Welfare, *Working with Older People. Vol. III. The Aging Person: Needs and Services,* and *Vol. IV Clinical Aspects of Aging.* Washington, D.C.: Government Printing Office, April 1970 and July 1971.

Wilkiemeyer, Diana S., "Affection: Key to Care for the Elderly," in *American Journal of Nursing,* 72 (December 1972) 2166-68.

Health of Minority Groups and the Poor

Baca, Josephine Elizabeth, "Some Health Beliefs of the Spanish Speaking," in *American Journal of Nursing,* 69 (October 1969) 2172-76.

Campbell, Teresa, and Betty Chang, "Health Care of the Chinese in America," in *Nursing Outlook,* 73 (April 1973) 245-49.

Coles, Robert, *Children of Crisis: A Study of Courage and Fear.* Boston: Little, Brown and Company, 1967.

Dumas, Rhetaugh G., "This I Believe . . . About Nursing and the Poor," in *Nursing Outlook,* 17 (September 1969) 47-49.

Forbes, J.D., ed., *The Indian in America's Past.* Englewood Cliffs, N.J.: Prentice-Hall, 1964.

Froh, R.B. and R. Galanter, "The Poor, Health, and the Law," in *American Journal of Public Health,* 62 (March 1972) 427-30.

Glazer, N., and D.P. Moynihan, *Beyond the Melting Pot: The Negroes, Puerto Ricans, Jews, Italians and Irish of New York City.* 2nd ed. Cambridge, Mass.: The M.I.T. Press, 1970.

Grebler, L., J.W. Moore, and R.C. Guzman, *The Mexican-American People: The Nation's Second Largest Minority.* New York: The Free Press, 1970.

Group, Thetis M., "If a Nurse Is To Help in Ghettos," in *American Journal of Nursing,* 69 (December 1969) 2635-36.

Humphrey, Patricia, "Learning about Poverty and Health," in *Nursing Outlook,* 22 (July 1974) 441-43.

Kane, Robert L., and Rosalie A. Kane, *Federal Health Care (with reservations!).* New York: Springer Publishing Company, 1972.

Kelly, Cynthia, "Health Care in the Mississippi Delta," in *American Journal of Nursing,* 69 (April 1969) 759–63.

LaRue, Mary T., "Head Start in a Tennessee County," in *American Journal of Nursing,* 70 (January 1970) 114-16.

Lewis, Margaret D., "Health Care for Denver's Poor," in *American Journal of Nursing,* 69 (July 1969) 1469-71.

Lewis, O., "The Culture of Poverty," in *Scientific American* (October 1966) 19–25.

Liston, R.A., *The American Poor: A Report on Poverty in the United States.* New York: Dell Books, 1970.

Milio, Nancy, "Untouched in the Holocaust," in *American Journal of Nursing,* 68 (March 1968) 508-9.

Mumford, Emily, "Poverty and Health," in *Nursing Outlook,* 17 (September 1969) 33-35.

Nolan, Robert L., and Jerome L. Schwartz, *Rural and Appalachian Health.* Springfield, Ill.: Charles C. Thomas, 1973.

Rainwater, L., *Behind Ghetto Walls.* Chicago: Aldine, 1970.

"The Sick Poor"—a series of articles on poverty. *American Journal of Nursing,* 69 (November 1969) 2424–54.

Standeven, Muriel, "What the Poor Dislike about Community Health Nurses," in *Nursing Outlook,* 17 (September 1969) 72-75.

White, Earnestine, "Health and the Black Person: An Annotated Bibliography," in *American Journal of Nursing,* 74 (October 1974) 1839-41.

Sickle Cell Anemia

Cerami, A., and J.M. Manning, "Potassium Cyanate as an Inhibitor of the Sickling of Erythrocytes in Vitro," in *Proceedings of the National Academy of Sciences USA,* 68 (June 1971) 1180-83.

Diggs, L.W., "Sickle Cell Crisis," in *American Journal of Clinical Pathology,* 44 (July 1965) 1-19.

Fielding, Jon, et al., "A Coordinated Sickle Cell Program for Economically Disadvantaged Adolescents," in *American Journal of Public Health,* 64 (May 1974) 427-32.

Foster, Sue, "Closing the Gap Between Theory and Therapy," in *American Journal of Nursing,* 71 (October 1971) 1952-56.

Herrick, J.B., "Peculiar Elongated and Sickle Shaped Red Blood Corpuscles in a Case of Severe Anemia," in *Archives of Internal Medicine,* 6 (1910) 517.

Marlow, D.R., *Textbook of Pediatric Nursing.* 2nd ed. Philadelphia: W.B. Saunders Co., 1965.

Murayama, M., "Molecular Mechanism of Sickled Erythrocyte Formation," in *Nature,* 202 (April 18, 1964) 258-60.

Nalbandian, R.M. et al. *Molecular Aspects of Sickle Cell Hemoglobin: Clinical Applications.* Springfield, Ill.: Charles C. Thomas, 1971.

Trouillot, Lenore, "Brooklyn Screens for Sickle Cell Anemia," in *HSMHA Health Reports,* 87 (January 1972) 9-11.

Lead Poisoning

Barltrop, D., "Prevalence of Pica," in *American Journal of Disturbed Children,* 112 (August 1966) 116-23.

Challop, Robert, M.D., Edward McCabe, M.D., and Robert Reece, M.D., "Breaking the Childhood Lead Poisoning Cycle—A Program for Community Case Finding and Self-Help," in *American Journal of Public Health,* 62 (May 1972) 655-57.

Chisolm, J.J., "Increased Lead Absorption: Toxicological Consideration," in *Journal of Pediatrics,* 76 (September 1971) 48 ff.

———, "The Use of Chelating Agents in the Treatment of Acute and Chronic Lead Intoxication in Childhood," in *Journal of Pediatrics,* 73 (July 1968) 30-38.

———, and E. Kaplan. "Lead Poisoning in Childhood: Comprehensive Management and Prevention," in *Journal of Pediatrics,* 73 (December 1968) 942-50.

De la Burde, Brigitte, and Betty Reames, "Prevention of Pica, the Major Cause of Lead Poisoning in Children," in *American Journal of Public Health,* 63 (August 1973) 737-43.

Goyer, R.A., "Lead Toxicity: A Problem in Environmental Pathology," in *American Journal of Pathology,* 64 (July 1971) 167-79.

Lin-Fu, Jane S., "Undue Absoption of Lead among Children—A New Look at an Old Problem," in *New England Journal of Medicine,* 286 (March 1972) 702-10.

———, "Childhood Lead Poisoning: An Eradicable Disease," in *Children,* 17 (1970) 2-9.

———, *Lead Poisoning in Children.* Washington, D.C.: Government Printing Office, 1970, (DHEW Publication Number HSM 70-2108).

"Medical Aspects of Childhood Lead Poisoning: Statement approved by Surgeon General, U.S. Public Health Service," in *Journal of Pediatrics,* 48 (1971) 464 ff.

U.S. Department of Health, Education and Welfare, *Increased Lead Absorption and Lead Poisoning in Young Children* (A Statement by the Center for Disease Control.) Atlanta, Georgia: Center for Disease Control, March 1975.

Health of the Working Population

Occupational Health

Brown, Mary Louise, "Trends for the Future of Occupational Health Nursing," in *Occupational Health Nursing,* 21 (August 1973) 7-11.

Cipolla, Josephine, and Gilbeart Collings, Jr., "Nurse Clinicians in Industry," in *American Journal of Nursing,* 71 (August 1971) 1530-34.

Gallaher, H., and G. Wyatt, "The Occupational Health Nurse and the Patient with Trauma," in *Nursing Clinics of North America,* 5 (December 1970) 609-19.

Goldstein, David H., "The Occupational Safety and Health Act of 1970," in *American Journal of Nursing,* 71 (August 1971) 1535-38.

Henriksen, Heide, "Health Care of Workers in the United States," in *Nursing Outlook,* 16 (May 1968) 32-35.

Howe, Henry, "Preventing Occupational Health and Safety Hazards in Small Employee Groups," in *American Journal of Public Health,* 61 (August 1971) 1581-82.

Keller, Marjorie, "The Occupational Health Nurse and Short-Term Illness Absences," in *Nursing Outlook,* 16 (September 1968) 32-34.

Kerr, Lorin E., "Occupational Health—A Discipline in Search of a Mission," in *American Journal of Public Health,* 63 (May 1973) 381-85.

Key, Marcus M., and Stanley J. Reno, "Occupational Health Programs at the Federal Level for the Next Ten Years," in *American Journal of Public Health,* 61 (August 1971) 1583-85.

Lindquiste, Paul, and Maxine Hurley, "Community Health Nursing for People Who Work," in *American Journal of Public Health,* 61 (October 1971) 2015-17.

Noel, Charlotte C., "Occupational Health Nursing Made Meaningful," in *Occupational Health Nursing,* 20 (August 1972) 13-15.

Rasmussen, Donald L., "Black Lung in Southern Appalachia," in *American Journal of Nursing,* 70 (March 1970) 509-11.

Rieke, Forrest E., "Industrial Clinic Services to Small Industries," in *American Journal of Public Health,* 62 (January 1971) 69-71.

Tinkham, Catherine, "The Plant as the Patient of the Occupational Health Nurse: A Survey Guide," in *Nursing Clinics of North America,* 7 (March 1972) 99-107.

Migrant Workers

Afek, Luella B., "A Health Referral System for Migrants," in *Health Service Reports,* 88 (January 1973) 31-33.

———, and Jane Hickey, "Health Classes for Migrant Workers' Families," in *American Journal of Nursing,* 72 (July 1972) 1296-98.

Cervantes, Robert A., "The Failure of Comprehensive Health Services To Serve The Urban Chicano," in *Health Services Reports,* 87 (December 1972) 932-40.

Fuentes, Jose Angel, "The Need for Effective and Comprehensive Planning for Migrant Workers," in *American Journal of Public Health,* 64 (January 1974) 2-10.

Johannsson, M.S., "A Migrant Referral System for Continuity of Health Care," in *Nursing Clinics of North America,* 7 (November 1972) 133-41.

McConnell, Beverly, "Group Care of Infants in Migrant Day Care Centers," in *American Journal of Public Health,* 61 (July 1971) 1330-34.

Moses, Marion, "Viva La Causa," in *American Journal of Nursing,* 73 (May 1973) 842-48.

"United States Government Expands Migrant Health Program," in *American Journal of Nursing,* 68 (July 1968) 1405-6.

Chapter 10
Health Care Delivery: Organization and Financing

"The health of the people is really the foundation upon which all their happiness and all their powers as a state depend."[1]

INTRODUCTION

The health care delivery system in our country is so vast and complex that it almost defies description. In the growing body of professional and popular literature on this subject, you will often find health care equated with medical care. In actuality these terms are not identical, and must be differentiated. Medical care is provided by physicians whose major concern is diagnosis and treatment of pathology. Health care is broader in scope and includes treatment of pathology as well as the promotion of health of all individuals with or without pathology. Public health and nursing, as was pointed out earlier, are concerned with health care in this broader sense.

In this chapter, we will discuss the patterns of organization in public health, the powers of government in matters of health, international health activities, and health care financing. We will begin with a brief look at the overall framework of health care delivery. First of all, we can identify two categories of service—private and public. Public health is an integral part of the public sector, but it does have many points of articulation with the private sector.

Health Care Delivery—Private Sector

The traditional entry into the health care delivery system in our country has been through the private sector, in which individual care is provided by a family physician on the basis of "fee-for-service" in a one-to-one relationship.

This type of private practice is primarily disease-oriented with emphasis on medical therapy. In recent years, with the growth of medical and health insurance plans—individual, industrial, government-sponsored—as well as government-supported medical assistance programs, third party participation has increased in the arena of private care. Group medical practice has grown.

The private sector of the health care delivery system can be broken down into three components:

Personnel—nurses, physicians, dentists, social workers, psychologists, nutritionists, physiotherapists, speech therapists, occupational therapists, chiropractors, laboratory technicians, X-ray technicians, pharmacists—some are engaged in private practice; others are salaried employees of health care institutions.

Facilities—institutions or agencies, which are classified as private or proprietary (that is, operating for profit), such as general and specialized hospitals for acute and subacute care; extended care facilities; custodial care homes; diagnostic clinics; medical laboratories; proprietary home health agencies.

Suppliers—distributors of pharmaceutical supplies, hospital equipment, prosthetic appliances, general supplies, and so forth.

Health Care Delivery—Public Sector

In the public sector we find various public health agencies—official and voluntary—operating at the local, state, federal and international level. Official agencies are tax supported; nonofficial or voluntary agencies are those nonprofit organizations that depend on voluntary contributions and/or fee-for-service. Some of the distinctions are listed in Table 10-1. Third party payments for direct services have grown in the public sector with the emergence of voluntary medical and health insurance plans as well as government-sponsored medical insurance and medical assistance programs. Health promotion and disease prevention are emphasized to a far greater extent in the public sector than in the private sector.

FEDERAL, STATE, AND LOCAL POWERS
IN MATTERS OF HEALTH

The delineation of federal, state, and local authority in health matters reflects the separation of power embodied in our Constitution; as the Tenth Amendment specifies, "the powers not delegated to the United States by the Constitution, nor prohibited by it to the States, are reserved to the States respectively, or to the people." The word *health* is not used in the Constitution, nor

Table 10-1   Health Agencies in the Public Sector—Characteristics and Examples

Voluntary (or Nonofficial) Health Agencies	Official Health Agencies
1. Supported by voluntary contributions and/or fee for service.	1. Tax supported.
2. Accountable to the supporters of the agency and to third party payment sources; attuned to public opinion.	2. Accountable to the citizenry (and the government) through an officially appointed or elected board.
3. Free to experiment and support research.	3. Duties more strictly prescribed or mandated by law.
4. Examples: American Heart Association; Visiting Nurse Associations; American Cancer Society; nonprofit community hospitals; American Lung Association; community health and welfare councils.	4. Examples: United States Department of Health, Education, and Welfare; state health departments; local health departments (county, city, municipality, township, etc.); federal, state, or municipal hospitals.

is there any reference to public health. Nevertheless, under the document's broad mandate "to promote the general welfare," the federal government has increased the quantity and scope of health legislation and expanded its role in health care. Also, it has acted in health matters through its power to regulate interstate and foreign commerce, to levy taxes, and to raise and support armed forces.

Each state has the sovereign power to make its own laws and regulations regarding health protection of the people within its jurisdiction. The legal responsibility for safeguarding the health of the general public is derived essentially through a state's police power and is assigned to the authority of the state board of health, whose members are appointed rather than elected. Regulations and policies adopted by the state boards of health are implemented by state and local health agencies. State governments delegate power to local governments for the establishment and maintenance of local boards of health and health departments.

Broadened federal health legislation in the mid-1960s had the effect of expanding the federal government's role in the field of health care. For example, with Medicare and Medicaid (established by the 1965 amendments to the Social Security Act) the federal government entered as a third party, providing funds to pay for needed services. Similarly, other legislation, in attempting to strengthen the nation's health services, made possible the establishment of Regional Medical Programs, Comprehensive Health Planning, Maternity and Infant Care Projects, and Children and Youth Programs.

One of the goals set forth by the federal government was regional planning to solve health problems. The concept of regionalization recognizes that many health problems—air pollution, water pollution, food sanitation, the efficient use of health resources—cut across city, township, county, and state lines. Therefore, regional programs do not necessarily coincide with established geographic and political boundaries. Planning at the regional level calls for coordination and cooperation among groups and communities, which must work together in seeking new ways to meet the complex health needs of contemporary society.

Another effect of the legislation of the 1960s was increased federal involvement in local areas. In some of the programs, notably Maternity and Infant Care (MIC) and the Office of Economic Opportunity (OEO), the federal government took a direct route to local agencies, bypassing the traditional approach of channeling categorical grants-in-aid through the states. Thus, local agencies negotiated directly with the federal government for financial support and consultation. The proponents of this approach declared that it allowed the federal government to respond directly to the needs of the people at the grass roots level. Those who disagreed felt that bypassing the states chipped away some of their sovereign power. Throughout these federally funded programs, the government sets forth guidelines, such as the Medicare requirement of utilization review; however, local and state health agencies responsible for implementation function independently of federal control.

Though basically determined by the United States Constitution, the interrelationships of federal, state, and local powers in matters of health are nonetheless affected by the prevailing political philosophy. The New Deal philosophy of the 1930s gave the federal government a prominent role in health care. This role has swung back and forth like a pendulum with succeeding administrations. During the Kennedy and Johnson era, there was much greater involvement at the national level in providing health care than at any other time. The tenor set under those administrations was one of "responsiveness to social needs" by the federal government. With the Nixon and Ford administrations, we saw a movement away from some of this federal participation in health care. A new tone was introduced, responding to the feelings that there had been "wasteful spending," "inefficient administration," and federal encroachment into states' responsibilities. This "New Federalism" called for greater responsibility on the part of state and local governments, tied in with the introduction of revenue sharing. The pendulum, in all likelihood, will continue to swing back and forth.

Official Health Agency Services at the Local Level

A local health unit exists as a health department of a city, county, township, or combination of these to form a district. This is the unit closest to the population and is in the first line of responsibility for community health. A health officer, serving as chief administrator, may be appointed by a mayor, or county governing body, or board of health; or he may be named from a civil service list.

The role and functions of a local health department depend on the kind of mandate it has from the state and on the quantity and quality of resources in the community. A typical organization chart is shown in Figure 10-1. In

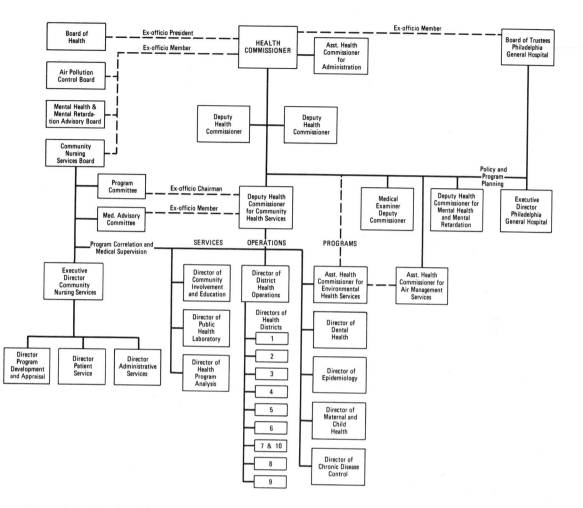

Figure 10-1 A local health department organization chart.

Source Courtesy of the Philadelphia Department of Public Health, Community Health Services.

providing community health services, a local health department may perform any or all of the following functions:

(1) investigate communicable diseases;

(2) maintain free clinics for the early diagnosis of tuberculosis and venereal disease;

(3) provide laboratory service to assist physicians;

(4) supervise milk and water supplies;

(5) conduct clinics for administration of protective biological agents—diphtheria, pertussis, tetanus, poliomyelitis, typhoid, etc.;

(6) collect vital statistics;

(7) provide maternal and child health care;

(8) maintain a public health nursing service;

(9) supervise quality and safety of meat and other foods;

(10) inspect and supervise the production, pasteurization and distribution of milk;

(11) investigate and supervise general sanitary conditions in public eating places;

(12) conduct a continual system of health education; and

(13) provide preventive and rehabilitative services in chronic disease control.

Hanlon discusses the future for local health departments, predicting that "truly comprehensive health services will soon be made available to the American people."[2] He points out that as a consequence of this and other changes, the health department functions and responsibilities cited above might be subject to change. Some of the new roles he suggests that would evolve for local health departments are listed as follows:

To serve as the community health conscience, the community health analyst, the community health counselor, and the community health catalyst

To become a key component of community health planning

To participate in the development of community health policy

To develop health criteria, standards, and qualifications

To promote necessary health legislation

To work with other components of local government whose work or resources may affect community health

To lead with new techniques, programs, and alignments

To conduct or promote research and demonstration in health program management, manpower development and use, clinical medicine, and the like

To insure involvement of community groups and the public in the decision-making process

To coordinate the efforts of various health resources in the community

To maintain surveillance over the activities of private or public agencies or institutions which may affect the public's health

To educate all components of society—the public, professions, business and industry, elected officials and others—in the fundamentals of community health.[3]

Official Health Agency Services at the State Level

Each state organizes its own public health services. There is often wide variation from one state to another. Typically there is a state health officer or commissioner, who serves as chief administrator, usually appointed by the governor upon recommendation by the state board of health. In all states, more than one agency has responsibilities in health care, but one agency, generally the state health department, is charged with primary responsibility in matters of community health.

The major functions of the state health department are as follows:

(1) statewide planning through assessment of health needs and resources;
(2) establishing policy;
(3) maintaining liaison with other state health departments and with the federal health program;
(4) encouraging and assisting the development of local health departments; and
(5) collecting vital statistics.

State health departments usually do not provide direct personal services, but assist local communities by offering consultative, supervisory, and financial assistance. Activities are usually organized within divisions such as Public Health Nursing, Communicable Disease Control, Health Education, Laboratory Service, Maternal and Child Health, Vital Statistics, and others. A typical breakdown is depicted in Figure 10-2.

Freedman expresses concern over what he describes as a disturbing trend toward fragmentation of health services at the state level. He feels that this fragmentation has manifested itself "by the way many legislatures keep diverting the administration of new health programs away from the traditional health agencies."[4] Furthermore, he is concerned by the actions of some state legislatures which, he feels, have downgraded the image of state health departments and deprived them of their autonomy by subordinating them to other state agencies. He sees this as a serious setback to coordinating and administering health services at the state level.

Official Health Agency Services at the Federal Level

The principal federal body concerned with the nation's health activities is the United States Department of Health, Education, and Welfare. Established in 1953, it absorbed and expanded the functions and responsibilities of the Federal Security Agency. The major component for health matters within HEW is the Public Health Service (PHS), or United States Public Health Service, which has had a long and distinguished history going back to 1798 when Congress had created its predecessor, the Marine Hospital Service. In 1973 the Department of Health, Education, and Welfare reorganized its Health component. Within the revised structure there are six agencies, as follows: Health Services Administration, Health Resources Administration, Center for Disease Control, National Institutes of Health, the Food and Drug Administration, and the Alcohol, Drug Abuse, and Mental Health Administration. These agencies comprise the Public Health Service, under the direction of the Assistant Secretary for Health (see organization chart, Figure 10-3).

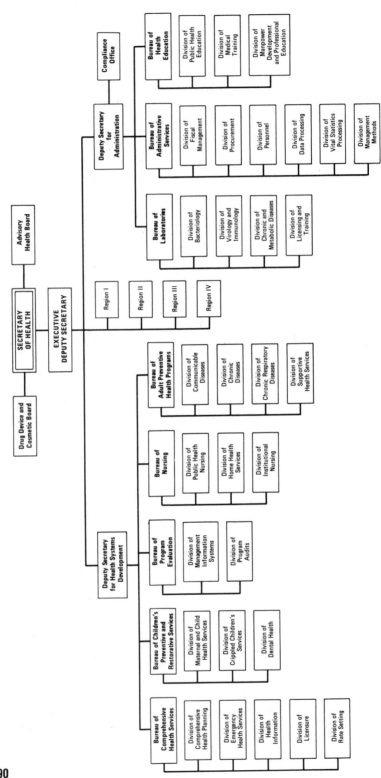

Figure 10-2 A state health department organization chart.

Source Courtesy of the Commonwealth of Pennsylvania.

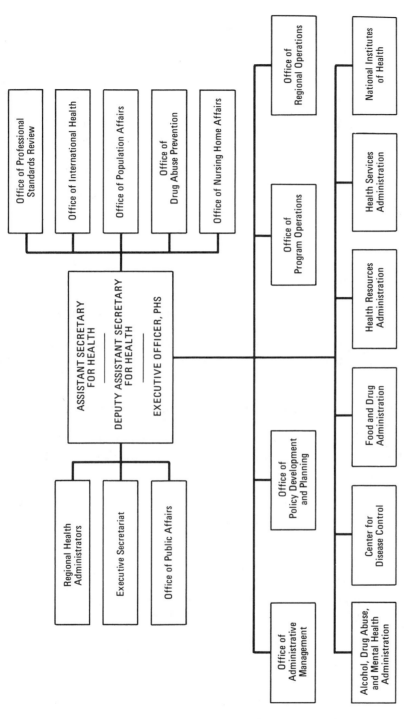

Figure 10-3 Department of Health, Education, and Welfare, Public Health Service.

Source Courtesy of Publications & Communications Branch, OPM, PHS, Department of Health, Education, and Welfare.

The major functions of the Public Health Service are:

to stimulate and assist states and communities with the development of local health resources and to further development of education for the health professions;

to assist with the improvement of the delivery of health services to all Americans;

to conduct and support research in the medical and related sciences and to disseminate scientific information;

to protect the health of the nation against impure and unsafe foods, drugs, cosmetics, and other potential hazards; and

to provide national leadership for the prevention and control of communicable disease and other health functions.

INTERNATIONAL HEALTH ACTIVITIES

World Health Organization (WHO)

In matters of health, the United States participates in the community of nations through its membership in the World Health Organization. The liaison body is the United States Department of Health, Education, and Welfare. The World Health Organization, a specialized agency of the United Nations, established as a permanent body in 1948, is a directing and coordinating authority in international health. Though not the first attempt at international health work, it does have greater prestige and responsibility than any previous international health body. The admission of East Germany in 1973 brought the total membership to 137 nations. A country may belong to WHO without being a member of the United Nations. WHO drafts its own budget made up of contributions from member states, which are assessed according to their national incomes and ability to pay.

From its inception the World Health Organization, which is headquartered in Geneva, Switzerland, has kept to the principle of regionalization. There are six regions:

Region	Location of Regional Office
Africa	Brazzaville, People's Republic of the Congo
Americas	Washington, D.C.
Southeast Asia	New Delhi, India
Europe	Copenhagen, Denmark
Eastern Mediterranean	Alexandria, Egypt
Western Pacific	Manila, Philippines

The World Health Organization was built on the premise that no nation can isolate itself from disease vectors by means of purely defensive barriers such as quarantine. Disease must be attacked at its source. In a world of rapidly shifting environment, optimum health for all people is essential in achieving international security, peace, and freedom.

The objective of WHO as defined in its constitution is "the attainment by all peoples of the highest possible level of health." Health has been defined as a "state of complete physical, mental, and social well-being and not merely the absence of disease or infirmity." Implied in this definition of health are both a right and a duty; that is, health so defined is "one of the fundamental rights of every human being without distinction of race, religion, political belief, economic or social conditions." Finally, the constitution declares "the health of all peoples is fundamental to the attainment of peace and security and is dependent upon the fullest cooperation of individuals and states."

The World Health Organization offers a program that is truly worldwide in its scope, and directly or indirectly benefits everyone. Upon the request of governments, it will assist in strengthening health services and furnish technical assistance. It encourages and coordinates international scientific research on health problems that cannot be solved by isolated efforts. Some of the WHO activities are listed as follows:

(1) To meet the danger of epidemics, it has established international sanitary regulations and it operates an epidemiological intelligence service. For example, it played an active role in the smallpox epidemics in Yugoslavia (1972) and in India (1974). In 1967, the World Health Organization launched an intensive program to wipe out smallpox. About that time, the disease was endemic in thirty countries throughout the world; by 1975 the number was reduced to three—India, Bangladesh, and Ethiopia.

(2) It has worked out international standards for biological products; it publishes an international pharmacopeia, and has provided international lists of diseases and causes of deaths for uniformity in reporting.

(3) It offers fellowships for postgraduate study to nurses, physicians, and other health workers.

(4) It assists member nations in the control of specific communicable diseases such as yaws, tuberculosis, malaria; its concern extends to noncommunicable health problems as well.

(5) It is concerned with environmental health and supports the fight against water, soil, and air pollution.

(6) It provides assistance to member states in the improvement of their health administration and services.

(7) It supports and coordinates research in the development of vaccines, in the control of heart disease and cancer, in human reproduction, and in other areas.

Agency for International Development (AID)

The United States supports international health through its foreign assistance program under the Agency for International Development. Established under the Foreign Assistance Act of 1961, it took over the work of its predecessors, the International Cooperation Administration and the Economic Cooperation Administration. A component of the Department of State, AID provides economic and technical assistance to other countries. Public health is included in technical assistance, and numerous cooperative programs have been established around the world. High on the list of priorities has been the training of health workers from abroad, for which fellowships and study grants have been awarded.

HEALTH CARE FINANCING

A basic tenet in nursing is that every patient is entitled to the highest quality of care, irrespective of his ability to pay. Traditionally, the fee status of the patient was something that did not concern the nurse, and nursing students were not expected to become involved in the financial aspects of health care. However, as nursing continues to move into the community, and as "third party" payments become more widespread, it is essential for nurses to acquire an understanding of health care financing and how it affects the patient and the family. For example, in many situations today, the plan of treatment calls for expensive equipment, medications, or other supplies. A nurse who is aware of the cost can assess the situation, and through her knowledge of community resources, will be able to help the patient plan for continued care.

Current literature abounds with descriptions of various methods of health care financing. Some of the prevailing methods have been summarized by Dr. Milton Roemer, as follows:

WAYS OF FINANCING HEALTH CARE

There are hundreds of ways of financing health services if we consider all the ramifications at different times and social settings. They can, however, be generally classified in a half dozen types:

Personal Payment private purchase of service, from the individual's personal resources, including those he may have borrowed or received from another source (a relative, friend, loan company, and so on). It could also include payment by barter.

Charity support from funds donated by persons who may or may not become beneficiaries of the service.

Industry provision of services at the expense of an enterprise, supported from its earnings.

Voluntary Insurance support of services from funds raised through periodic contributions by groups of persons. These funds may be variously sponsored, but the services are supported only for contributors or their dependents.

Social Insurance insurance required by law to support certain services to designated beneficiaries. Statutory requirements may set up governmental trust funds or may mandate contributions to various nongovernmental bodies.

General Revenues support through taxation by local, provincial, or national governmental authority on incomes, land, sales, corporation profits, and the like. Services are not confined to tax payers.

Milton I. Roemer, "Health Care Financing and Delivery Around the World," American Journal of Nursing, 71:1158-63, June 1971. Copyright June 1971, The American Journal of Nursing Company. Reprinted from American Journal of Nursing.

One or another of these methods may predominate in any one nation, but often all of them may be found in varying degrees in most of the countries of the world. In reviewing these methods in the United States, we find that existing financing mechanisms are often geared to medical care for treatment of illness rather than for health care in its broader scope.

Until a few years ago, the predominant method of financing health care in the United States was personal payment, that is, fee for service from patient to physician or hospital. This method still carries most of the cost of ambulatory medical care, dental care, and medications.

Charity continues to play an important role in American society's participation in financing health care. The neighborhood drive for the cancer association, the mothers' march for dimes to fight birth defects, the annual United Way campaign—these are very much a part of the American scene and are stimulated by the humane force of voluntarism. Sometimes people show signs of irritation from the many mail and door-to-door solicitations for funds. They throw up their hands in annoyance and wish that all the organizations would get together and have a single, unified drive for funds. However, it just has not worked that way because of the many diversified interests and the complexity of the problems that require financial help. These same people often grumble or shout with alarm when government steps in to legislate funds for needed services that, unfortunately, charity alone is unable to provide. Charity's role is important for the emotional, psychological, and public support, but it cannot cope unaided with the health care financial burden.

In this country many industrial firms finance preventive health services for their workers through their occupational health programs. Examples of comprehensive health and medical care programs supported by industry may be seen in certain Latin American countries where foreign companies producing sugar and coffee are required to provide such services. Another illustration would be programs operated in some of the large oil companies in the Middle East.

Voluntary health insurance consitutes a major source of health care financing in the United States today. In the last few decades, Blue Cross, Blue Shield, and various other insurance plans have gained wide acceptance. Although the majority of our population has some form of voluntary health insurance, many people—especially the poor, the aged, and those who dwell in rural areas—are not covered by this kind of insurance. Voluntary health insurance has done very little to change the health care delivery system or to rectify its inequities. Notable exceptions in this category are those consumer- or employer-sponsored plans, for example, the Health Insurance Plan of Greater New York and the Kaiser-Permanente Health Plan, which provide comprehensive health service through group medical practice and health maintenance organizations.

Health care financing from social insurance and general revenues are now an accepted part of our health care delivery system. Medicare, which covers hospitalization and home care for the elderly, is a form of social insurance, derived from Social Security funds the individual has been obliged to pay during his years of employment. Medicaid, or medical assistance, is derived from general revenues and provides financial support for medical care to those who are in need.

Table 10-2 illustrates the benefits provided by Medicare and Medicaid.

Medicare

Title 18 of the amendments to the Social Security Act offered a vast new program of medical insurance for the aged. On July 1, 1966, certain provisions of the Health Insurance for the Aged Act, *Medicare,* went into effect. Congress, in enacting Medicare legislation, sought to protect the elderly against the catastrophic financial debts often incurred in the treatment of chronic illness. The program was open to all persons sixty-five years of age and older. Thus, for the first time, federal legislation was enacted to remove financial barriers to medical care for a vulnerable segment of society, the elderly.

Under Medicare, certain nonprofit health insurance groups, for example Blue Cross, are designated as fiscal intermediaries. These intermediary groups are charged with the responsibility of interpreting the conditions of participation to providers and recipients of service. Providers are accountable both to their fiscal intermediaries and to the recipients of service. This accountability factor has moved agencies to evaluate their total operation and to take appropriate measures to upgrade the quality of patient care.

Ongoing evaluation has had the effect of bringing about changes in the Medicare Act to increase coverage and provide additional service. As of January 1, 1973, outpatient diagnostic and treatment services became fully reimbursible except for the first $60 in each calendar year. As of July 1, 1973, the "homebound" status was eliminated as a requirement for speech, occupational, and physical therapy—patients may now go to a private therapist's office or to a rehabilitation center for treatment. In July 1973 Medicare coverage was further extended to include disabled persons under sixty-five years of age who qualified for Social Security cash disability benefits (for at

Table 10-2 Medicare-Medicaid—Which is Which? Both Medicare and Medicaid help pay medical bills, are part of the Social Security Act, and work together; they both insist on high standards, support expansion of facilities, encourage innovation in medical care delivery, require review of care. But Medicare and Medicaid are not the same.

Medicare

Medicare is for people 65 or older.

Medicare is an insurance program.

Money from trust funds pays medical bills for insured people.

Medicare is a federal program.

Medicare is the same all over the United States.

Medicare basic hospital insurance covers the costs of:

   (a) inpatient hospital care,
   (b) post-hospital extended care,
   (c) post-hospital home health services.

Medicare medical insurance provides supplemental coverage for:

   (a) physicians' and surgeons' services,
   (b) home health services,
   (c) outpatient hospital services,
   (d) other medical and health services (e.g. walkers, crutches, canes, commodes, hospital beds).

Medicare pays part, but not all, of hospital and medical costs.

Medicare paid medical bills for over 10 million people in 1971. Altogether, about 20 million people in the United States (or 10% of the population) have the protection of Medicare.

The Bureau of Health Insurance of the Social Security Administration of HEW is responsible for Medicare.

Medicaid

Medicaid is for needy and low-income people.

Medicaid is an assistance program.

Money from federal, state, and local taxes pays medical bills for eligible people.

Medicaid is a federal-state partnership.

Medicaid may vary from state to state.

Medicaid provides for these services:

   (a) inpatient hospital care;
   (b) outpatient hospital services;
   (c) other laboratory and X-ray services;
   (d) skilled nursing home services;
   (e) physicians' services;
   (f) screening, diagnosis, and treatment of children;
   (g) home health care services;
   (h) family planning services.

In many states Medicaid pays for such additional services as dental care, prescribed drugs, eye glasses, clinic services, and other diagnostic, screening, preventive, and rehabilitative services.

Medicaid can supplement the services of Medicare for people who are eligible for both programs.

Medicaid paid medical bills in 1971 for more than 18 million people who were aged, blind, disabled, under 21, or members of families with dependent children.

The Medical Services Administration of the Social and Rehabilitation Service of HEW is responsible for federal aspects of Medicaid; however, each state is responsible for its own program.

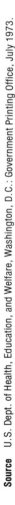

Source U.S. Dept. of Health, Education, and Welfare, Washington, D.C.: Government Printing Office, July 1973.

197

least twenty-four consecutive months) and persons under sixty-five who require hemodialysis or kidney transplantation. The Medicare benefits provided to these disabled persons are the same as for persons sixty-five years of age and older.

Home health agencies providing service under Medicare must adhere to conditions of participation under the Social Security Act. The patient's homebound status, establishment of a plan of treatment, medical certification, and other conditions of eligibility specified by the Social Security Administration must be met before services to the patient can be approved. Applying these guidelines, the providers of service are required to make a professional judgment to determine the patient's eligibility. In the home setting skilled nursing care is a service which, according to Medicare requirements, must be furnished by or under the direct supervision of a licensed professional nurse to assure the safety of the patient and to achieve medically desired results. Thus, nursing is charged with the responsibility of assuring high quality care to our senior citizens.

Though medical care for the aged has become more readily accessible through Medicare, many barriers to health care have not been removed under the terms of this law. For example, the designation of "skilled" nursing and the interpretation that restricts such service to "sick" care have had the effect of depriving the elderly of nursing services for health maintenance. Nurses, as the largest single professional group providing health care, must take a more active role in supporting legislation that will help to eliminate these barriers. The Council of Home Health Agencies of the National League for Nursing has actively worked for a change in federal legislation so that elderly people might receive needed services not provided through Medicare.

Medicaid (Medical Assistance)

Title 19 of the amendments to the Social Security Act provided medical assistance for both the indigent and the medically indigent. Families and individuals classified as indigent are those receiving cash grants from the Department of Welfare. This group receives medical benefits under the welfare system in addition to cash grants for support. Federal guidelines for 1975 state that the medically indigent are those families and individuals whose gross annual income does not exceed:

> $2000 per year for one person;
> $2500 per year for a two-member family;
> $ 750 per year for each additional dependent member.

Eligibility for medical assistance is not hampered by ownership of a home; assets other than a home, furniture, and car for a single person must be less than $2,400 and for a family, $3,840. Services covered under medical assistance include hospital and physician fees, certain outpatient services, and home health care. Payments are made directly to the hospital, agency, or person who supplied the medical care. In addition to the medical and regular benefits under Medicaid, the Department of Welfare provides information and referral services to help the family or individual with problems that may arise from illness.

By April 1, 1973, the federal government required participating states to establish and maintain a program of early and periodic screening, diagnosis, and treatment (EPSDT) for persons under twenty-one years of age (see p. 155). Certain states exercised the option of phasing in the program gradually by age levels. By 1975, EPSDT was operational at varying levels throughout the United States. The 1972 amendments to Title 19 signal a significant and official recognition of the need for a more positive approach to health care through health maintenance programs.

REFERENCES

1. Benjamin Disraeli, from a speech given on July 24, 1877.

2. John J. Hanlon, "Is There a Future for Local Health Departments?" *Health Services Reports,* 88 (December 1973) 898-901.

3. Ibid.

4. Ben Freedman, "What Is and What Must Be Done," *American Journal of Public Health,* 62 (June 1972) 759-64.

ADDITIONAL READINGS

Anderson, C.L., *Community Health.* 2nd ed. St. Louis: C.V. Mosby, 1973.

Anderson, Odin W., and Ronald M. Andersen, "Patterns of Use of Health Services," in Freeman, Howard, Sol Levine, and Leo G. Reeder, *Handbook of Medical Sociology.* 2nd ed. Englewood Cliffs, N.J.: Prentice-Hall, 1972.

Blum, Henrik L., and Alvin R. Leonard, *Public Administration: A Public Health Viewpoint.* New York: The Macmillan Co., 1963.

Brockington, C. Fraser, *World Health.* Boston: Little, Brown, 1968.

Bullough, Bonnie, "The Medicare-Medicaid Amendments," in *American Journal of Nursing,* 73 (November 1973) 1926-29.

Burton, Lloyd E., and Hugh H. Smith, *Public Health and Community Medicine.* Baltimore: Williams and Wilkins Co., 1970.

Buzzell, Harold O., "A New National Strategy To Make Health Services Flexible and Responsive," in *Health Services Reports,* 88 (December 1973) 894-97.

Carter, Richard, *The Gentle Legions.* New York: Doubleday and Co., 1961.

Coe, Rodney M., and Kevin R. Andrews, "Effects of Medicare on the Provision of Community Health Resources," in *American Journal of Public Health,* 62 (June 1972) 854-56.

Gossert, Daniel J., and C. Arden Miller, "State Boards of Health, Their Members and Commitments," in *American Journal of Public Health,* 63 (June 1973) 486-93.

Hanlon, John J., *Public Health: Administration and Practice.* 6th ed. St. Louis: C.V. Mosby, 1974.

Hess, Arthur, "Through Government Action: Medicare Begins," in *American Journal of Nursing,* 66 (June 1966) 1295-97.

Howard, Lee M., "Three Key Dilemmas in International Health," in *American Journal of Public Health,* 62 (January 1972) 73-78.

Leavell, Hugh R., and E. Gurney Clark, *Preventive Medicine for the Doctor in His Community.* 3rd ed. New York: McGraw-Hill, 1965.

Mytinger, Robert E., *Innovation in Local Health Services.* U.S. Department of Health, Education, and Welfare, 1968.

Roemer, Milton I., "Health Care Financing and Delivery Around the World," in *American Journal of Nursing,* 71 (June 1971) 1158-63.

Rogers, David E., "A Private Sector View of Public Health Today," in *American Journal of Public Health,* 64 (June 1974) 529-33.

Sartwell, Philip E., ed., *Maxcy-Rosenau Preventive Medicine and Public Health.* 10th ed. New York: Appleton-Century-Crofts, 1973.

U.S. Department of Health, Education, and Welfare, *Selected Vignettes on Activities of Regional Medical Programs.* Washington, D.C.: Government Printing Office, July, 1971.

Wilner, Daniel M., Rosabelle Price Walkley, and Lenor S. Goerke, *Introduction to Public Health.* New York: Macmillan Co., 1973.

Chapter 11
Reform of the Health Care
Delivery System

"The concept that comprehensive health opportunities are the right of all people, and not a privilege of a few, has long been supported by the nursing profession."[1]

NATIONAL CONCERN ABOUT HEALTH CARE

With total expenditures over the $100 billion mark, health care delivery has become one of our nation's largest "industries," employing over 4 million persons. Since the early 1960s, the health care delivery system has been subjected to intense scrutiny and criticism from many segments of our society. There is growing concern about the lack of an adequate system for providing health care to all who need it. Those who have seriously studied the situation have described it as a "crisis." In looking at some of the reasons behind this crisis, we can cite three major problems: the high cost of care, the uneven accessibility of health resources, and the shortage and maldistribution of personnel.

In the wave of a general economic inflation, health care costs have skyrocketed, rising more sharply than other consumer prices. Since 1950 health expenditures increased from $13 billion by more than 600 percent to over $94 billion in 1973.[2] The nation as a whole has been unable to economize and put brakes on this galloping inflation. Specific measures adopted under the government's Economic Stabilization Program, launched in November 1971, could not stem the tide. With termination of economic controls on the health care industry in April 1974 costs continued to rise. A leading expert in the field of health care had estimated that national health expenditures would climb to over $103 billion in 1974 and "if there are no new forces of escalation or de-escalation, these totals will go to about $115 billion in fiscal 1975 and to about $127 billion in fiscal 1976.''[3]

In spite of these vast outlays of money, many people simply have no financial protection against catastrophic illness nor do they have the means to provide themselves with necessary health maintenance and preventive services. This is true even though private health insurance has grown in the last twenty-five years, so that now between 80 and 90 percent of the population have some kind of coverage. This coverage, however, has serious limitations, for premiums are constantly increasing, without any increase in benefits, and many essential services are not covered. Estimates vary, but it is believed that over 25 million persons have no protection whatsoever, and many of these are children who live in poverty.

There has been increasing public dissatisfaction with the poor accessibility of health services. The supply of manpower and facilities is both limited and inadequately distributed. Marked technological advances have brought about new methods and techniques of care. Through the mass media, people have become much better informed about these innovations. The concept of health as a right of all people, and not merely a privilege for a few, has spread. There are growing demands, on the part of the consumers, for better health care and for a greater voice in planning health programs.

The organization of health care in our country has been unsparingly characterized by some critics as a ''nonsystem'' that fails to respond to the needs of the public and gives rise to two different classes of care—one for the rich and one for the poor. An oft-repeated criticism is that we lack national planning and coordination, a fact that has led to fragmented services and disjointed programs. Dr. Herman Hilleboe, for example, has pointed out that there is an urgent need for a long-range comprehensive health plan that would look at the nation as a whole—the private and public sectors; personal, environmental and social needs; and the total resources at our command.[4]

Indeed, both providers and consumers of health care are evincing a growing acceptance of the fact that reform of the entire health care system is a necessity, and they are looking to the federal government for leadership and support. As a first step in response to this need, the United States Department of Health, Education, and Welfare in 1971 issued a *White Paper* on the delivery of health care entitled ''Towards a Comprehensive Health Policy for the 1970s.''

The findings of the *White Paper* might be summarized as follows:

HEALTH CARE STATUS OF THE NATION

Strengths   Gross measures indicate a long-term trend of improvement.

(1) Life expectancy has increased (people who are 45 have already lived almost as long as the average person born in 1900 could have expected to live, and, today, they have about 30 more years of life remaining.)

(2) Infant mortality and maternal mortality rates have dropped.

(3) Disability days have also declined.

These trends may be attributed to such factors as rising level of income, better nutrition and housing, higher levels of educational attainment, general improvement in sanitation, control of infectious diseases, improvements in treatment and rehabilitation in chronic disease.

Weaknesses   The gains are offset by great disparities in health status.

(1) Among the subgroups in our population, particularly the poor and the racial minorities, we find more illness, higher death rates, less access to health services.

(2) In certain sensitive measurements (e.g., infant mortality rate) we, as a nation, compare unfavorably with other countries, notably Sweden, Netherlands, Norway, Finland, Denmark, Japan, Switzerland, France, New Zealand, Australia, United Kingdom.

HEALTH CARE RESOURCES

Strengths   Main health care resources have been growing faster than the population, especially in recent years.

(1) Number of hospital beds per 1,000 people increased from 12.4 (1963) to 13.5 (1968).

(2) Between 1950 and 1966, the number of people in health occupations increased by more than 90% (the population increase was 29%).

(3) In 1960, 2.9% of the civilian work force were in health occupations; by 1966 there were 3.7%.

(4) The supply of nurses and physicians has increased.

Weaknesses   Health care resources are inadequately distributed, improperly managed, and poorly utilized.

(1) There are great disparities in geographic location and accessibility.

   (a) There are 82 active physicians per 100,000 people in Mississippi, but 228/100,000 in New York.

   (b) A study of 1,500 cities and towns in the upper midwest in 1965 found 1,000 towns without a physician, and 200 others had only one.

   (c) Large metropolitan areas average 185 physicians per 100,000 people, while the average is only 76 per 100,000 in nonmetropolitan areas.

   (d) Cities, particularly ghetto areas within them, fare worse than the suburbs in the supply of physicians.

   (e) In 9 out of 10 Appalachian states, there are fewer physicians in the poorer counties than in the wealthier counties.

(2) Although the numbers of physicians have increased, there has been a decline in the ratio of primary care physicians (general practitioners, pediatricians, and internists)—94 per 100,000 population (1931) to 73 per 100,000 population (1967).

(3) Other health care personnel who could provide primary health care are poorly utilized because of a traditional insistence that the primary care provider be a physician.

(4) Health care facilities are often inappropriately used.

(a) Patients have been hospitalized for X-ray and laboratory services that could be performed in outpatient care.

(b) Hospital beds have been used in cases where extended care facilities were more appropriate.

(c) Hospitals have been found to maintain expensive facilities that are rarely used (e.g., in 1967, 31% of the hospitals that had open-heart surgery facilities had not used them for a year).

As a response to these problems, the *White Paper* sets forth a "comprehensive health strategy" within the framework of our "capitalistic, pluralistic, competitive" political economy. More specifically, solutions are sought within the existing limits of national priorities and within the present structure of the health insurance industry. As such, the strategy does not go far enough to satisfy those who see a need for broad health and social planning, including complete reform of health care delivery with greater public responsibility in health matters. At the same time it exceeds the wishes of those who see nothing wrong with the status quo and who shout "welfare state" at every new piece of social legislation.

The *White Paper* identified four general areas for its health strategy proposals—prevention; innovation and reform in health care; health manpower; and improving the financing of health services.

HEALTH STRATEGY PROPOSALS—WHITE PAPER

(1) **Prevention** The area of prevention includes welfare reforms, nutrition, family planning, occupational health and safety, automobile accidents and alcoholism, pollution control, health research, prevention of communicable diseases, lead paint poisoning, product safety, Indian health, personal responsibility for health, financial incentives for preventive health care.

(2) **Innovation and Reform in Health Care: Health Maintenance Organizations (HMO)** HMOs are organized systems of health care, providing comprehensive services for enrolled members for a fixed, prepaid annual fee; they emphasize prevention and early care, provide incentives for holding down costs, offer opportunities for improving the quality of care, and provide a means for improving the geographic distribution of care. (HMOs are not new. There are several well-known privately sponsored plans built on the HMO concept, e.g., the Health Insurance Plan of Greater New York and the Kaiser-Permanente Health Plan of the West Coast.) The government has committed various existing authorities to stimulate the development of HMOs for the general population, especially in areas where health care resources are scarce.

(3) **Health Manpower** The following proposals have been made:

(a) improve the distribution of manpower resources;

(b) improve the utilization of health manpower;

(c) provide student assistance;

(d) improve the financial stability of health professional schools;

(e) increase the supply of health manpower.

(4) Improving the Financing of Health Services The government proposes a national health insurance program providing some financial protection for everyone; as a partnership between the public and private sectors, it does not require the federal government to assume the entire national health care bill.

NATIONAL HEALTH INSURANCE PROPOSALS

National health insurance is not a new topic. An accepted part of the health care system in many countries, it goes back to the 1880s in western Europe. In the United States, it has captured wide public interest since the 1960s. Earlier attempts to introduce it here can be traced to the report of the Committee on Costs of Medical Care in the 1930s and the Wagner-Murray-Dingell Bills which failed to pass in four successive Congresses—1943, 1945, 1947, and 1949. In the late 1940s, the issue of national health insurance precipitated one of the major battles of the Truman administration.

Long a controversial issue, national health insurance in some form is almost certain to become an accepted part of our system in the future. Those who favor national health insurance feel that it would be effective in easing the financial burden of health care. In the opponents' camp are those who object to national health insurance because they are against any kind of government financing, as well as those who feel that the only remedy would be outright public subsidization of health care through taxation.

Proponents of national health insurance generally agree on the following:

1. Alone, it cannot solve all health problems.

2. It must be accompanied by a sincere effort to reform and reorganize the health care delivery system.

3. It should be developed as part of a national health policy, "directed toward increasing the comprehensiveness of health care, reducing the inequalities in distribution of health resources, improving the quality of care, and increasing the efficiency of the delivery system." [5]

With the advent of the 1970s, the resurgence of interest in national health insurance was reflected by the fact that in every congressional session (since the 91st Congress, 1969-70), national health insurance was a key issue. Each of the numerous plans introduced for consideration in the 91st, 92nd, and 93rd Congress mirrors the political philosophy of its sponsors, and each differs in its approach to such key issues as:

1. Whom should national health insurance cover?
2. What benefits should be offered?
3. How should the program be financed?
4. What should the role of the federal government be in administering and financing a health insurance program?
5. How extensively, if at all, should private health insurers be involved?
6. What methods of reimbursement should be used?
7. How should the overall organization and delivery of health care be modified, if at all?

By the end of 1974 there were many proposals, from which several emerged as leading contenders. These could be grouped into four categories, according to the measures provided in the plans. To illustrate these four groups, we have summarized some of the major proposals introduced into the 93rd Congress (1973-74), as follows:[6]

1. Legislation that would make the federal government responsible for financing health care only for the "high risks" in society—the aged, poor, disabled, and persons experiencing catastrophic illness costs. An example is the *Catastrophic Illness Insurance Act* introduced by Senator Russell Long. It builds catastrophic benefits into the Medicare program, coverage applies to all persons insured under Social Security, and all contributions would be in a federal Catastrophic Health Insurance Fund. (This bill was later re-introduced as the *Catastrophic Health Insurance and Medical Assistance Reform Act* by Senators Long and Abraham Ribicoff).

2. Legislation that would provide federally financed economic incentives toward the purchase of private health insurance plans. Example: *The Health Care Insurance Act of 1973*—"Medicredit" — introduced by Senator Vance Hartke and Congressman Richard Fulton, and endorsed by the American Medical Association. Coverage would be on a voluntary basis through allowance of tax credits to encourage purchase of health insurance from private carriers. This bill does not call for changing or improving any segment of the nation's health care system.

3. Legislation that would mandate employers to purchase adequate private health insurance plans for employee groups (special provision would be made with government support for unemployed persons). Example: *The Comprehensive Health Insurance Act of 1974* (Administration Bill) introduced by Senator Robert Packwood and Congressmen Wilbur Mills and Herman Schneebeli. In many ways it was similar to the Administration's earlier National Health Insurance Partnership and Family Health Insurance Plan which had been under consideration in the 92nd Congress. The new comprehensive health insurance plan—CHIP—kept the underlying principles of mixed public-private financing and administration, reliance on states for carrying out the program, and encouraging coverage through HMOs. CHIP would assure all Americans affordable health insurance through employer–employee plans and subsidization of insurance for persons who are not covered through employment plans; it would rely on the private health insurance industry and on deductibles and coinsurance to help control costs.

4. Legislation that would entitle all Americans to federally financed and administered comprehensive health benefits. Example: *The Health Security Act of 1973* introduced by Senator Edward Kennedy and Congresswoman Martha Griffiths and endorsed by the Committee for National Health Insurance and the AFL-CIO. This is probably the broadest-based proposal with the most far-reaching coverage. It would cover the entire population and offer a comprehensive range of services without cut-off dates, coinsurance, deductibles, or waiting periods. The program would be federally administered and financed—50 percent from general federal revenues with the remainder from payroll and self-employed taxes. The plan would call for reforms and innovations in the health care delivery system, e.g., the use of HMOs.

Other leading proposals were introduced in the 93rd Congress which combined some of the features described above, as follows:[7]

The National Catastrophic Illness Protection Act of 1973 (Senator Glenn Beall and Congressman Robert Roe) provided for coverage on a voluntary basis with government support for purchase of health insurance from the private insurance industry.

The National Health Care Act of 1973 (Senator Thomas McIntyre and Congressman Omar Burleson), endorsed by the Health Insurance Association of America, called for coverage through private insurance on a voluntary basis to include an employer–employee plan, an individual plan, and a plan for the poor and uninsurable; the latter would be financed primarily by federal and state governments.

The National Health Care Services Reorganization and Financing Act of 1973—"Ameriplan"—(Congressman Al Ullman), endorsed by the American Hospital Association, called for a reorganization of the health care delivery system. The basic unit offering service would be a health care corporation as a community-based, non-profit organization to provide comprehensive health services to all residents in defined geographic areas.

The National Health Insurance and Health Services Improvement Act of 1973 (Senator Jacob Javits) would have extended Medicare to the general population. It would have provided for mandatory coverage of all citizens, with direct federal administration using private insurance carriers, intermediaries, and state health agencies.

This wide array of legislative proposals reflected the divergent forces which would have to be reconciled before effective compromise on national health insurance could be reached. During the 93rd congressional session, it began to appear that opposing sides might be moving closer to some kind or workable agreement. For example, Senator Kennedy, withdrawing support from his Health Care Security Bill, joined with Congressman Mills in introducing a new bill, *The Comprehensive National Health Insurance Act of 1974.* The Mills-Kennedy plan combined features of some of the other leading proposals, including the Administration plan, and was offered as a compromise bill. However, a series of compelling events combined in such a way as to prevent any decisive action: It was a time when the nation was beset with serious problems—rampant inflation, the energy crisis, the "Watergate" episode. The final period of the 93rd Congress witnessed a state of affairs previously unknown to this country: An elected president had resigned rather than face impeachment; moving in to fill the vacancy was a vice-president who had been appointed rather than elected; and a new vice-president was appointed and sworn in after one of the most exhaustive Congressional investigations of a potential officeholder.

In January 1975, the 94th Congress began its session, preoccupied with problems such as rising unemployment, spiraling cost of living, and the continuing energy crisis. These conditions had the effect of moving national health insurance into the background; however, this effect is probably temporary, since most major NHI legislation has been reintroduced in the 94th Congress. As 1975 draws to a close, no one can forecast with any certainty how the issue will be resolved. Some observers predict an incremental approach to national health insurance, with legislation for catastrophic protection as the next step, rather than a single all-encompassing bill.[8]

EMERGING PATTERNS AND INNOVATIONS IN HEALTH CARE DELIVERY

National health insurance can provide the means to remove financial barriers in health care, and it can help to alleviate "crisis" situations in the lives of individual persons. Most experts agree, however, that the many problems in the delivery of health care will continue to exist unless some attention is given to a reorganization and restructuring of the overall system. Needed reforms in our health care system would include proposals from the *White Paper,* and might be summarized as follows:

(1) A reorientation in the philosophy of health care for consumers and providers; health must be viewed as a right, not a privilege. Emphasis belongs on positive health promotion and prevention. Dr. Charles Hoffman as President of the AMA has spoken of the need to create a whole new atmosphere in our country where health would come to be regarded as a "status symbol."

(2) Removal of financial barriers to health care for all citizens;

(3) Formulation of a national health policy;

(4) Comprehensive health planning on a regional basis;

(5) Wider consumer participation in establishing priorities and administering the health care system;

(6) More effective use of health manpower with recognition of nursing's unique contribution as a primary provider of health care;

(7) Specific provisions for a step-by-step expansion of needed health services, including care outside hospitals and other institutions:

(a) expanded ambulatory or outpatient care, including HMOs and community health centers;

(b) improved emergency services;

(c) home care;

(d) centers for multiphasic screening and patient education;

(8) Coordinated planning for the utilization of high cost facilities or complicated technological equipment;

(9) Provisions for training health personnel, with opportunity for professional practice, advancement, and reasonable compensation;

(10) Built-in mechanisms for evaluation and accountability at every level.

As time goes on, there is increasing federal involvement in meeting health needs. Since 1966 many new developments have been initiated through governmental action. In Chapter 10 we described government efforts to remove financial barriers through Medicare and Medicaid, as well as efforts to stimulate communities to consider regional and comprehensive health planning. We also mentioned categorical health programs such as family planning, sickle cell anemia, lead poisoning, nutrition for the elderly, and others. Often these programs have been directed toward meeting specific health needs, and, within their specialized framework, have been able to demonstrate successful results. On the whole, however, we have watched these developments at times appear to add to the fragmentation and duplication of services, in the absence of an overall coordinated policy.

Now let's discuss some of the emerging patterns—health maintenance organizations, comprehensive neighborhood health services, home care programs, emergency health services, peer review programs—which the government is encouraging to help eliminate some of the inequities in the delivery of health care. Once again, in the absence of a national health policy, they may appear to be piecemeal and uncoordinated. However, they are intended to help fill the gaps in the existing framework and to provide basic elements in a reorganized framework for the health care delivery system. These approaches are being evaluated for their efficacy. All of them have implications for nursing in planning, organizing, implementing, and evaluating needed services for the population. At the same time nursing has a responsibility to work toward the eventual goal of an equitable health care system for all our citizens.

Health Maintenance Organization (HMO)

A new stimulus to the establishment of prepaid comprehensive health care organizations through federal aid was provided through the Health Maintenance Organizations legislation, enacted in 1973. Health maintenance organizations, which have been in existence for more than forty years, provide comprehensive health care services on a prepaid, capitation basis with emphasis on primary care, preventive services, and efficiency of operations. The HMO is not a panacea; it is but a first step in the direction of eliminating fragmentation. HMOs offer ambulatory, inpatient, and home care. The patient is guided through the system for health or sick care by a person qualified to provide primary care—a nurse practitioner, primary care physician, or other allied health personnel. There is an ongoing record, facilitating continuity of services, clinical auditing, and peer review. There are built-in measures for efficiency, economy, and eliminating duplication of services.[9]

Persons who enroll in an HMO pay a fixed sum each month, whether they use the services or not. Under this system, traditional incentives are turned around; that is, prepayment becomes an incentive to treat people efficiently. The objective is to keep people well so as to prevent the need for costly therapeutic services, and if they do become ill, to treat them early in the most economic site. One of the results of this system is cost consciousness. Health providers become aware of the need to give quality health care within the financial limitations of the organizations.

Third party insurance payments are eliminated. The risk of illness is borne by the provider—the HMO. In effect, good primary care is rewarded because savings accrued by preventing the need for hospitalization go back into the organization. Supply is related to need—personnel and facilities are acquired as dictated by needs of the enrollment. Accountability is an integral part of the system.

One added feature about the HMO is that it offers an alternative to the consumer and provides a means of competition within the present system. HMOs could be public, private, profit, or nonprofit. They could be built upon group medical practice or individual practices with an overseer body. The form is not rigid; HMOs need only embody three basic elements: (1) integrated care of the whole person, (2) efficient incentives of competition, and (3) prepayment.

In addition to the Kaiser-Permanente Plan and Health Insurance Plan of Greater New York, other HMO-like organizations include the Group Health Cooperative of Puget Sound in Seattle, Washington, the Physicians' Association of Clackamas County of Portland, Oregon, and more recently the Harvard Community Health Plan, Boston, Massachusetts, and the Health Services Plan of Pennsylvania in Philadelphia. One widely publicized model, based on the experience of the Kaiser-Permanente program, separates health-care from sick-care.[10] The heart of this system is the health testing and referral service. Data are processed by computer, thus providing a basic sorting out for services to be rendered—health-care, preventive-maintenance, or sick-care.

Comprehensive Neighborhood Health Services Program

The concept of comprehensive health care at the neighborhood level is not new. District health centers and neighborhood health stations are built-in features of the health care systems of other countries where they work efficiently to serve all segments of the population. In the United States, it was traditionally the family physician who fulfilled this service. However, as the population has grown, shifting from rural to urban or suburban, and as the supply of family physicians in critical areas has dwindled, a vacuum has been created. To help solve this problem, Neighborhood Comprehensive Health Centers have been developed through the anti-poverty program of the Office of Economic Opportunity. These centers were designed expressly for the poor with the recognition that some way had to be found to break the vicious cycle of sickness and poverty. The Comprehensive Neighborhood Health Services Program has attempted to rectify the inadequate, inaccessible, impersonal, and fragmented services available to the millions who live in poverty or who are considered to be medically indigent.

Guidelines set up by the Office of Economic Opportunity (OEO) determined which communities would be eligible for funding. Communities were considered eligible when they were characterized by unemployment or underemployment, a large number of welfare recipients, poor housing, high incidence of disease, disability, infant mortality, crime and juvenile delinquency, and inadequate and inaccessible existing health services. A wide array of ambulatory services is offered to all eligible individuals and members of families at a single, conveniently located setting. These services include diagnosis and treatment, preventive health services, family planning, home care of the chronically ill and other home health services, rehabilitation services, dental care, and mental health services. Specialized services that cannot be provided at the center, such as inpatient hospital and highly specialized diagnostic procedures, are provided elsewhere.

Many centers have been developed where nurses are in the forefront as providers of primary care (see pp. 18, 38). Two centers which have gained wide recognition are cited as examples—Boston's Columbia Point Health Center,[11] and Chicago's Mile Square Health Center.[12] At Columbia Point patients, who come in without an appointment, are evaluated by the triage nurse, who handles many of the problems herself or makes appropriate referrals to a physician or another nurse. She also handles telephone calls from patients and determines what action is necessary. At Mile Square the nurse provides the entree to health care, serves as family health counselor, is responsible for follow-up of the patient in the center, the community, and the hospital, and coordinates the care process.

The OEO has helped to fund special health projects initiated by other community agencies (see page 18). For example, the visiting Nurse Society in Detroit, in collaboration with the Mayor's Committee for Human Resources and Development, initiated a maternal and child health center, which became known as the "Mom and Tots" center and offered comprehensive services to young mothers and their children, including prenatal care, family planning, day care, cooperative baby sitting, and sex education.[13]

The year 1974 was the last year of operation for the Office of Economic Opportunity. Plans for the systematic dismantling of the organization were drawn up and during the course of the year many OEO programs were placed under newly designated administrative units. The health programs under OEO were transferred to the Department of Health, Education, and Welfare, and many of the health services funded by OEO as demonstration projects have continued with support from other sources.

In addition to the OEO comprehensive neighborhood health services, other ambulatory health services to the poor have been provided through the maternity and infant care projects (see p. 152), children and youth projects (see p. 153), Volunteers in Service to America (VISTA), and through grass roots efforts of diverse community groups, such as the Salvation Army. In response to the need for better health care, these groups, by themselves or with help from others, have organized free clinics, offering services with "humanity and dignity and primary concern for the patient rather than the convenience of the provider."[14] Operating on a shoestring, they are usually staffed by volunteers, often socially conscious professional practitioners and students in the health sciences.

Home Care Programs

In recent years home care programs have assumed a prominent position in the delivery of health care. Although we tend to look upon these programs as another innovation in health care delivery, they have, in fact, existed in one form or another for quite some time. Initially the major purpose was to provide care for the sick poor in their homes. This was the motivating factor in the establishment of visiting nurse programs which began to appear in the nineteenth century. Indeed, for many years, visiting nurse programs were the sole providers of professional home health services. Then, in 1946, with the inception of a hospital-based home care program (Montefiore Hospital, New York), another purpose was served, namely, to extend hospital care to patients who were inappropriately hospitalized and could be cared for at home.[15] In today's context both of the foregoing purposes are accepted, and a new one has been added. Home care has become not merely a substitute for institutional care, but rather a vital preventive and therapeutic service in a system that seeks to provide appropriate care as needed, to the patient in his own home.

Home health services have grown rapidly with the advent of Medicare. The leading factors currently influencing the development of home care programs across the country may be identified as follows:

(1) continued rise in cost of hospital days;
(2) federal legislation such as the 1972 Social Security Act amendments;

(3) growing concern of third party payment groups (both government and voluntary) about the appropriate utilization of hospital beds;

(4) demand for accountability of health service providers by consumers through officially designated government agencies or voluntary groups;

(5) extension of government and voluntary third party payment coverage for home care services;

(6) continued emphasis on health maintenance, specific protection, early diagnosis, and treatment; and

(7) consumer demands for comprehensive health care.

A major change in the delivery of home health services has come about with the development of the *coordinated home care program*. In 1955, the Public Health Service and the Commission on Chronic Illness, in their joint study of home care programs, defined a coordinated home care program as "... one that is centrally administered, and that through coordinated planning, evaluation, and follow-up procedures provides for physician-directed medical, nursing, social, and related services to selected patients at home."[16] This aspect of health delivery offers an integrated service with a team approach organized to meet the health needs of selected patients. These multiple service programs have been designated under Medicare as "home health services" and are required to include nursing plus at least one additional service.

Coordinated home care programs may be organized and administered by any one of several sponsoring groups as follows:

(1) Building on their experience with home care, visiting nurse agencies have moved into the administration of coordinated home care programs; e.g.. the Detroit Visiting Nurse Association acts as the administering body of a coordinated home care program.[17] It contracts with numerous hospitals to establish units that seek out patients, develop the plan of treatment, and then refer those patients back to the Visiting Nurse Association for direct service.

(2) Using the Montefiore Hospital home care program as a model, other hospitals across the country have developed their own coordinated home care programs.

(3) Other agencies which have a total community outlook are getting involved in starting home care programs. Some are health departments; others are freestanding agencies such as the Home Care Association of Rochester and Monroe County, Inc. [18]

Advantages to patients under coordinated home care programs are summarized as follows:

(1) Patients often recover more comfortably and quickly in their own homes where they are more at ease than they are in the unfamiliar and regimented hospital milieu.

(2) Patients are assured continuity of needed care through a system that assists physicians to plan and arrange for the delivery of medical services outside the hospital.

(3) The prompt admission or transfer of patients to home care, when 24-hour professional nursing and other inpatient services are not needed, releases hospital beds for more acutely ill patients.

(4) The cost of providing home care services is about one-third the cost of inpatient care on a daily basis.

Emergency Health Services

Emergency health services are an essential component of the health care delivery system. The mounting toll from accidents and sudden heart failure have focused attention on the need to improve these services. "Today's inadequate emergency medical care accounts for a minimum 60,000 premature deaths annually, plus untold disability."[19] The general public and professional health care personnel must realize that the medical care provided during the first hour after onset of sudden illness or injury may be more important than the entire subsequent regimen of care. Emergency health services include accident prevention, first aid care, resuscitation measures, and disaster preparedness.

Numerous problems and deficiencies in emergency care have been identified. One major problem is apathy of the general public and insensitivity to the magnitude of the problem of accidental death and injury. Local political authorities have neglected their responsibility to provide optimal emergency medical services. Emergency departments of hospitals are overcrowded and archaic. Fundamental research in shock and trauma is inadequately supported. There is a lack of personnel trained in first aid, as well as trained personnel for the advanced techniques of cardiopulmonary resuscitation, childbirth, or other life-saving measures. Medical and health-related organizations have failed to join forces to apply knowledge already available to advance the treatment of trauma, or to educate the public and inform the responsible legislative bodies.

The federal government has recognized the problem and, through the Division of Emergency Health Services of the Public Health Service, has offered guidance and assistance to local communities in establishing emergency health care services. At the local level, coordinated community action is required for the establishment and maintenance of an emergency care program. In each community, lay and professional responsibilities should be centralized in a council on emergency services. This council would serve to coordinate the activities of the various agencies; for example, a council would coordinate teaching programs on basic and advanced first aid of the Red Cross, the medical self-help program of the Public Health Service, cardiopulmonary resuscitation of the American Heart Association, and others.

Peer Review

Among the Social Security amendments enacted by Congress in 1972 is one that provides a means for peer evaluation of patient care through the establishment of Professional Standards Review Organizations (PSRO). Representing the nation's practicing physicians (M.D. and D.O.), these PSROs are responsible for comprehensive and continuing review of services covered by Medicare and Medicaid. [20]

In order to qualify as a PSRO, an organization must be a nonprofit professional association, or a component thereof, which is made up of practicing physicians. These PSROs function in geographic areas designated by HEW. The Secretary of HEW must establish statewide professional standards review councils and appoint members to these councils.

In evaluating health care practices, PSROs pose the following questions:

(1) Are the services and items medically necessary?

(2) Does the quality of the services meet professionally recognized standards of health care?

(3) Could the services and items, provided in a hospital or other health care facility on an inpatient basis, be provided either more economically in another type of health facility or be provided on an outpatient basis and still be consistent with the provision of appropriate medical care?

Peer reviews initially will cover inpatient care, but eventually will be extended to cover ambulatory service, drug utilization, extended care facilities, and home health services. PSRO's chief control mechanism is economic, and it is indirect. If the PSRO considers services inappropriate or unnecessary, it can recommend that payment for services be suspended by Medicare or Medicaid. The law provides channels for appealing such decisions.

Though PSROs are physician-oriented and physician-controlled, sixteen months of experience in a program of peer review of patient care in Utah demonstrated the necessity for nurses to play a major role in the process. The Utah program has recognized the nurse's expertise in interpreting and coordinating the delivery of medical care services, as well as evaluating patient needs and assembling information for professional review. [21]

Nurse participation in peer review organizations was called for in a resolution passed at the ANA 1972 House of Delegates, as follows: that in every health care facility there be provision for nurses to participate in utilization review activites related to facilities, personnel and services, and other arrangements for monitoring health care practices. [22]

The National Health Service Corps

Under the Emergency Health Personnel Act of 1970, the National Health Service Corps was established to provide medical and health services directly to communities where such services are inadequate because of critical shortages in health manpower. (See Figure 11-1). Public Health Service commissioned officers and civil service personnel are assigned to local areas, and their salaries are paid directly by the federal government.

The National Health Service Corps, operating a short-range, limited program, is not meant to solve the problem of the nation's overall shortage of health personnel. It is an attempt to begin to redistribute nationally some of the scarce health manpower resources into shortage areas. NHSC hopes to stimulate local development of health care services by introducing a small number of health workers as a catalytic effect.

Established health groups in surrounding areas, for example, a county health department, a county medical society, a district nurses association, may take part in developing health care systems with "Corps" personnel, and, together with the local government, certify to the Corps that the personnel requested are needed. State and areawide comprehensive health planning agencies, regional medical programs, other health and welfare organizations, and community representatives, including consumers of health services, may also be involved.

The Corps attempts to match health personnel to particular locales. One of the goals of the Corps is to find ways to increase the number of communities where the health care workers become professionally and economically integrated and stay there on their own in the private or quasi-private sector. It hopes to develop incentives to induce top-quality people to stay beyond their two-year contracts and continue to meet the long overdue health requirements of people in underserviced parts of the country.

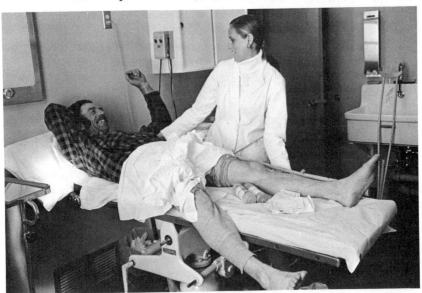

Figure 11-1 A National Health Service Corps nurse in Jackman, Maine, prepares a patient for the application of a full leg cast.

Source Reproduced by permission of the National Health Service Corps.

Consumer Involvement

One of the characteristics of the health centers funded through the Office of Economic Opportunity was the requirement that consumers participate in the health center program. A basic change was involved here, for the consumer was no longer regarded as a passive recipient of health care. He became involved as part of an organized group and had a voice in shaping policies that would ultimately affect him and the health care he would recieve.

Regarding consumer involvement, the National Health Council has stated the following principles:

WHY INVOLVE CONSUMERS?

Involvement of a person in determining the types of health services he will receive and how these should be provided is a contribution to human dignity and provides a sense of meaning and control of one's own life. . . .

Consumer involvement helps to find ways that health resources may be applied to meet health needs of the intended consumers with increasing effectiveness....

Consumer involvement helps to gain acceptance of priorities of need important to most persons affected by a health service and support for maintenance of a quality of performance that is usually effective . . .

Consumer involvement is a sound business practice for health organizations and professional societies . . .

Consumer "input" helps in recruitment of additional manpower for provision of health services. . . .

Involving consumers in health services planning and evaluation may contribute to minimizing the need for governmental intervention in the delivery of health services. . . .

Source   from National Health Council, Consumer Input—Why? (New York: The Council, 1972), pp. 5–7.

Patient's "Bill of Rights"

In the interest of "more effective patient care and greater satisfaction for the patient, his physician, and the hospital organization," the American Hospital Association has adopted a "Patient's Bill of Rights" as a national policy statement. Copies have been distributed to member hospitals throughout the country. The document indicates that it cannot guarantee the kind of treatment the patient has a right to expect in a hospital. It declares, however, that the hospital's functions of preventing and treating disease, educating members of health professions and patients, and conducting clinical research should all be conducted with an overriding concern for the patient, and above all, the recognition of his dignity as a human being.

THE PATIENT'S BILL OF RIGHTS

(1) The patient has the right to considerate and respectful care.

(2) The patient has the right to obtain from his physician complete current information concerning his diagnosis, treatment, and prognosis in terms the patient can be reasonably expected to understand.

(3) The patient has the right to receive from his physician information necessary to give informed consent prior to the start of any procedure and/or treatment . . . Where medically significant alternatives for care or treatment exist, or when the patient requests information concerning medical alternatives, the patient has the right to such information . . . (and) to know the name of the person responsible for the procedures and/or treatment.

(4) The patient has the right to refuse treatment to the extent permitted by law, and to be informed of the medical consequences of his action.

(5) The patient has the right to every consideration of his privacy concerning his own medical care program.

(6) The patient has the right to expect that all communications and records pertaining to his care should be treated as confidential.

(7) The patient has the right to expect that within its capacity a hospital must make reasonable response to the request of a patient for services.

(8) The patient has the right to obtain information as to any relationship of his hospital to other health care and educational institutions insofar as his care is concerned . . . (and) any professional relationships among individuals, by name, who are treating him.

(9) The patient has the right to be advised if the hospital proposes to engage in or perform human experimentation affecting his care or treatment . . . (and) has the right to refuse to participate.

(10) The patient has the right to expect reasonable continuity of care.

(11) The patient has the right to examine and receive an explanation of his bill regardless of source of payment.

(12) The patient has the right to know what hospital rules and regulations apply to his conduct as a patient.

REFERENCES

1. Jessie M. Scott, R.N., Assistant Surgeon General; Director, Division of Nursing, Public Health Service, Department of Health, Education, and Welfare, from a speech at the Pennsylvania League for Nursing Annual Meeting, April 3-5, 1972, Hershey, Pa.

2. Casey Crawford (ed.), *National Health Insurance Reports,* Washington, D.C., vol. 4, no. 1 (January 14, 1974).

3. I.S. Falk, member of the executive committee, Committee for National Health Insurance. As quoted in *National Health Insurance Reports,* Washington, D.C., vol. 4, no. 11, (June 3, 1974).

4. Herman E. Hilleboe, "Public Health in the United States in the 1970s," *American Journal of Public Health,* 58 (September 1968) 1588-1610.

5. Howard J. Brown, "National Health Insurance—Some Vital Issues," *Nursing Outlook,* 19 (January 1971) 24-25.

6. Kathleen S. Cavalier, *National Health Insurance Issue Brief Number IB 73015* (Washington, D.C.: Library of Congress, Congressional Research Service, April 29, 1975), p. 3. Kay Cavalier and Richard Price, *National Health Insurance: A Summary of Major Legislative Proposals Introduced into the 93rd Congress.* (Washington, D.C.: Library of Congress, Congressional Research Service, April 12, 1974), *passim.*

7. Ibid.

8. Casey Crawford, ed. *National Health Insurance Reports,* 2814 Pennsylvania Avenue, N.W., Washington, D.C. Vol. 4, no. 10, May 20, 1974, p. 1; vol. 5, no. 13, July 7, 1975, p. 10.

9. Walter McClure, "National Health Insurance and HMOs," *Nursing Outlook,* 21 (January 1973) 44-48.

10. Sidney R. Garfield, "The Delivery of Medical Care," *Scientific American,* 222(4) (April 1970) 15-23.

11. Ann Stokes, David Banta, and Samuel Putnam, "The Columbia Point Health Association: Evolution of a Community Health Board," *American Journal of Public Health,* 62 (September 1972) 1229-34.

12. Iris R. Shannon, "Nursing Service at the Mile Square Health Center of Presbyterian-St. Luke's Hospital," *American Journal of Public Health,* 60 (September 1970) 1726-32.

13. Nancy Milio, "Project in a Negro Ghetto," *American Journal of Nursing,* 67 (May 1967) 1006-9.

14. Irene R. Turner, "Free Health Centers: A New Concept?" *American Journal of Public Health,* 62 (October 1972) 1348-53.

15. E.M. Bluestone, et al., *Home Care: Origin, Organization, and Present Status of the Extra-Mural Program of Montefiore Hospital* (New York: Montefiore Hospital, 1949).

16. U.S. Department of Health, Education, and Welfare, Public Health Service, *Home Care, What It Is* (Washington, D.C.: Government Printing Office, 1966, reprinted 1967), p. 1.

17. S. Peabody, "The Home Care Program of the Detroit Visiting Nurse Association," *American Journal of Public Health,* 51 (November 1961) 1681-87.

18. Dorothy Watts White, "A Community-Based Home Care Program," *Hospitals,* 37, Feburary 1, 16, 1963.

19. U.S. Department of Health, Education, and Welfare, "Proceedings of Second National Conference on Emergency Health Services, December 2-4, 1971," Division of Emergency Health Services.

20. "PSRO," *Pennsylvania Medicine,* 76 (3) (March 1973) 35-37.

21. *The American Nurse,* The Official Newspaper of the American Nurses' Association, 5 (3) (March 1973).

22. Ibid.

ADDITIONAL READINGS

National Concern about Health Care

Breslow, Lester. "Role of the American Public Health Association in the Decade Ahead," in *American Journal of Public Health,* 58 (September 1968) 1611-19.

Brown, Douglas R., "Community Health Planning or Who Will Control the Health Care System?" in *American Journal of Public Health,* 62 (October 1972) 1336-39.

Burns, Eveline M., "Policy Decisions Facing the United States in Financing and Organizing Health Care," in *Public Health Reports,* 81 (August 1966) 681 ff.

Citizens' Board of Inquiry into Health Services for Americans. *Heal Yourself.* 2nd ed., rev. Washington, D.C.: American Public Health Association, 1972.

Cohen, Wilbur J., "What Makes an Effective National Health Program?" in *American Journal of Nursing,* 72 (October 1972) 1828-30.

Committee on the Costs of Medical Care, *Medical Care for the American People.* Final Report of the Committee. Chicago: University of Chicago Press, 1932.

Echeveste, Dolores W., and John L. Schlacter. "Marketing: A Strategic Framework for Health Care," in *Nursing Outlook,* 22 (June 1974) 377-81.

Hilleboe, Herman E., "Preventing Future Shock: Health Developments in the 1960s and Imperatives for the 1970s," in *American Journal of Public Health,* 62 (February 1972) 136-45.

Interdepartmental Committee To Coordinate Health and Welfare Activities, Technical Committee on Medical Care, *The Need for a National Health Program.* Washington, D.C.: The Committee, 1938.

Jeffers, James, and Mario F. Bognanno, "Medical Economics: An Introduction," in *Inquiry,* 7 (March 1970) 4-14.

Kerr, Lorin, "The Poverty of Affluence," in *American Journal of Public Health,* 65 (January 1975) 17-20.

Kisch, Arnold I., "Planning for a Sensible Health Care System," in *Nursing Outlook,* 20 (October 1972) 640-42.

Leininger, Madeleine, "An Open Health Care System Model," in *Nursing Outlook,* 21 (March 1973) 171-75.

Moxley, John, "The Predicament in Health Manpower." *American Journal of Nursing,* 68 (July 1968) 1486-90.

National Commission on Community Health Services, *Health Is a Community Affair.* Cambridge: Harvard University Press, 1966.

National Urban Coalition, *RX for Action.* Washington, D.C.: The Coalition, 1970.

United States President's Commission on the Health Needs of the Nation, *Building America's Health.* Washington, D.C.: Government Printing Office, 1967-68.

National Health Insurance Proposals

Bodenheimer, Thomas S., "The Hoax of National Health Insurance," in *American Journal of Public Health,* 62 (October 1972) 1324–27.

"The Comprehensive Health Insurance Plan," in *Nursing Outlook,* 22 (April 1974) 248–50.

Gorman, Mike, "The Impact of National Health Insurance on Delivery of Health Care," in *American Journal of Public Health,* 61 (May 1971) 962–71.

Silver, George A., "National Health Insurance, National Health Policy and the National Health," in *American Journal of Nursing,* 71 (September 1971) 1730–34.

Wolfe, Samuel, "Health Care for the Poor: When Oh When?" in *American Journal of Public Health,* 62 (October 1972) 1313–14.

Emerging Patterns and Innovations in Health Care

Amenta, Madalon, "Free Clinics Change the Scene," in *American Journal of Nursing,* 74 (February 1974) 284-88.

ANA Division on Community Health Nursing Practice, "HMO Statement—Nursing in Health Maintenance Organization," in *American Journal of Nursing,* 73 (November 1973) 1925.

Annas, George J., and Joseph Healey, "The Patient Rights Advocate," in *Journal of Nursing Administration,* 4 (May-June 1974) 25-31.

Bates, Barbara, "Nursing in a Health Maintenance Organization—Report on the Harvard Community Health Plan," in *American Journal of Public Health,* 62 (July 1972) 991-94.

Billings, Gloria, "NHSC Carries Health Care to the Community," in *American Journal of Nursing,* 72 (October 1972) 1836-38.

Callow, Betty M., "An R.N.'s View of the Health Maintenance Organization," in *Journal of Nursing Administration,* 3 (September-October 1973) 39-41.

Campbell, John, "Working Relationships between Providers and Consumers in a Neighborhood Health Center," in *American Journal of Public Health,* 61 (January 1971) 97-103.

Chapman, Larry S., "The Neighborhood Health Center Foundation for Health Care: A Portend for the Future or a Necessity for Survival?" in *American Journal of Public Health,* 63 (October 1973) 841-45.

Collen, Frances Bobbie, Blanche Madero, Krikor Soglukian, and Sidney R. Garfield, "Kaiser-Permanente Experiment in Ambulatory Care," in *American Journal of Nursing,* 71 (July 1971) 1371-74.

DeGeyndt, Willy, and Betty J. Hallstrom, "The Role of the Nurse in a Comprehensive Health Care Services Delivery Structure," in *Journal of Nursing Administration,* (July-August 1971) 8-16.

Dustan, Laura, "Community Health Services—Forward Planning." in *Community Health—Strategies for Change* (New York: National League for Nursing, 1973).

Ellwood, Paul M., "Concept, Organization, and Strategies of HMOs," in *Journal of Nursing Administration,* 3 (September–October 1973) 29–34.

Gold, Harold, Marjorie Jackson, Barbara Sachs, and Margie J. Van Meter, "Peer Review—A Working Experiment," in *Nursing Outlook,* 21 (October 1973) 634–36.

Gray, Pat Perry, "National Health Service Corps Teams Filling Health Manpower Void," in *Health Services Reports,* 87 (June-July 1972) 479-90.

Hanlon, John J., "Emergency Medical Services—New Program for Old Problem," in *Health Services Reports,* 88 (March 1973) 205-12.

Harding, Elizabeth, Charlene Harrington, Gloria Jean Manor, "The Berkeley Free Clinic," in *Nursing Outlook,* 21 (January 1973) 40-43.

Hess, Gertrude, "Broadening Our Approach to Emergency Nursing Care," in *Nursing Clinics of North America,* 5 (December 1970) 599-607.

"HMOs—A Special Section" (collection of articles on HMOs), in *Public Health Reports,* 90 (March-April 1975) 99–112.

Kramer, Marlene, "The Consumer's Influence on Health Care," in *Nursing Outlook,* 20 (September 1972) 574-78.

Levin, Lowell S., "Time To Hear a Different Drum," in *American Journal of Nursing,* 72 (November 1972) 2007–10.

Mengers, Gunnar, "How's the Health Service Corps Doing?" in *RN,* 35 (September 1972) 46-49.

Milio, Nancy, "Dimensions of Consumer Participation and National Health Legislation," in *American Journal of Public Health,* 64 (April 1974) 357-63.

Miller, Albert G., "Health Care Delivery—Changing Patterns," in *Organizational*

Behavior—Conflict and Its Resolution. New York: National League for Nursing, 1974.

Mulligan, Joan E., "There's an HMO in Your Future: Is Your Future in the HMO?" in *Journal of Nursing Administration,* 3 (September-October 1973) 35-38.

Munier, Sandra, and Aldean Richardson, "Development of New Nursing Roles in a Comprehensive Health Center," in *Journal of Nursing Administration,* 4 (July-August 1974) 44-49.

Murphy, Donna, and Eleanor Dineen, "Nursing by Telephone," in *American Journal of Nursing,* 75 (July 1975) 1137-39.

Murphy, Stephen P., "San Diego Plan for Emergency Services," in *American Journal of Nursing,* 72 (September 1972) 1615-19.

Myers, Beverlee A., *Health Maintenance Organizations: Objectives and Issues.* Washington, D.C.: Government Printing Office, 1972 (HSM 73-13002: 1-7).

Nicholls, Marion E., "Quality Control in Patient Care," in *American Journal of Nursing,* 74 (March 1974) 456-59.

O'Boyle, Catherine, "A New Era in Emergency Services," in *American Journal of Nursing,* 72 (August 1972) 1392-97.

Orme, June Y., and Rosemary S. Lindbeck, "Nurse Participation in Medical Peer Review," in *Nursing Outlook,* 22 (January 1974) 27-30.

Policy Statement (Working Draft), "Nursing in Health Maintenance Organizations," in *American Nurses' Association, Executive Committee of the Division on Community Health Nursing Practice* (April 1972).

Quinn, Nancy K., and Anne R. Somers, "The Patient's Bill of Rights: A Significant Aspect of the Consumer Revolution," in *Nursing Outlook,* 22 (April 1974) 240-44.

Ramphal, Marjorie, "Peer Review," in *American Journal of Nursing,* 74 (January 1974) 63-67.

Roemer, Ruth, "Legal Regulation of Health Manpower in the 1970s," in *HSMHA Health Reports,* 86 (December 1971) 1053-63.

Romano, Teresa, "Trauma Nurse Specialist," in *American Journal of Nursing,* 73 (June 1973) 1008-11.

Ryder, Claire F., "In-Home Care—Towards a National Policy and Strategy," from *Community Health—Strategies for Change.* New York: National League for Nursing, 1973.

Saward, Ernest W., *The Relevance of Prepaid Group Practice to the Effective Delivery of Health Services.* Washington, D.C.: Government Printing Office, 1972.

Slater, Reda R., "Triage Nurse in the Emergency Department," in *American Journal of Nursing,* 70 (January 1970) 127-29.

Story, Donna, "A Mock Disaster on a Rural Road," in *American Journal of Nursing,* 72 (December 1972) 2222-24.

Swan, Lionel F., "Group Approach to Medical Care," in *Nursing Outlook,* 18 (January 1970) 56-57.

U.S. Department of Health, Education, and Welfare, *Accidental Death and Disability: The Neglected Disease of Modern Society.* Washington, D.C.: Government Printing Office, 1970, (Public Health Service Publication 1071-A-13).

U.S. Department of Health, Education, and Welfare, Community Health Services, *Selected Annotated Bibliography on Health Maintenance Organizations.* Washington, D.C.: Government Printing Office, May 1971.

Wagner, Doris L., "Issues in the Provision of Health Care for All," in *American Journal of Public Health,* 63 (June 1973) 481-85.

Waller, Julian A., "Rural Emergency Care—Problems and Prospects," in *American Journal of Public Health,* 63 (July 1973) 631-34.

Waterhouse, A.M., et al., *A Study of Selected Home Care Programs.* Public Health Monograph 35. Washington, D.C.: Government Printing Office, 1955 (Public Health Service Publication 447).

Waters, John M., "Jacksonville's Emergency System," in *American Journal of Nursing,* 72 (July 1972) 1289.

Welch, Cathryne A., "Health Care Distribution and Third Party Payment for Nurses' Services," in *American Journal of Nursing,* 75 (October 1975) 1844-47.

UNIT IV
NURSING INTERVENTION
IN THE COMMUNITY

Chapter 12
Care of the Patient and the Family in the Home Setting

"Public health nurses have long believed that the family is the unit of community nursing service; there is nothing new about this concept."[1]

INTRODUCTION

The concept of nursing and community health nursing was discussed in Chapter 3. We subscribe to the prevailing philosophy of nursing that recognizes the person as a unified whole—who exists as an individual and as a member of a family within a community. We also hold to the philosophy that nursing is family centered. The family as the unit of service has always been a working model in community health nursing agencies, where we find that services are family centered and they are documented in family records. The realization has grown that professional nursing practice in any health care setting requires expertise in family nursing. Indeed, if it is to move ahead in an independent way and not exist merely as an ancillary to medicine, nursing must broaden its responsibility to include the family in providing care to the patient. Thus, as a practitioner of nursing, in any setting—hospital, school, clinic, industry, physician's office—you will find that you cannot plan effective nursing care unless you consider the individual patient in relation to his family. Nowhere is this more evident than in caring for the patient in his own home. Unlike other health care settings, where family members may or may not be present, the home is a place where the family is a visible entity which must be taken into consideration in the overall plan of care.

The home presents a whole new set of circumstances and conditions that are totally unlike those encountered in the traditional hospital setting. When you are providing "nursing service without walls"[2] you step out beyond the protective environment of the hospital and meet the patient on his own "turf." You present yourself in a new, free-flowing situation in unfamiliar surroundings, without the built-in institutional controls of the hospital. In the hospital setting, the practitioner of nursing is confronted by the "patient in the bed" who is assigned to a medical diagnostic category. The patient's plan of care depends upon (1) the prescribed medical treatment, (2) his general needs such as food, warmth, and restorative therapy, and (3) hospital policies. In many instances the climate for care is established according to the "doctor's orders," and nursing service is provided to the patient in conformance with hospital rules. Organization of treatment schedules around the daily hospital routine leaves little incentive for family and patient participation in the plan of care. The services that are offered may be helped or hindered by the presence or absence of the family. Family members may spend most of the day with the patient, or in some cases, they may never appear during the entire hospitalization.

Without participation of the family, can traditional hospital routines and practices really prepare a patient for a return to health? To what avail is the prescribed institutional regimen if it is unable to alter the factors in the patient's way of living that had necessitated his hospitalization in the first place? Consider, for example, the alcoholic victim who has been hospitalized for acute pancreatitis. During a lengthy hospitalization period, he receives expert medical and nursing care. His disease process has been arrested, and he has been sent back into the community in "good health." He returns to his home in a neighborhood where there is a bar on every corner, and drinking is a way of life. Through the use of outreach services, an attempt must be made to involve the family in helping the patient alter his life style. If not, the technologically superb hospital care he has received will have been to no avail.

Recognizing the need for more family involvement in the patient's treatment program, some hospitals have changed their routine. They have extended visiting hours and encouraged families to take a more active role in the patient's nursing care and medical therapy. In those institutions where policies have become more flexible, the nurse has greater opportunity to talk with patients and their families, to interpret the treatment, and to explain plans for follow-up care. Thus, when the patient is ready to be discharged, the family may be better prepared to continue the plan of care in the home setting.

WHAT IS A FAMILY?

In this chapter we will describe the family as the basic unit of society and we will discuss the family forces and interactions that influence the health needs of its members. We will also point out how as nurses we must relate this knowledge to our plan of care. To begin with, what is a family? Let us review some basic concepts about the family that have been derived from the social sciences:

(1) The family is a collection of individuals who form a primary group. As such, they should be viewed in the context of group behavior.

(2) The family is the basic unit of a society.

(3) The family is the main unit of the social system and the agency for the transmission of cultural values.

(4) The family is the most important medium for the development of its members—it is a potent force in promoting their health or in generating their illness.

(5) The family group dwells in a particular geographic location, which may influence the family structure and function.

The family, as a social institution, has existed from the beginning of time in every corner of the world. It is the most stable, enduring, and universal cultural form. There is historical evidence that entire civilizations have survived or disappeared depending on the strength or weakness of family life. Family life style and behavior are profoundly influenced by the economic and political shifts in our society. The industrialization of society brought forth new jobs and monetary rewards, providing a stimulus for people to "get away from the farms." The Industrial Revolution, in effect, hastened the passing of the joint family system and the emergence of the nuclear family system. This type of family organization—married man and woman with offspring living in a common household—is the predominant form in western society. However, the traditional, patriarchal nuclear family of the early twentieth century has undergone further change especially since the end of the second world war.

There are many variations of the traditional nuclear family, some of which we are listing here. Most people move through several family structures in their lifetime. Often there is overlapping, and the divisions outlined here are not always clear cut.

VARIATIONS OF THE TRADITIONAL NUCLEAR FAMILY STRUCTURE

(1) Husband and wife

Early years (establishing the household)—childless; expectant parents; with first child; with growing children (infant, preschool, school age).

Early middle years—childless; with dependent children (all ages, some now entering adolescence or young adulthood).

Later middle years—childless or no children living at home; children living at home (young adults—dependent, self-supporting, or supporting their parents).

Late years—childless or no children living at home; adult children living at home—dependent, self-supporting, or supporting their parents; dependent or independent members of a three-generation household.

(2) Single parent—widowed; separated, divorced, or deserted; out-of-wedlock
   (a) living alone with one or more dependent children;
   (b) living in a three-generation household.

(3) Single adult living alone
    (a) independent young adult with or without ties to a nuclear family;
    (b) single parent whose children have become independent; or
    (c) aging adult—never married, widow or widower, childless or children with their own households.

Old established values, associated with a sense of family solidarity and stability, have been assaulted from all directions by many forces. Scholars and scientific observers of the contemporary scene feel that the nation is undergoing a social revolution which erupted with the violence of the 1960s. The disruptive events and turbulent changes that followed have left their mark on all social institutions, especially the family. We refer to events such as the riots, confrontations, and demonstrations; the nationwide frustration, bitterness, and polarity that gained momentum in the wake of the controversial military commitment in southeast Asia; the upsurge in the use of dangerous drugs, including alcohol; spiraling and uncontrolled inflation; "credibility gap" with national problems such as the energy crisis; and the "Watergate" affair.

ALTERNATE LIFE STYLES

Family identity and kinship have been challenged by the current quest for self-fulfillment and the pursuit of individual happiness. In highly individualistic ways, people are making their own decisions about when and whom to marry, or not to marry at all. (See page 146.) This approach to life has fostered greater permissiveness, which has led to experimentation with new life styles. Many of these modes of living do not conform to traditional societal norms and have not been sanctioned by contemporary social institutions. Nevertheless, we must recognize that communal living, group marriage, homosexual and heterosexual cohabitation, and other variant family forms are a reality and exist side by side with the traditional nuclear family. All these family groups have one thing in common—at some time or other, health problems are bound to arise, and nursing intervention may be required. The nurse who can operate with a nonjudgmental approach is better equipped to evaluate the strengths and weaknesses in any family group. The formulation of an effective family-centered plan of care should not be contingent upon the nurse's approval or disapproval of the particular lifestyle she may encounter.

EXAMPLE

    Put yourself into the following situation. A visiting nurse service received a request to teach a family member to administer a narcotic every four hours as needed to a fifty-five-year-old man in the terminal stage of cancer. The information from the referring agency stated that he lived alone but that there were family members in the area. As the nurse in the district, you made contact with a family member to arrange a meeting in the patient's home. The response was "Don't ask me to help my father; he walked out on my mother years ago." Upon entering the home on your first visit, you discovered that the patient was not living alone. You were greeted at the door by a middle-aged woman who apologized for the appearance of the home and stated she had been injured in an auto accident and was recuperating. You assumed that she was the patient's present wife, and you proceeded to address her as Mrs. Smith. She promptly informed you that "I am not Mrs. Smith, but we've been together for the last five years and we're very happy." Obviously this couple has chosen, without any pretense, to "flaunt" the "socially accepted" rules of behavior. Their life style might offend you if you have been brought up according to certain social and religious standards. Certainly the man's family had turned against him, and, even though he was dying, would have nothing to do with him. Nevertheless, you must operate in a nonjudgmental way and determine the strengths in the relationship between the two persons in this household. As it turned out, there were many strengths—the woman was a warm and compassionate person who was committed to the well-being of the patient. Working together, you were able to set up an effective nursing plan with realistic goals. The woman willingly assumed the responsibility of learning to take care of the patient and to help alleviate the pain that accompanied his illness.

The nurse, in planning health care with the family, whether traditional or otherwise, must take into consideration the adaptability of the individuals within the group and examine their commitment to the group as a whole.

EXAMPLE

Let us say that you are a visiting nurse going in to care for a patient paralyzed as the result of a motor vehicle accident, one of our most common public health problems. The patient's treatment calls for range of motion, skin care, and positioning every two hours throughout the day and evening. This patient may be part of a traditional nuclear family, or he may be a member of a motorcycle gang living in a commune, or a single parent with several dependent children. As the nurse, you must identify the degree of commitment of the group members toward the injured person. If you expect to establish a realistic plan of care, you must determine who in the group seems most amenable to accepting the responsibility for carrying out the treatment program. Is he or she physically and mentally capable of performing these tasks? Are other members of the family group willing to assist by assuming part of the responsibility?

FAMILY ROLES

In any family group, traditional or experimental, the roles of its constituent members are an integral part, if not the determining factor, of the overall living pattern. What do we understand by "role," and how is the knowledge of role theory useful for effective nursing intervention? Let us review some basic concepts about role. Sargent describes an individual's role as the patterns or types of social behavior that seem to him to be appropriate in a given situation, in view of the demands and expectations of those in his group.[3] Various definitions of role have been set forth by students and scholars in the behavioral sciences. Certain common elements emerge as follows:

(1) Role may be viewed as a set of behavior patterns;
(2) These behavior patterns are learned through the process of socialization;
(3) A role does not exist in isolation;
(4) Role implies status or position;
(5) Status or position is characterized by a set of expected behaviors.

An individual in society plays many roles. A man is a father to his children, but he is a son to his parents. He is a consumer of services, a provider of economic security for his family, and a citizen in the political system. An individual acts out his role in a given situation, and he expects certain reciprocal action from the other persons, based on prescribed role expectations. If he perceives that his behavior has not evoked the expected response, he may experience role strain. He may or may not alter his role, depending on the amount of disequilibrium created by the situation.

EXAMPLE

Let us say that an elderly woman moves into her married daughter's home and at times communicates in a manner reminiscent of a former relationship where she, the grandmother, was the mother of the household. The daughter can maintain a homeostatic relationship by subtly shifting her role relationships, responding when the need arises, as child to her mother, while maintaining her role relationships as wife to her husband and mother to her own children.

You will have a better understanding of family dynamics, if you are familiar with role theory. As you begin to work with families, you must develop an inquiring mind, seeking answers to questions which will help you sort out role relationships. How are decisions made in the family group? Who handles the money? Where does responsibility lie for family discipline? What are the family's priorities and who sets them? Who is the mother figure? the father figure? What is the feeling tone of the family group in general? These are questions through which you may discover some of the subtle forces operating within the family group. An astute nurse with a working knowledge of role relationships was able to circumvent the pitfalls in the following situation by reevaluating the family dynamics and identifying the major decisionmaker.

EXAMPLE

The nurse was called in to care for a seventy-five-year-old woman who was recovering from a stroke that left her with some weakness of the left side. Her physical and functional abilities were affected to a degree that she required retraining in the following areas: stair climbing; bathing, dressing, and grooming; bladder control; standing balance; self-feeding activities. The patient, Mrs. T., eager to regain her former independence, understood and accepted the rationale of the care plan. Six months earlier, her husband had died. Following his death, Mrs. T. had continued to maintain her own home, which she shared with her forty-year-old unmarried daughter. This daughter held a responsible position in a local firm, which required frequent travel and long hours away from home. The nurse's only contact with Miss T. was by phone. Another daughter, Mrs. Q., who lived nearby, came in daily to help her mother with her exercises, and to prepare the noon meal for her. It was this daughter, and, of course, the patient herself, with whom the nurse worked out the plan of care.

Within a short time, the patient began to walk independently with the aid of a straight cane; she had established a satisfactory degree of bladder control; she was largely independent in her bathing, dressing, grooming, and feeding activities; and she was ready to begin stair climbing. At this point, the agency began to receive frantic calls from Miss T. (Figure 12-1) demanding immediate help for her mother. "My mother is a sick woman; she can't take care of herself; someone's got to come, and give her a bath, and feed her; she's wetting the bed at night, and she needs her catheter back in." The district nurse, knowing that the patient was doing well, and puzzled by this report, made an unscheduled visit. Upon entering the home, she found the elderly Mrs. T. in tears, and her daughter, Mrs. Q., visibly upset and making rash statements, such as "I don't think I'll be coming any more; somebody else will have to look after my mother; nothing I do pleases my sister." As the nurse continued to listen to the complaints, she began to realize that the major decisionmaker was neither the patient nor the daughter who provided most of her care. It became obvious that the "invisible" daughter was the family member who made all the major decisions, but had never involved herself in the plan of care. After careful consideration of all the factors, the nurse scheduled a family conference at a time when Miss T. could be present. Goals were redefined, and some minor changes were made which were acceptable to all. The patient continued to move toward independent living.

When working with a family which is attempting to cope with the illness of one of its members, we as nurses must be aware that the family may assign us a role they perceive as being abdicated by another member. This may be the role of any member of the family, sick or well, present or absent. In the case of the elderly stroke victim just cited, it is possible that Mrs. T. and Mrs. Q., left

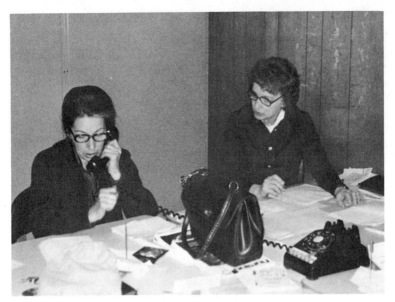

Figure 12-1   A frantic call "My Mother is a sick woman . . ."

on their own because of Miss T.'s continued absence from the home, had assigned her role to the nurse. There are other situations where family members assign roles in more obvious ways. For example, if the mother becomes ill, the children may look to the nurse as a mother surrogate. If the husband becomes ill, the wife may look to the nurse for guidance in decisions formerly made by the husband. Nursing intervention will be more effective in such situations if we understand this type of role transference and continue to identify our own role in the overall health care plan.

HEALTH AS A FAMILY VALUE

In working with families, you will be seeking answers to questions such as: what is their concept of health? where do they place health in their order of priorities? For instance, do they have a plan for medical care? Are they covered by health insurance? If so, does it include preventive health services? What are their health practices? What is their form of recreation? Does it include physical activity and exercise? When do they seek medical help—on a routine, periodic basis? for crisis care only? Do they take their children in for immunizations? Are the immunization schedules current? Do they keep a record of immunizations? What part of the food budget goes for highly nutritious foods as compared with less nutritious sweets and treats? Will the television repair come ahead of Jackie's new glasses and Amy's dental work? A family's values with regard to health may not coincide with your values. This you must take into consideration, and look for family strengths upon which to build, if you wish to succeed in establishing realistic goals for family health care.

EXAMPLE

> You have been called in to plan nursing care for an elderly woman who had been hospitalized with a diagnosis of myocardial infarction. She has just returned home from the hospital and is on anticoagulant therapy. She lives with her son and daughter-in-law and their three young children, ages two, three and one-half, and five. During your family assessment, you observe that the middle child walks with a decided limp. In planning the total family health care, you include a counseling session with the parents of this child. In speaking to them about their child's defective gait, you realize that neither of the parents has ever recognized that this is a health problem requiring medical evaluation. "Oh, yes, we've noticed that, but he's still pretty young, and we're sure he'll outgrow it when he starts to walk better." In addition, you find that the children's immunization program is incomplete. "Oh, well, they got most of their shots when they were babies, but they haven't been sick and we've had no need for a doctor until just now when Mom had her heart attack."

Do you begin to form an impression about this family's health values? It would appear they they do not equate their child's defective gait with ill health, and they might not readily accept an immediate recommendation for orthopedic evaluation. What is your approach in this situation? Certainly you will be looking for the positive aspects and the strengths in this family. You observe a loving relationship among family members. The children are well nourished and are protected from environmental hazards. The young parents are concerned about their mother's illness and they fully participate in her plan of care. They come to accept you as a skilled provider of care, and to respect your judgment in matters related to the "sick" member of the family. The family's confidence in your ability grows, and you become their health consultant. With patience, skill, and proper timing, you may be able to help them change their attitude and behavior so that they will seek appropriate health care for their children. You will be more likely to function as a "change agent" if you demonstrate, by your actions, that you respect the values and that you recognize the strengths of the families with whom you work.

Many forces help to shape a family's attitude toward health—social and ethnic background, traditions handed down from earlier generations, environmental conditions and community influences, level of education, and economic status are but a few. An individual's or family's concern for health is often secondary to the achievement of the primary needs—food, shelter, sex drive. Concern may not be shown until the physical or mental condition of a family member becomes impaired and the achievement of primary goals is threatened.

EXAMPLE

> Let us look at the man in his early middle years who is overweight and overfed, gets little or no exercise, smokes excessively, and holds a demanding job where tension never lets up. Alert and well-informed, he is intellectually aware that he is a high-risk candidate for a coronary attack. However, he takes no steps to alter his way of living. He is much too busy, trying to make ends meet for himself, his wife, and four young children. He suffers a coronary attack that sends him to the intensive care unit, and he requires a prolonged period of treatment for recovery. During this time he realizes that he is facing a crisis whereby his achievement of primary goals is threatened, and he is now willing to consider the necessary changes in his life style that will enable him to go on providing for himself and his family.

ILLNESS AS A FAMILY "CRISIS"

The situation we have just described depicts a man who has been faced with a crisis, precipitated by illness. Illness, generally, is a crisis-producing event in the life of an individual. In family nursing practice, you see the individual as a member of a family, and you view his illness within the context of the family system. What happens in a family when illness strikes one of its members? Does the illness constitute a crisis for the family as it does for the individual? How are the activities of the family affected? How does the family react to the situation? What factors determine their behavior? How well do they respond to the total needs of their afflicted member? These are the kinds of questions you should consider as you begin to look at the family dynamics in relation to the crisis of illness. To interpret these dynamics, you need a working knowledge of crisis theory. The considerable body of literature on crisis theory provides a frame of reference for nursing practice. Let us review some of the basic concepts and see how they might be applied to family nursing.

To begin with, what do we mean by "crisis"? Miller defines crisis as the "experiencing of an acute situation where one's repertoire of coping responses is inadequate in effecting a resolution of the stress."[4] Caplan defines crisis as a condition occurring "when a person faces an obstacle to important life goals that is, for a time, insurmountable through the utilization of customary methods of problem solving. A period of disorganization ensues, a period of upset, during which many abortive attempts at solution are made."[5] Two types of crises have been identified as follows: (1) normal, maturational crises, as defined by Erikson,[6] and (2) accidental or situational crises, as described by Caplan.[7] Crisis disrupts the dynamic equilibrium of a person, and brings about a shift in his homeostatic balance. There is a rise in inner tension, an increase in emotional discomfort, and a disorganization of functioning. To cope with these unpleasant manifestations, the person must instantly mobilize his defense mechanisms. His ability to select and utilize coping mechanisms effectively will depend on his previous life experiences, personality make-up, and environmental influences.

At times, the changes in the life situation of an individual are such that his usual methods of problem solving are inadequate. Faced with the "crisis" he either finds a way to reduce his conflict or he must adapt to a "nonsolution." In either case, some form of equilibrium must be restored. In seeking to restore equilibrium, the person may look to his family or significant others in his "life space" to come to his rescue. The problem-solving techniques utilized by a person facing a crisis may be modified in constructive ways through the intercession of family members or significant others during the resolution phase. The family's ability to respond to the affected member depends on several factors, as follows:

(1) the degree to which they recognize the existence of the crisis;
(2) their capacity to withstand stress and maintain balance;
(3) the degree to which they are able to organize effective coping mechanisms to deal with the disruption of the equilibrium.

Ackerman places great emphasis on the family's ability to act as a stabilizing force and to provide emotional support in times of stress. "In the meeting of new problems and crisis, some families are weakened and others grow in solidity and emotional strength. Some families grow and learn from experience; others seem unable to do so because they are too inflexible and tend to disintegrate."[8] Much of the family's response to stress is based on memories of past behavior. The adaptive mechanisms that resulted in restoration of family function in the past may be recalled and, if utilized, will probably have a positive result. If a supportive emotional framework exists within the family, the family members should be able to organize effective coping mechanisms in times of stress to help them adapt. Families may hinder the resolution of a crisis if they are ineffective in functioning as a family group. Poorly defined role structure, poor communication, and lack of a leadership figure contribute to family disorganization and hamper their ability to work together effectively.

When illness is the crisis-precipitating event, the way in which a family responds will be determined by the factors mentioned above, that is, recognition of the crisis, capacity to withstand stress, and ability to mobilize effective coping mechanisms. The family-oriented nurse will understand that family members react to the impact of illness in highly individual ways. She will evaluate the appropriateness and effectiveness of the behaviors selected by the family to meet the crisis of illness.

The nurse, recognizing that a crisis exists, tries to relieve the immediate tension-producing conditions and the threat of loss the patient is experiencing. At the same time she is concerned with the long-term effects of the crisis on the individual and the family. In planning her intervention, she must determine whether the patient and family also recognize that a crisis exists. When the patient or family avoids or denies the problem of illness, a barrier to effective nursing intervention may develop. This kind of avoidance behavior is not unusual when the crisis-precipitating event is one which does not cause immediate curtailment of daily activity.

EXAMPLE

Mrs. W. is a fifty-seven-year-old woman who lives in a modest, single dwelling in a middle-income suburban area. The mother of three grown sons, she was widowed at an early age and has been working for many years in a large, reputable, nationwide underwriters' firm. She supervises the work activities of twenty-five men and women. She is an outgoing person with considerable charm, well-liked by all her coworkers. Neat, attractive, and always well-groomed, Mrs. W. is moderately overweight, but watches her diet very closely and tries to control further weight gain. In addition to her business career, she maintains close ties with her children and grandchildren, leads an active social life, belongs to several philanthropic organizations, and is involved in various fund-raising activities.

Shortly before her scheduled annual physical examination, Mrs. W. begins to experience periods of drowsiness, excessive thirst, and a most uncomfortable vulvar pruritis. She develops a pronounced frequency of urination. An unusual craving for carbohydrates causes her to become careless about her normally well balanced diet. She adds doughnuts to her morning coffee break and rich desserts to her lunch. At about the same time, her coworkers notice a change in her behavior from a stable, well-organized pattern to an erratic, demanding, and unpredictable one. A trusted friend takes her aside, and urges her not to wait for her scheduled annual physical exam, but to report her symptoms immediately to the firm's occupational health nurse. Following the friend's suggestion, Mrs. W. consults the nurse. After an assessment of the patient's condition and symptoms, the nurse, suspecting maturity onset diabetes, suggests a postprandial blood sugar and a complete urinalysis. Mrs.W. agrees, and the tests are done. The nurse schedules Mrs. W. for a complete physical examination by the physician the next morning.

After her physical examination, Mrs. W. is informed that her blood sugar is 310 mg. percent, and the urinalysis report shows "4+ sugar, trace of acetone." The physician informs Mrs. W. that she has diabetes, maturity onset type, which can be managed with a carefully planned diet and weight control. He refers her back to the nurse for health counseling and diet instruction. Mrs. W. seems to accept the stated diagnosis; for the next several weeks she follows the therapeutic regimen. Her symptoms subside, and as she begins to feel better, she tells her closest friend, "You know that time you talked me into seeing the nurse, she and that doctor tried to tell me I had sugar diabetes. But I'm perfectly fine now, and I don't believe I ever had that in the first place." Soon Mrs. W. begins to disregard her dietary restrictions. Ignoring the counseling of the nurse who sees her periodically, Mrs. W. continues to deny the whole idea that she has a diabetic condition. Her daily pattern of living and her total life style are unchanged.

One morning as Mrs. W. is getting out of the shower, she feels a stabbing sensation in her left foot as though she had stepped on something sharp. When she looks down she notices that her left great toe has a small cut and is bleeding a little. She then recalls that on the previous evening she had dropped a bottle of shampoo on the bathroom floor, which she thought she had cleaned up thoroughly; but now she wonders if perhaps she had missed some small pieces of glass. She washes off her toe and tries to see or feel if there are any bits of glass under her skin. She even takes a needle and pokes around to try to dig them out. The bleeding stops and although her toe is painful she feels confident that all is well. She goes about her usual routine at work. Two days go by, the pain persists, and she notices that there is some redness and swelling on her toe that does not go away. On the third day, the inflammation comes to a head, and she "pops" it open, squeezing out some yellow suppurative material, along with bits of glass. She feels certain now that she has gotten rid of the problem. Three more days go by, and the pain gets worse. The redness and swelling do not subside, and she becomes concerned when she notices a red streak going up her leg. By this time, she is having difficulty in walking, and when she gets to work, she stops at the health unit for advice. The nurse examines Mrs. W.'s toe, elicits all the essential data, and realizes that the situation could be serious in view of the patient's history of diabetes. The nurse calls the physician aside, describes the urgency of the situation, and asks him to work Mrs. W. into his busy schedule of appointments, as she feels that there is a need for an immediate evaluation.

After examining Mrs. W., the physician informs her that she has a serious infection that is complicated by her uncontrolled diabetes, and that she must be hospitalized at once. A prolonged period of treatment and follow-up interrupts Mrs. W.'s full and busy life. During this time, she has ample opportunity to reflect on her situation. With the continued care of the physician, the counseling from the nurse, and the support of her other friends, she begins to accept her diabetic condition as a reality. She realizes for the first time that it is up to her to work along with the plan of treatment in order to control her diabetes, to maintain her health, and to continue to enjoy a fulfilling and active life.

PRINCIPLES OF SYSTEMS THEORY
APPLIED TO FAMILY HEALTH

As community nurses we must be aware of the family dynamics operating in illness and recognize that conflict within the group should not be viewed as a signal of complete disorganization. On the contrary, some sociologists feel that "a certain degree of conflict may actually help reinforce solidarity"[9] within the family system. "Like other institutions the family also may be described as a system of conflict management."[10] To interpret the forces working within the family, the nurse should observe how its members work together to manage the elements of conflict that feed into the system. As disharmony arises because of the additional responsibility of an ill member, the nurse must be alert to any change in the division of labor (wife assuming the role of breadwinner; husband taking on additional responsibilities of household maintenance), and monitor the level of functioning. If interpersonal relations within the system move toward disequilibrium, the nurse should be formulating alternative plans to relieve the growing tension.

Some families are able to survive extreme periods of stress, but the cost to their members' physical and mental health may be expensive. However, illness may not be the event that precipitates the family crisis. Other factors of long duration may be the primary source of disharmony among members. The degree of disruption of family life, which may appear to be caused by illness, should be carefully monitored over several visits before a plan of intervention is implemented. Input into the system by family members cannot be measured accurately without interviewing each individual. For example, if the father works during the day, the nurse should make some effort to see him at his place of employment if indicated, or visit the home on the father's day off. A guiding principle that the nurse must keep in mind when involved with family groups is that complete and accurate assessment is achieved through a planned interview with the total family group.

In formulating nursing care plans, we may consider the family within the framework of general systems theory. Systems analysis, which is based on probability theory and concepts, can be applied to the study of complex problems. "A whole which functions as a whole by virtue of the interdependence of its parts is called a system, and the method which aims at discovering how this is brought about . . . has been called general systems theory."[11] A system is a set of units or series of events that are functionally related to each other. It has a life history spread out over time and is made up of separate steps that occur in sequence. In this sequence each event "occurs when it does or how it does according to how or when the previous event in the sequence occurred, and this event in turn has a determining influence on how or when the next event occurs."[12] A system exists in an environment with identifiable physical, biological, and social characteristics, all of which will have an impact on how that system will function. The environment for any given system is the field of effective stimulation and interaction for the units of that system. In studying living, behavioral, or social systems, we find that it is difficult to differentiate between system and environment. "A system, together with its environment, makes up the totality of what is to be studied in a given situation, and the division into system and environment depends on the intention of the person studying the phenomena."[13]

In this context we can view the family as an open social system that receives input from the environment and depends on interaction with the environment for change. The family consists of interrelated "parts"—parents, siblings, and other family members—who interact with the environment. The environment is characterized by physical, biological, and social conditions that influence the family. As we look at the family in relation to the overall environment, we can begin to identify the factors of input, output, and feedback. Input is anything that enters the system from the environment and influences what happens next. Output is the end result of the operation of any part of the system and it goes out into the environment. Feedback is that portion of output that is fed back with the input and affects succeeding outputs.

Feedback may be positive or negative, depending on how it interacts with the system.

To illustrate how this may operate, let us say that you are the nurse assigned to a family with a recently diagnosed diabetic patient. The event of this illness has precipitated a crisis in the family. You are going to try to help the patient and the family understand and accept what it means to live with this condition, and what must be done to curb related potential hazards. All members of this family want to resolve the crisis and to help the patient regain and maintain optimal health. If you consider the family as a system functioning within its given environment, input may come from the plan of care that you formulate jointly with the members of the family. Let us say you have established a good relationship with the patient and the family, and you have effectively taught principles of positive health promotion. This is your input. As a result of your input, you will look for output in the form of certain expected behaviors from family members. Through their behavior, the patient and family demonstrate whether they can and will perform those functions that would help the stricken member to attain optimal health. For example, will the patient or some member of the family administer insulin? test urine routinely? apply principles of diet control? Will the patient take proper care of his skin and nails? take appropriate measures to prevent infection? follow up under medical supervision? Will the members of the family provide the emotional support needed in this time of crisis? Such outputs, when fed back into the system, are regarded as negative feedback, as the effects of the disease process are diminished. If the output, in the form of some identifiable behavior, is fed back into the system so that the effects of the disease process are increased, we regard this as positive feedback. If no output is fed back, and if there is no effect on the disease process, there is no feedback.

In this way we are able to perceive and understand the operative ongoing mechanisms through which balance is restored. The situation never remains static and is always changing. When balance is restored there is a new set of circumstances, objects, or events, so that the system changes, readjusts, and is something different from what it was before.

EXAMPLE

Let us look again at the T. Family, where the nurse was called in for help when the aging Mrs. T. was recovering from a stroke. Let us go back to the point six months earlier when Mr. T. passed away. The loss of the husband/father in this family disrupted the balance in the family "system," so that it became necessary for the other members to make adjustments in their pattern of living. The event of his passing may be regarded as "input" that influenced the behavior of his survivors. The children came together ("output") to comfort each other and to console their mother ("output," some of which was fed back into the system as negative feedback). Thus, through the support from her loved ones ("negative feedback") added to her own inner strength ("input"), Mrs. T.

was able, after a period of grieving, to pick up and go on. Her behavior may be regarded as output fed back as negative feedback with other inputs, which helped to restore balance to her family system. That is, she continued to maintain the home for herself and her daughter. Thus, though balance had been restored to the family system, the situation was no longer the same as it had been before. The system was once again disturbed when Mrs. T. became ill. Her illness might be regarded as input that brought about imbalance. When balance was restored with the help of the input of nursing intervention, the situation was again changed.

The systems approach to family nursing is an attempt to make the study of people scientific and meaningful. In applying systems theory, we are able to perceive wholes rather than parts—we can look at individuals and their families in their totality, as they exist on the health-illness continuum. The systems approach serves as a tool enabling us to determine, if not predict, the effect of nursing intervention as an environmental component. It provides a framework for the problem-oriented method of assessing family health needs, planning nursing care, recording our findings, and evaluating our services. We close this chapter with an editorial comment. Although we have liberally used the commonly accepted terminology in describing the family as a "system," we caution against any connotation that reduces human beings to mechanical elements suitable for "programming into computers." Such a view would certainly jeopardize the humanistic approach and the element of caring that are the very essence of nursing. "The nurse's commitment will continue to be that aspect of good nursing care that cannot be programmed into any system."[14]

REFERENCES

1. Jayne A. Tapia, "The Nursing Process in Family Health," *Nursing Outlook,* 20 (April 1972) 267-70.

2. From the title of the book by Edith Wensley, *Nursing Service Without Walls* (New York: National League for Nursing, 1963).

3. S.S. Sargent, "Conception of Role and Ego in Contemporary Psychology," in J.H. Roherer and M. Sherif, eds. *Staff Psychology at the Crossroads* (New York: Harper and Brothers, 1951).

4. Kent Miller, "The Concept of Crisis: Current Status and Mental Health Implications," *Human Organization,* 22 (1963) 195-201.

5. Gerald Caplan, *An Approach to Community Mental Health* (New York: Grune and Stratton, 1961), p. 18.

6. Erik H. Erikson, *Identity and the Life Cycle. Psychol. Issues Monog. No. 1.* (New York: International Universities Press, 1959).

7. Gerald Caplan, *Principles of Preventive Psychiatry* (New York: Basic Books, 1964).

8. N.W. Ackerman, "Psychological Dynamics of the Family Organism," *Public Health Reports,* 71 (October 1956) 1017-19.

9. Jetse Sprey, "The Family as a System in Conflict," *Journal of Marriage and the Family,* 31 (November 1969) 699-706.

10. Ibid.

11. Anatol Rapoport, "Foreword" to W. Buckley, *Modern Systems Research for the Behavioral Scientist* (Chicago: Aldine, 1968) pp. xiii-xxii.

12. Charles E. Goshen, "Your Automated Future," *American Journal of Nursing,* 72 (January 1972) 62-67.

13. Mary E. Hazzard, "An Overview of Systems Theory," *Nursing Clinics of North America,* 6 (September 1971) 385-93.

14. Joyce Finch, "Systems Analysis: A Logical Approach to Professional Nursing Care," *Nursing Forum,* 8 (1969) 176-90.

ADDITIONAL READINGS

Aguilera, Donna, Janice Messick, and Marlene Farrell, *Crisis Intervention Theory and Methodology,* St. Louis: C.V. Mosby Co., 1970.

Backscheider, Joan, "Self-Care Requirements, Self-Care Capabilities, and Nursing Systems in the Diabetic Nurse Management Clinic," in *American Journal of Public Health,* 64 (December 1974) 1138-46.

Barrell, Lorna Mill, "Crisis Intervention: Partnership in Problem-Solving," in *Nursing Clinics of North America* (9) 1 (March 1974) 5–16.

Bronfenbrenner, Urie, "The Origins of Alienation," in *Scientific American,* 131 (August 1974) 53-61.

Burgess, Ann Wolbert, and Lynda Lytle Holmstrom, *Rape: Victims of Crisis.* Bowie, Maryland: Robert J. Brady Co. (Prentice-Hall, Inc.) 1974.

Carlson, Carolyn E., et al., *Behavioral Concepts and Nursing Intervention.* Philadelphia: J.B. Lippincott Co., 1970.

Chinn, Peggy L., *Child Health Maintenance: Concepts in Family-Centered Care,* St. Louis: C.V. Mosby Co., 1974.

Christopherson, Victor A., Pearl Parvin Coulter, and Mary Opal Wolanin, *Rehabilitation Nursing, Perspectives and Applications.* New York: McGraw-Hill, 1974.

Clavan, Sylvia, and Ethel Vatter, "The Affiliated Family: A Device For Integrating Old and Young," in *Nursing Digest,* 1 (October 1973) 16-23.

Cohn, Helen, and William M. Schmidt, "The Practice of Family Health Care," in *American Journal of Public Health,* 65 (April 1975) 375-83.

Cohn, Helen, and Joyce E. Tingle, *Manual for Nurses in Family and Community Health.* 2nd ed. Boston: Little, Brown and Co., 1974.

Costello, D., "Communication Pattern in Family Systems," in *Nursing Clinics of North America,* 4 (December 1969) 721-29.

Daubenmire, M. Jean, and Imogene M. King, "Nursing Process Models: A Systems Approach," in *Nursing Outlook,* 21 (August 1973) 512-17.

Duvall, Evelyn, *Family Development.* 4th ed. Philadelphia: J.B. Lippincott Co., 1974.

Epstein, Charlotte, *Effective Interaction in Contemporary Nursing.* Englewood Cliffs, N.J.: Prentice-Hall, 1974.

Erikson, E.H., *Childhood and Society.* 2nd ed. New York: W.W. Norton, 1964.

Fagin, Claire M., *Family-Centered Nursing in Community Psychiatry.* Philadelphia: F.A. Davis Co., 1970.

Freeman, Howard E., Sol Levine, and Leo G. Reeder, *Handbook of Medical Sociology.* 2nd ed. Englewood Cliffs, N.J.: Prentice-Hall, 1972.

Freeman, Ruth, *Community Health Nursing Practice.* Philadelphia: W.B. Saunders Co., 1970.

Gaspard, N., "The Family of the Patient with Long-Term Illness," in *Nursing Clinics of North America,* 5 (March 1970) 77-83.

Hall, Joanne E., and Barbara R. Weaver, *Nursing of Families in Crisis.* Philadelphia: J.B. Lippincott Co., 1974.

Haller, Linda Lacey, "Family Systems Theory in Psychiatric Intervention," in *American Journal of Nursing,* 74 (March 1974) 462-63.

Hartmann, Kathleen, and Mary Bush, "Action-Oriented Family Therapy," in *American Journal of Nursing,* 75 (July 1975) 1184-87.

Hill, Reuben, "The American Family," in Alfred Katz and Jean S. Felton, *Health and the Community.* New York: The Free Press, 1965.

Hymovich, Debra, and Martha U. Barnard, *Family Health Care.* New York: McGraw-Hill, 1973.

Jaco, E. Gartly, *Patients, Physicians and Illness.* 2nd ed. New York: The Free Press, 1972.

Leahy, Kathleen, Marguerite Cobb, and Mary C. Jones, *Community Health Nursing.* 2nd ed. New York: McGraw-Hill, 1972.

Levine, Myra E., "The Pursuit of Wholeness," in *American Journal of Nursing,* 69 (January 1969) 93-98.

Lindemann, Erich, "The Meaning of Crisis in Individual and Family Living," in *Teachers College Record,* 57 (1956) 310-15.

Linton, R., *The Cultural Background of Personality.* New York: Appleton, 1945.

Martin, Leonide, " 'I Like Being an FNP'," in *American Journal of Nursing,* 75 (May 1975) 826-28.

Mayers, Marlene, "Home Visit—Ritual or Therapy?" in *Nursing Outlook,* 21 (May 1973) 328-31.

McBride, Angela Barron, "Can Family Life Survive?" in *The American Journal of Nursing,* 75 (October 1975), pp. 648–53.

McGrath, Eileen, "Guidelines for New Community Nurses," in *Nursing Outlook,* 19 (July 1971) 478-80.

Murata, Jo Ellen, "The Nurse As Family Practitioner," in *American Journal of Nursing,* 74 (February 1974) 254-57.

Parad, H.J., ed., *Crisis Intervention: Selected Readings.* New York: Family Service Association of America, 1965.

Pavenstedt, Eleanor, "To Help Infants Weather Disorganized Family Life," in *American Journal of Nursing,* 69 (August 1969) 1668-73.

Pender, Nola J., "A Conceptual Model for Preventive Health Behavior," in *Nursing Outlook,* 23 (June 1975) 385-90.

Pierce, Lillian, "A Patient-Care Model," in *American Journal of Nursing,* 69 (August 1969) 1700–04.

Pollak, Otto, "The Outlook for the American Family," in *Journal of Marriage and the Family,* 29 (February 1967) 193-205.

Purinton, Lynn R., and Helen F. McGrane, "A Survey of Sterilization Procedures Recommended to Diabetic Patients," in *Health Services Reports,* 87 (April 1972) 357-65.

Reinhardt, Adina M., and Mildred D. Quinn, *Family-Centered Community Nursing.* St. Louis: C.V. Mosby, 1973.

"Re-Thinking Stroke," a collection of articles in *American Journal of Nursing,* 75 (July 1975) 1140-47.

Robischon, Paulette, "Challenge of Crisis Theory for Nursing," in *Nursing Outlook,* 15 (July 1967) 28-32.

Robischon, P., and Diane Scott, "Role Theory and Its Application in Family Nursing," in *Nursing Outlook,* 17 (July 1969) 52-57.

Rubin, Reva, "Food and Feeding: A Matrix of Relationships," in *Nursing Forum,* 6 (1967) 195-205.

Saba, Virginia K., *Management Information Systems for Public Health/Community Health Agencies.* New York: National League for Nursing, 1974.

Sager, Clifford J., and Helen S. Kaplan, *Progress in Group and Family Therapy.* New York: Brunner/Mazel Inc., 1972.

Schwartz, Lawrence H., and Jane Linker Schwartz, *The Psychodynamics of Patient Care.* Englewood Cliffs, N.J.: Prentice-Hall, 1972.

Sobol, Evelyn G., and Paulette Robischon, *Family Nursing: A Study Guide.* St. Louis: C.V. Mosby, 1970.

Stewart, Dorothy M., and Pauline A. Vincent, *Public Health Nursing.* Dubuque, Iowa: Wm. C. Brown Co., 1968.

Sutterly, Doris Cook, and Gloria Ferraro Donnelly, *Perspectives in Human Development.* Philadelphia: J.B. Lippincott Co., 1973.

"Symposium on a Systems Approach to Nursing," in *Nursing Clinics of North America,* 6 (September 1971) 383-462.

Tinkham, Catherine W., and Eleanore F. Voorhies, *Community Health Nursing.* New York: Appleton-Century-Crofts, 1972.

Toman, Walter, *Family Constellation.* 2nd ed. New York: Springer Publishing Co., 1969.

Tyzenhouse, Phyllis S., "Myocardial Infarction," *American Journal of Nursing,* 73 (June 1973) 1012-13.

Vincent, Pauline, "Do We Want Patients To Conform?" in *Nursing Outlook,* 18 (January 1970) 54-55.

Vincent, Pauline, "The Sick Role in Patient Care," in *American Journal of Nursing,* 75 (July 1975) 1172-73.

Walker, Lorraine O., "Every Patient is Unique," in *Nursing Outlook,* 16 (September 1968) 39.

Wallace, Mary A., and Wilbur E. Morley, "Teaching Crisis Intervention," in *American Journal of Nursing,* 70 (July 1970) 1484-87.

Yauger, Ruth Anne, "Does Family-Centered Care Make a Difference?" in *Nursing Outlook,* 20 (May 1972) 320-23.

Zacha, Margaret C., "Nursing Goals in Working with Families under Multiple Stress," in *Nursing Clinics of North America,* 4 (March 1969) 69.

Chapter 13
Mobilizing
Community Resources
for Family Health

"Society exists for the benefit of its members; not the members for the benefit of society."[1]

INTRODUCTION

Now that we have looked at the individual in relation to the family, let us turn to the individual and family in relation to the community. Just as family members interact in their efforts to maintain dynamic equilibrium, so do individuals and families interact with society and its institutions. People live together in a community they have helped to create, and which, in turn, modifies their health and behavior. A community is constantly undergoing change—deterioration in one neighborhood, a new housing development in another, industry moving in or out, population shift in size or composition, depletion of natural resources, and so forth. These events are interrelated and do not occur in isolation. Change is an unremitting force built into community life. In nursing we say that in order to relate ourselves and our work to the community, we must learn to accept change as a normal part of the dynamic society in which we live.

Nursing practice in the community may be a new experience for you, quite different from that which you expected from your own perception of the traditional nursing role. You are quickly brought into close contact with people in the world outside of the hospital. Furthermore, you may find yourself in situations that bear no resemblance to your own life style. However, you can begin to develop a feeling of familiarity and identification when you look at the sum total of your own experiences, which have helped to determine how you react to people and to new situations. The study of the community begins with an understanding of yourself. You are an individual, a member of a family, and you have come from a community that has helped to shape your outlook on life. A community is dynamic—you are dynamic; you are part of the community—you look at the community.

WHAT IS A COMMUNITY?

Whatever its size, nature, or location—city, suburb, town, village, rural area, New England, Middle Atlantic, South, Midwest, Pacific-Northwest, Mountain States, West Coast, Southwest—your community has a flavor all its own. At the same time, it shares many common characteristics with all other communities. The answer to "what is a community?" would be different today from what it was one or two generations ago. There have been many changes in community life in America in the last few decades. The small town and well-defined city of yesteryear have made way for the sprawling megalopolis with its ever-widening tentacles of suburbia. There is a startling sameness on the superhighways that link one area with another. Interspersed with shopping centers, covered malls, and industrial parks, these roads provide one means for the ever-increasing speed in transportation and com-community? What has your community done to help you and what have you done to help it? The basic functions of a community might be summarized as follows:

In today's context, legal boundaries or geographic continuity are often not the major criteria for defining a community. A community is seen as a social unit wherein we find transaction of a common life among the people who compose the unit. A community may be defined as a group of inhabitants living together in a somewhat localized area under the same general regulations and having common interests, functions, needs, and organizations. It goes beyond city, village, county, and is defined by relationships between people as well as by physical contours. By this definition, a whole country may be viewed as a community. In this chapter we will describe the dynamics of the community in relation to the health of individuals and families. We will also discuss the use of community resources in meeting the health needs of the inhabitants.

FUNCTIONS OF A COMMUNITY

What are the functions of a community? Think of your own community. How have you, as an individual and a member of a family, interacted with your community? What has your community done to help you and what have you done to help it? The basic functions of a community might be summarized as follows:

(1) to determine the use of space for living and other purposes;

(2) to make available the means for production and distribution of necessary goods and services;

(3) to protect and conserve the health, life, resources, and property of individuals;

(4) to educate and acculturate newcomers—children and immigrants;

(5) to transmit information, ideas, and beliefs;

(6) to provide opportunities for interaction between individuals and groups.

The community is basically the medium for the development of its inhabitants. It provides the means whereby society imposes its expectations on people. The environment of the home or the neighborhood is influenced by the character of the community, and, in turn, influences the community. Ultimately, a community is judged by the kinds of people it produces. Whether it expands and grows, or dries up and withers away, will be determined by many factors. What are its educational and employment opportunities? What is the caliber of its schools, religious institutions, health and welfare facilities? Are there cultural and recreational centers? Does it generate a "healthy" environment where people strive for excellence? Or does it provide a breeding ground for multiple social problems? Is there a recognizable "community spirit" that encourages community development and improvement? Does the community act to protect the most vulnerable persons in its midst—the very young, the very old, the ill, the abandoned, the homeless? What steps does it take to correct the conditions that foster serious problems such as poverty, unemployment, drug abuse, child neglect, alcoholism, accidental deaths and injuries, crime, juvenile delinquency, environmental pollution?

In studying a community, we try to identify those forces that positively or adversely affect the health of its inhabitants. There are so many factors closely interrelated that it would not be possible to list them all. However, let us look at some of these conditions and see how they may affect health.

CONDITIONS IN A COMMUNITY THAT AFFECT HEALTH

In the epidemiological approach (see Chapter 5), three major environmental components are identified—physical, biological, and social. In order to conduct a scientific investigation of the conditions in a community that affect health, you must gather information related to these three broad categories. We suggest the following questions as a useful guide for such a systematic assessment.

Physical

What is the geographic location of the community? Is the community located in a rural or semirural area where a safe water supply and sewage disposal may pose a problem? Is the community isolated and far away from needed resources? Is it in an urban or suburban setting, where social and psychological isolation may pose a serious problem in spite of physical proximity? Are neighborhoods crowded and congested? Are there any wide open spaces? Are the air and water clean and free of pollution? Is the community in a mountain region? a valley? a plateau? Is it surrounded by living foliage and forests or is it at the edge of a desert? Is there soil suitable for growth of food plants? Is it in a low-lying, marshy area, which may serve as a breeding ground for insect-borne diseases? Are there seasonal changes in the climate that have a direct bearing on the spread of certain diseases?

Biological

What is the prevailing system of plants and animals? How does it affect health? Are the food plants rich in nutrient value? Have they been contaminated by environmental wastes, which in turn harm higher forms of life? Are rats and rodents rampant? Are there wild animals nearby serving as reservoirs of infection that may be transmitted to man? Is there a large population of domestic animals and are they subject to hygienic control? Is there a large number of people who are highly vulnerable from the standpoint of genetic risks?

Social (Demographic, psychological, cultural, economic, political, educational)

What are the prevailing social norms? Are local customs in conformance with or contrary to well-established principles of health promotion? How are illness and health defined? Where does health fit into the community's order of priorities? What is the power structure of the community? Does power lie within the hands of the elected officials? Or is power held by a nonelected but potent political, socioeconomic, religious, or ethnic group? What are the principal means of livelihood in the community? Do community industries—for example, coalmining, steel production, asbestos manufacturing—pose health hazards for the workers? Is there industrial waste which pollutes the environment? What is the educational level of the community? What is the age distribution of the population? Is this a stable community where the inhabitants have a sense of belonging? a transient community? one that has been unable to adapt to change and has begun to deteriorate? Are there well-developed means of transportation and communication? Are there deep rooted prejudices or traditions or strong religious influences that affect health practices? Are voluntary efforts made for the development of health programs? (Such as illustrated by Figure 13-1.) Are political officials willing to take the leadership in raising taxes for needed health services and are the people willing to pay such taxes?

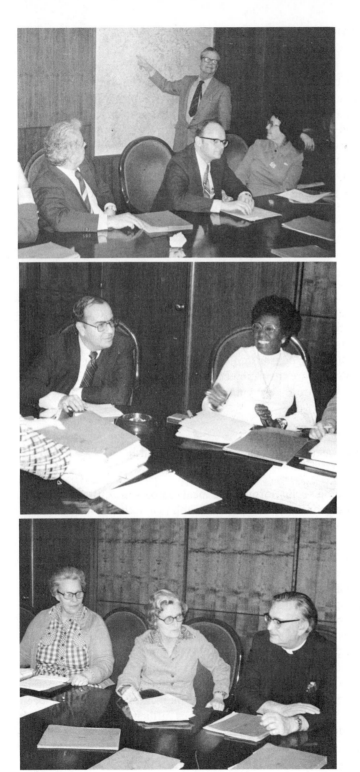

Figure 13-1 Voluntary efforts for the development of health programs: Interested citizens representing the community serve on the board of directors of a voluntary home health agency. Here they are shown meeting with the executive director (far left).

As a nurse practicing in the community, you must consider these conditions and their relationship to the health status of a community. They determine not only the kinds of health problems that arise, but also the action programs taken to alleviate these problems. In an earlier chapter we looked at the components of the health care system and found a vast array of persons and institutions involved. There is no overall, unified, organized network, but rather a melange of fragmented parts that may create confusion for the consumer in his pursuit of health care. Much of the confusion stems from the fact that there are so many types of health planning, financing, and service organizations within the total system. In community nursing practice, one of your major responsibilities is to look at all of these organizations and see what they are doing for the benefit of the community.

COMMUNITY HEALTH SERVICES AND FACILITIES

Begin by viewing the community as a whole. You must find out what kinds of facilities and services are available for health promotion and disease prevention, as well as for treatment and rehabilitation. To do this, you look at the entire range of outpatient, ambulatory, home health, emergency, and institutional facilities and services. You may find it useful to seek answers to the following questions:

(1) Are there adequate clinics and outpatient facilities in the community? Are they within easy reach of most community residents? Do they provide a full complement of services—e.g., sick and well child care, immunization, adult health, maternal and infant care including family planning, community based mental health units, alcohol and drug abuse units? Are there comprehensive neighborhood health centers? Health Maintenance Organizations (HMOs)? Are there enough well-qualified nurses and physicians to staff these ambulatory facilities?

(2) Who provides home health care in the community? Do the home health agencies meet the conditions of participation to provide services under Medicare and Medicaid? Is home nursing offered by a voluntary agency, official agency, a combination of these? Or is the community dependent on proprietary agencies for home health services? Is there a full range of services available in the home, i.e. nursing, homemaker, home health aide, physical, occupational, speech therapy, social service?

(3) Does the community have a hospital with a well-qualified staff of nursing and medical practitioners, so that most care can be provided on the premises? Is the hospital equipped to handle most situations, i.e., diagnostic tests, acute and elective care, and rehabilitation? Or, is the facility set up primarily to provide only simple diagnostic and treatment services, with more comprehensive services available elsewhere? Is the staff capable of administering emergency life-saving measures in cases of severe shock and trauma? Are there available resources—orthopedic expertise and equipment—for emergency management of fractures? Is there a full range of laboratory services, including a blood bank or provisions for obtaining blood immediately? Are there maternity services available on a 24-hour basis? Where are the nearest hospitals that provide special services to the community, e.g., intensive coronary care, rehabilitation, mental

illness and mental retardation, pediatric, orthopedic? Is there transportation available to reach these facilities?

(4) Does the community have extended care facilities? Are posthospitalization beds available for continued treatment and rehabilitation? Are there nursing home beds available for those persons who can no longer be maintained in their own home because of increasing disability? If so, do these facilities meet state and local criteria for personal safety, sanitation, and fire protection? Are extended care facilities proprietary, state or county operated, voluntary (non-profit, church-related or other philanthropic)? Do they recognize the value of and do they provide skilled rehabilitation nursing for the prevention and limitation of disability?

(5) What services are available for emergency health care? Does the community have a coordinated ambulance and rescue squad? Are the ambulances properly equipped for on-the-spot emergency care? Is there an ongoing in-service training program to keep rescue personnel up to date?

A community may be blessed with the most sophisticated health care facilities—hospitals, clinics, and extended care institutions. Health manpower supply may pose no problem. However, none of this will have any impact unless you reach out to find the people who need help. And then, you must go one step further; having found these people, you must assess their needs, and offer appropriate supportive services. What agencies are responsible for providing these supportive services? Are people aware of services offered? Do they know how to use them? Who is responsible for assessing the social needs of the target population? Are there agencies that offer counseling for social and psychological problems? Are there treatment services available if such problems are identified? People with health and social problems often need financial assistance, not necessarily in the form of a cash grant, but perhaps as a third party mechanism to pay for needed health care. Does your community have a well-organized department of public welfare with a full complement of supportive services? How does the patient or client apply for services under the welfare program? Would you be able to assess his eligibility for such services? If not, would you know the resource person who could assist you in these matters?

As you become familiar with the services and facilities which are available, you will begin to get a picture of the community's response to its health needs. In some communities, you will find adequate services, well established and efficiently coordinated, capable of growing and expanding as the need arises. In others you may find few or no resources other than yourself, as, for example, in an isolated area with a small, county health department where you are the only nurse on the staff. There are some communities that have inadequate health care despite an abundance of facilities and services because of overlapping and duplication of efforts and competition for prominence among the providers. You may wonder about how community resources are developed; who decides whether they should be continued, dissolved, expanded, or curtailed. How does the community determine what health facilities it needs, and how comprehensive they should be? How does the community establish priorities for services? With these questions in mind, you should look at the community's health planning and health financing activities.

HEALTH PLANNING

Health planning is an integral part of the total health care system. In most communities you will find a local Health and Welfare Council, or some other central coordinating body that concerns itself with health planning. Such councils have existed in our country for more than six decades. Originally they were formed to organize the fund raising efforts of many voluntary agencies into one annual drive, but have broadened their functions to include areawide planning. As voluntary, nonprofit organizations, they are usually supported by the United Fund or "community chest." Voluntary and official community nursing agencies work very closely with these councils, which you will find indispensable as you plan, coordinate, implement, and evaluate family nursing care. For example, check in your local area for the directory of social agencies. You will find that virtually every community in the country will have some kind of directory that has been compiled, issued, and made available by the local health and welfare council.

The Hill-Burton Hospital Survey and Construction Act of 1946 was the nation's first major venture into health facilities planning. An important landmark in federal legislation for health, the Hill-Burton Act provided grants-in-aid to the states for partial financing of hospital construction. Under this program, each state was expected to formulate a statewide plan for regional organization of hospitals and related health facilities based on an analysis of the supply, distribution, and use of facilities within its area. At first there was a lack of financial support for such planning activities, but in 1962 some federal funding for planning councils became available. Thus, you may find another type of coordinated health planning body in the community you are studying—the areawide Health Care Facilities Planning Council.

Beginning with the mid-1960s, federal legislation provided considerable impetus to health planning as an organized and coordinated community activity. We refer specifically to the federal *Partnership for Health* legislation in 1966 and 1967, which introduced the concept of comprehensive health planning as a mechanism through which the planning activities of all health and health-related elements can be linked together. This legislation authorized comprehensive health planning on a state and areawide basis, bringing together, as operating partners, the federal and state governments with the local area. Further impetus was given to this approach with the enactment of the Health Planning and Resources Development Act of 1974. The federal government provides money and technical assistance to states and communities to help them organize and conduct comprehensive health planning. The states establish statewide Comprehensive Health Planning agencies that deal in broad terms with the health of their citizens. Local areas organize Comprehensive Health Planning bodies which are concerned with the health needs of the people in the area and with the specific facilities, services, and manpower to meet these needs.

Both state and local Comprehensive Health Planning bodies depend heavily on advisory councils for direction. These councils are made up of representatives of consumers and providers of health services, with the requirement that consumer representatives be in the majority. Nurses, individually and through their professional organizations, are often invited to serve on such advisory councils. If ever you are invited to serve on such a council, do not hesitate to seek information and become involved. If you are working in an area where you feel that the interests of the people are not being served because of the lack of nursing input, you have a responsibility to inform the appropriate authorities and request representation to these councils.

Federal guidelines for Comprehensive Health Planning groups include the following objectives: (1) to identify area health needs and problems; (2) to inventory health resources; (3) to consider alternative courses of action; (4) to develop priorities and recommendations for action; (5) to mobilize resources and coordinate activities for the resolution of health problems; (6) to evaluate the results of the actions taken.

HEALTH FINANCING

In Chapter 10 we discussed in a general way how health care delivery may be financed. Now we suggest that you look at the community where you are working to see how its financial resources are allocated for the delivery of health care. Secure financial backing is absolutely essential for the viability of an agency providing nursing service. This kind of support will not be forthcoming unless individual nurses take an active role in stimulating the community and its inhabitants to provide the necessary funds. These funds may come from voluntary contributions, public taxes, or a combination of both.

What kinds of action can nurses take to encourage financial support from the community? First, they can demonstrate that their service is a vital link in maintaining the health of the people by (1) identifying community health needs, (2) offering quality care to meet these needs, and (3) holding themselves accountable to the community they serve. They can seek wide citizen support so that the community can speak in a united voice when appealing to government authorities for financial allocations. They can look for input from interested citizens who are able to make financial contributions or who are willing to organize fund-raising campaigns. They can conduct their own campaign to reach the public. This approach was used by a public health nurse who worked alone in a small rural county health department. She carried the message throughout the county at public meetings, and through individual contacts with the people whom she served in a 400-square-mile area, where efforts were being made to enact a special levy to support the health department. Her county's health levy passed by a handsome margin, and many of the voters admitted that their support would not have been forthcoming without the convincing actions of their nurse.

No matter what type of agency you are working in, you will find that in order to plan effective nursing intervention, you will need to know something about the family's financial situation as it relates to the provision of their health care. Nurses often are reluctant to ask questions about their patients' finances. They consider this to be prying and outside the scope of nursing practice. However, in the best interest of the patient and his family, you must evaluate their financial status in order to formulate realistic health care plans within the framework of existing personal or community resources. A nonjudgmental approach on your part will help to allay the anxiety of families who may be reluctant to disclose their resources. The success of your nursing care to families will depend in part on your ability to assess their financial status and help them find the resources for their health needs. You will want to be familiar with local sources of payment that are available for family nursing care and for other supportive services.

Some families with whom you work will be recipients of health care benefits through third party sources such as Medicaid, Medicare, and the various types of voluntary health insurance, which provide payment for the use of facilities and services. You should develop an understanding of how these payment sources relate to individual consumers and their eligibility for services. You soon discover that these plans have helped many people by removing financial barriers to needed health services. However, these plans contain limitations that pose problems. For instance, a person over sixty-five, eligible for Medicare, will not be reimbursed for needed services until he meets the deductible requirement under the Medicare plan.

Many persons simply do not qualify for any of these methods of third party coverage. For example, they may be under 65, and not eligible for Medicare. Or, they may be ineligible for state aid to the medically indigent (Medicaid) because their income, though limited and fixed, may exceed the amount designated for eligibility under the state plan (see Chapter 10). What happens when individuals and their families find themselves in this "no-man's land" of financial coverage for health care? What are the options of a family faced with a catastrophic illness that may have exhausted their third party benefits and drained their own modest financial resources? Sometimes families are reluctant to relinquish their last small holdings in order to receive financial assistance. They will not tolerate any "intrusion" into their personal affairs by community agencies. They perceive the conditions for assistance imposed by the social system as humiliating and depersonalizing, and they prefer to maintain their financial independence, often with drastic consequences. The following case illustrates how one family, under such circumstances, became immobilized and suffered immeasurable misery.

A fifty-nine-year-old man was hospitalized for diabetes with gangrene of his right foot. During the course of a three-month hospitalization period he suffered a cerebrovascular accident that resulted in a paralysis of his left side. He received the full range of services including nursing, physical therapy, and medical care, and was discharged to the hospital Home Care program (see p. 212). The overall plan was directed toward increasing his independence and preparing him for eventual return to his job as a machine operator. Up to this point his financial worries were not critical, as his care was covered under the hospitalization insurance through his place of employment, and he continued to receive two-thirds of his usual salary. Approximately six weeks after he returned home, he was able to complete his activities of daily living (ADL) without assistance; he managed to get around the house with the aid of a walker; he could climb stairs to the second floor of his home and could negotiate the front steps to get into an automobile with minimum assistance. At this time he made a follow-up visit to the hospital so that the rehabilitation team could review his progress and assess his level of functioning. The outcome of the conference, although correctly complying with established guidelines, was nonetheless a dismal one for the patient. The following recommendations were made by the team:

(1) the patient was advised that the original goal to return to his job as a machine operator was no longer realistic because he was unable to achieve the function needed for this type of work;
(2) as he was now largely independent in his ADL, there was no further need for Home Care benefits;
(3) because of the patient's age and disability, he did not qualify as a candidate for vocational retraining;
(4) application for social security disability funds was advised because he was no longer eligible for his salary or medical benefits from his place of employment.

The community nursing agency had been active in this case under the Home Care program. The district nurse recognized that there was a need for further counseling and emotional support as well as ongoing rehabilitation therapy. The agency therefore continued to provide service to this patient who was suddenly left without any kind of health care benefits and could not expect to receive any under Medicare for at least eighteen months. The patient became depressed and began to regress in his functional abilities. He spent more time in bed, refused to eat, and was generally withdrawn. In counseling the patient and family the nurse suggested that they apply for state aid to the medically indigent (Medicaid) because of an anticipated need for health care. The family followed this suggestion in spite of their own strong feelings against accepting what they considered to be welfare. However, their application was turned down because their annual income was thirty dollars above the designated level and their personal savings were in excess of the allowable amount. The family reacted to this turn of events by doubling their efforts to help their disabled member become self-sufficient. The patient himself, determined not to become dependent on "welfare," resolved his mental depression, regained his functional independence, and was able to participate in many social activities with family and friends. Encouraged by the patient's progress, the district nurse and the family agreed that there was no further need for services at this time. The case was closed with the recommendation that if the family should need the nurse again they could call the agency. Six months went by, when one day the agency received a frantic call from the patient's wife saying "Oh, Ms. Martin, can you come right away, my husband is very sick, and I don't know where to turn; he would be furious if he knew I was calling you. He says we have no money for doctors or nurses or hospitals and he just won't take charity." When the nurse arrived in the home, she found the patient semicomatose. She made arrangements for immediate admission to the hospital, where the patient died several hours later.

The nurse's approach in helping this family was based on her knowledge of the community's financial resources and the family's interaction with the community. Her efforts to help alleviate their financial problems were stymied. This is not an uncommon situation—where a family is caught in the system. On one hand are the family's self-imposed barriers to accepting financial assistance they perceive as charity. On the other hand are the barriers imposed by the system, which squeeze out a family because of eligibility limitations. We have no answer to this dilemma; perhaps some aspects of this problem will be resolved if and when national health insurance becomes a reality.

USING COMMUNITY RESOURCES TO MEET HEALTH NEEDS

Gathering information about the community and its resources is but the first step. You then must apply this knowledge, so that individual persons and families in need may receive help which is available through community resources. Using this knowledge, you must also seek ways to improve existing services and initiate plans for new services in the community. In Chapter 3 we refer to the nurse's role of "patient advocate" and "change agent." We see the nurse functioning as a facilitator and coordinator in the use of community resources to meet family and community health needs. The efforts of the nurse and other members of the health team are built around the basic premise that personal responsibility of the patient or family is a key element, and the needs and rights of the individual can never be bypassed.

If individual rights interfere with public health or if public health interferes with individual rights, the situation must be reconciled. Sometimes the problem must be brought before a court of law for a solution. Or, a court might be petitioned if an individual becomes incapacitated and is unable to bear responsibility for his own actions. The whole team, working together, should make every effort to protect the rights of the individual. The following situation shows how staff members of various community agencies cooperated in their efforts to support a senior citizen in her desire to maintain independent living. It also points out that ultimately, when measures had to be taken for institutional care, the individual rights of this woman had to be safeguarded.

An elderly woman who had been living alone in back of an empty store had managed well for many years with help from interested friends and neighbors. Approaching her eighties, she began to find herself rather isolated. All her former neighbors and friends had died or moved away, and new residents in the neighborhood showed no interest. One of the "old-timers" became concerned about the poor health and increasing feebleness of the woman, and called in the Community Nursing Service.

On initial assessment the nurse found this elderly woman, physically weak and poorly nourished, living in deteriorating quarters behind her "penny-candy" store. The store had been closed for over a year, but the stock, which remained in open dishes in the display cases, became an enticing source of food for invading rodents and vermin. In view of these overwhelming conditions, the nurse recommended temporary care in a nursing home. When this suggestion was adamantly rejected, the nurse attempted to help the patient formulate alternate plans.

On further assessment, the nurse was able to identify some positive aspects in the dilapidated surroundings. Heat and light were in good supply, and indoor plumbing and cooking facilities were adequate for one person. The nurse referred the case to the local health department and department of safety, and with the cooperation of these two agencies, was instrumental in bringing the rodent and vermin problem under control. In this improved environment, the patient was able to continue as an independently functioning member of the community, with periodic health supervision from the nursing service.

Several months later the patient had to be hospitalized for an acute illness. In following through the nurse sent a complete report to the hospital social service department. Upon further contact, she was advised that the patient was being discharged from the hospital to an extended care facility. A short time later the nursing agency received an urgent call about the patient from the same concerned neighbor. Responding to the call, the nurse discovered that the woman, having refused nursing home care, had been returned to her home. Because of a breakdown in communication, the nursing agency had not been notified. Continuity of care had been interrupted, and, by this time, the patient's condition had deteriorated considerably. She was mentally and physically incapacitated. Her home and its surroundings had become an unsightly hazard to herself and the community. The nurse initiated an interagency conference, at which time the situation of this elderly woman was discussed. There was no longer any question about the fact that she required institutional care. Upon the entire team's recommendation, the court was petitioned, a legal guardian was appointed, and arrangements were made for admission of the patient to a nursing home where she would receive twenty-four-hour care.

How you proceed in using community resources will depend at first on the needs which you find. In facilitating and coordinating community resources, you must reach out to identify needs and bring them into focus. Since community nursing practice is family centered, you should look for those elements in a situation that directly affect the well-being of the family and in turn affect the whole community. Perhaps you will have a relatively uncomplicated situation such as you might find with a family, in modest circumstances, living in a clean and healthful environment. They are able to get along with minimal outside help, e.g., a request to the cancer society for surgical dressings and other supplies, or referral to another local agency for the use of a hospital bed or commode.

Or you may be involved in more complicated situations where you find environmental conditions, such as poor housing and sanitation, inadequate garbage and trash disposal, or rat and vermin infestation, which have a decidedly deleterious effect on the well-being of a family and a community. Families living under these conditions are often beset by so many other problems that they are extremely vulnerable. These are the high-risk families with multiple social and health problems—fatherless or motherless homes, poverty, out-of-wedlock births, child abuse, mental illness/retardation, alcoholism, drug abuse, malnutrition, and many others. In these situations health and social problems are so closely bound up together that you need to set priorities, confront the problems that can be handled through your specific expertise, and make referrals to appropriate agencies that can handle other problems. You must proceed with exceptional skill and tact, remembering that families with multiple problems are often beleaguered by a multitude of workers from many social agencies, with much overlapping, confusion, and duplication of services. Aware of this, you may be instrumental in bringing all the agencies together in an interagency conference to sort out the problems and goals. One of the agencies—often the one whose worker has established the best rapport in the home—might be designated to coordinate the services of all the other agencies. Many times the nursing agency is the one that provides this coordination, and you will be the coordinator.

Often there is much wasted effort from the duplication of services by the various agencies in their attempts to help the patient and family. Assistance is nearly always crisis-oriented and short term, especially in multiproblem situations. Consider the effect of multiple agency activities on the patient and family. Bombarded on all sides by agencies such as child protection, welfare, community nursing, housing, safety and health departments, the patient and his family may feel threatened. With pressure mounting on all sides, the family may resist or retreat from all efforts, especially in cases where there is suspected child neglect or abuse. When many agencies are involved you may find that you can help to facilitate the use of these resources without being directly involved in the care of the patient. The following case may illustrate this point.

You have received a referral from a childrens' clinic to evaluate the home of Susan, an eleven-year-old child who had been hospitalized during a crisis period in which she had reported that "voices are telling me to jump out a window and kill myself." In checking back with the referral source, you discovered that there were at least seven other agenices involved with this family—the children's clinic, the mental health clinic, the child protection agency, the school, the health department, the welfare department, and the hospital. With this information, you felt that it would be necessary to do some further checking before entering this "overcrowded scene." What services were all of these agencies providing in the home? What were the immediate needs of this family? Was a home evaluation appropriate at this time? Regarding the home environment, what information was available from these other agencies? Before charting your course of action, you felt that you needed to gather this information. You made contact with each of the agencies involved in the care of the family and formulated the family profile from the following data:

(1) *From the Children's Clinic*—when last seen, Susan was brought in by her parents, with complaints about her fear of public places. She had refused to go to school because voices were telling her to jump out a window and kill herself. When efforts were made to encourage her to return to school, she attempted suicide. A referral was made to the mental health clinic. After her second attempt at suicide, the child was brought back to the children's clinic, whereupon it was decided that she should be hospitalized.

(2) *From the School Nurse*—up until two months before the "voices" began, Susan had been doing well in school, had many friends, and was a leader in her class. One day, during a reading period, she informed her teacher that she heard "voices" telling her to jump out of the window. She became agitated and complained that there were too many people in the room. Examination by the school psychologist proved negative. At that point, she left school and did not return. Repeated attempts have been made to get her to return but they have not been successful.

(3) *From the Health Department*—the home was very dirty with the excreta of five dogs and numerous pigeons that shared the living quarters with the family.

(4) *From the Mental Health Clinic*—the parents had taken Susan to this clinic upon the recommendation of the pediatrician at the time of the suicide attempt. On their first visit the father told the psychiatrist that "my daughter is possessed by demons and I'm going to take her to a priest." The psychiatrist felt that the father was in need of psychiatric help, but could not get him to agree to accept family therapy. The next day the child ran away. When she was returned to her home three days later, she made a second attempt at suicide. A second visit to the clinic, upon the insistence of the child protection agency, was not fruitful because the social worker was unable to convince the father either to accept family therapy or to allow Susan to be removed from the unhealthy home en-

vironment. In fact the mother and father were "clinging" to Susan—three other siblings had been removed from their care in the past.

(5) *From the Child Protection Agency*—the family had been known to this agency over a long period of time. Within the last two years, three other children had been removed from the home. The parents felt threatened and they resented the involvement of so many agencies. The child protection agency, in their effort to help the child and family, supported the mental health clinic recommendation for family therapy. Upon the insistence of this agency, the parents made a return visit to the mental health clinic, but as already noted, were not amenable to therapy.

Having assembled these facts, you realize that the situation is at an impasse with a very grave outlook for the child. You arrange an interagency conference. During this conference it becomes obvious from all the reports that the children's clinic is the agency that has the best rapport with the family. You recommend that the nurse and the social worker at the children's clinic continue to urge the family to allow the child to be placed in a foster home. Your plan is to continue as a facilitator of services even though you have not had direct contact with the family. Several weeks later, you are informed that the family has voluntarily accepted the child's placement in a foster home. The child has now returned to school. You close the record in this case with the realization that you may be called upon again for your expertise.

We present the following case to illustrate the role of the nurse as the patient advocate.

In this situation we find an aging couple (Mr. and Mrs. B.) with numerous health and social problems—illness, disability, poverty, inadequate housing, and isolation are but a few. Mr. B., age 85, is physically active, mentally alert, and staunchly independent in spite of the fact that he is blind and has arteriosclerotic heart disease with some cardiac decompensation. He has assumed the responsibility for the care of his seventy-eight-year-old wife who, following a cerebrovascular accident, had been rehabilitated with assistance from the local community nursing service. They have no children and no other living relatives. With the exception of one other neighbor Mr. and Mrs. B. are the only remaining residents in an area that has been marked for redevelopment. They cling to their house, which is in deplorable condition; however, it is their "castle" and they are not going to leave it until the last possible moment. Their sole financial support comes from the aid-to-the-blind program through the local welfare department. While working with this family, the nurse has suggested the possibility of planning for admission to a nursing home, in view of the couple's advancing age, infirmity, poor housing, and other problems. The merest suggestion of such a plan is completely rejected by the couple. As time goes on, Mrs. B. suffers a series of strokes. After each of these episodes, she continues to deteriorate until she is paralyzed, bedfast, incontinent, and senile. And yet, Mr. B. continues to reject nursing home care, because he knows it means that he and his wife would be separated.

The nurse at this point calls upon other community agencies that are involved with this family. An interagency conference is arranged, where the nurse, along with representatives from the welfare department, the health department, homemaker's service, and the blind association, explore the couple's attitude toward nursing home placement. All parties agree that the couple would be better cared for in a nursing home environment. However, separation from each other at an advanced age after fifty years of marriage makes this alternative ethically and morally undersirable. The nurse as the patient advocate is committed to work out a plan that would be more acceptable to this elderly couple.

Alternatives to institutionalization are discussed, and it is decided that the nurse working with a representative from the welfare department will coordinate the services required for the couple's care. A major problem is the need for services beyond any of the community agencies' usual hours of operation. By special arrangement the homemaker service is able to cover a few hours each evening, five days a week. On the weekends, Mr. and Mrs. B.'s neighbor agrees to help out. Thus the agencies are assured that the couple will receive their evening meal and that Mrs. B. will be prepared for bed.

As the advocate of the patient and family, the nurse is able to maintain them as well as can be expected under prevailing conditions. The chosen course of action cannot be regarded as an ideal resolution of the problems, but rather as the best of several possible alternatives, and the only one that is acceptable to the family. The nurse continues to work toward the Bs.' accepting the plan for nursing home care.

The nurse as coordinator may work to bring about change in situations where the community resources may have proved inadequate. We cite as an example a situation where lines of communication among various community agencies had fallen down. Recognition of this problem came about only after the occurrence of a tragic event, and it was the community nursing service that prodded the agencies into action.

The situation involved a twelve-year-old girl who had been accused of killing her younger brother. Several months earlier this girl, Mae X., had been referred to the nursing agency for follow-up after treatment in a local hospital for attempted suicide. On her initial visit to the family, the nurse had learned from Mae that this had not been her first attempt. In response to the nurse's effort to explore the problem, the mother pointed out "My daughter is being taken care of through the psychology service of the school district and we go to the community mental health clinic. So you don't really have to come here anymore." Mrs. X. terminated the home visit leaving the nurse with many unanswered questions. Back at the agency the nurse made several telephone calls to check out the plan of care for the patient and the family, and she learned that the school had indeed referred the child to the local mental health center where psychiatric therapy had been recommended. The local mental health unit made it clear that they did their own follow-up and would be working with the patient and the family. With this as the appropriate referral, the nurse closed the case, after learning that a contact had been established between the family and the mental health unit, and after offering the services from the nursing agency for any future development. Several weeks went by, when one day an account of the little boy's death appeared in the local press.

After the initial shock of this tragic news item wore off, the nurse asked herself several compelling questions. Could this tragedy have been prevented? Was every possible resource utilized in the most effective way to help the patient get the required treatment? Were there other steps the nurse could have taken to facilitate and coordinate needed services? The conclusion she reached was that it was futile to speculate on whether the tragedy might have been pi ented. But was there some course of action that might bring about improvement for the future, so that young people with problems like Mae's might be helped? Certainly there had been gaps in service. The repeated suicide attempts should have been recognized as a call for help, and the child should have been referred directly from the hospital for psychiatric treatment. There had been a breakdown in communication among the various agencies involved with the family. This became painfully clear when it was learned that the mother had not followed through with the needed psychiatric treatment for her child at the mental health unit after the first posthospitalization visit. Yet no one had referred the case back to the community nursing agency. Nor did anyone make a referral to the child protection agency, which had no means of compelling the mother to bring the child in for treatment. The courts were frustrated in their efforts to help in similar cases of emotional neglect—there was little they could do "before the fact." There were no local facilities, such as a halfway house, to provide help. All these factors had combined to stultify positive action. After the terrible event occurred, it was impossible to pass it off as an unavoidable tragedy. The nurse initiated an interagency conference to review the situation. All persons involved in this case came together to determine what steps could be taken by the community as a whole to avert such extreme consequences. There were several positive outcomes, one of them being improved communication among the cooperating agencies, with a better understanding of the roles of the various disciplines involved. The hospital reviewed its policies in cases of attempted suicide and took steps to improve their mechanism of referral. Another positive outcome was the formation of a nucleus of workers whose interest remained high and helped to stimulate the development of a county mental health program.

Nursing can provide leadership as the agent of change in situations where community resources do not exist and are sorely needed.

In an industrialized, heavily populated area of the mid-Atlantic region there is a small, urban community (pop. 60,000). A thriving city for many years, with a proud heritage and rich historical background, it had reached its zenith around the era of the First World War, after which a period of slow stagnation set in. As the years went on it gradually became a tired, worn-out community whose inherent industrial wealth had been drained and removed by entrepreneurs who felt no responsibility to put back what they had taken out. It had further been ravished by unscrupulous public officials who grasped political power and used it to their own selfish ends. In the mid-1960s violence erupted; it came as no surprise. There was poverty, massive unemployment, poor schools, deteriorated housing unfit for human habitation, a serious rat infestation problem, malnutrition, drug abuse, and numerous other adverse conditions. The infant mortality rate was the highest in the entire state. Many elderly people were living in isolation in substandard housing without supportive services. Suddenly the community found itself without needed health services when its only hospital closed its doors, no longer able to exist with dwindling voluntary support. There was no local health department and most of the physicians who had practiced in the inner city had moved away. The only facilities and services within easy reach were those offered by the local voluntary nursing agency, which provided family nursing care and operated a network of child health centers. Over the years, the agency had gained the trust, respect, and confidence of the community it served.

Under the dynamic leadership of the agency's director and with the support of her progressive board, nursing took the initiative in trying to correct some of these serious problems. They applied for and received a federal grant to help them establish a network of neighborhood clinics to provide maternity care. Within a year, there was a dramatic decline in the infant mortality rate. They also mobilized community resources and stimulated the formation of a local health department. They served as a catalyst in bringing together various groups into a comprehensive health planning unit. They prodded professional and citizens' groups into placing needed outpatient health facilities within easy reach of the inner city inhabitants and spearheaded the community movement to establish a Maternity and Infant Care Program with support from the U.S. Department of Health, Education, and Welfare. They coordinated areawide efforts to provide nutritious meals to the elderly by establishing a group dining program as part of an overall health maintenance program for the elderly. These were but a few of the accomplishments of a nursing agency that perceived itself as an agent of change, and took positive action.

SUMMARY

To summarize, then, we would like to point out that in mobilizing community resources, you are a coordinator and facilitator of these resources and you serve as the patient's advocate. How you go about using these resources will depend on many factors:

your knowledge about the community and its resources;
the policies of your agency;
the kinds of relationships you have been able to establish with other agencies;

how you perceive your role in nursing;

how well you have interpreted your role to the families with whom you work;

how well you have interpreted your role to other agencies;

how well you have interpreted the role of other agencies to your patients and their families.

The community with all of its resources—health planning, health financing, health services and facilities—may be viewed as a system that serves as a medium for the development of its inhabitants. In nursing, you must go beyond simply understanding the mechanism of the overall system when it is described in impersonal terms. You must learn how to use the various components in providing family health care. When you observe individuals who are caught in the system, you must make a special effort to see that they receive needed services, and that they are treated fairly and with respect. And, finally, you must be ready and willing to provide leadership in bringing about desired change to establish or improve needed services.

REFERENCES

1. Herbert Spencer, *Principles of Ethics,* as cited by George Seldes, in *The Great Quotations* (New York: Pocket Books, May 1967), p. 883.

ADDITIONAL READINGS

Anderson, C.L., *Community Health.* 2nd ed. St. Louis: C.V. Mosby, 1973.

Bayer, Mary, "Community Diagnosis—Through Sense, Sight, and Sound," in *Nursing Outlook,* 21 (November 1973) 712-13.

Blum, Henrik L., *Planning for Health.* New York: Human Sciences Press, 1974.

Brown, Frances Gold, "Social Linkability," in *American Journal of Nursing,* 71 (March 1971) 516-20.

Burton, Lloyd E., and Hugh H. Smith, *Public Health and Community Medicine.* Baltimore: Williams and Wilkins, 1970.

Carl, Mary K., "Community Planning for Nursing and Nursing Education," in *Nursing Outlook,* 20 (August 1972) 507-9.

Corey, Lawrence, Steven Saltman, and Michael Epstein, *Medicine in a Changing Society.* St. Louis: C.V. Mosby, 1972.

Freeman, Ruth, *Community Health Nursing Practice.* Philadelphia: W.B. Saunders, 1970.

Helvie, Carl O., Ann E. Hill, and Charlotte F. Bambino, "The Setting and Nursing Practice, Part I," in *Nursing Outlook,* 16 (August 1968) 27-29. Part II, 16 (September 1968) 35-38.

James, George, "Competition in Providing Community Health Services," in *Nursing Outlook,* 18 (February 1970) 42-45.

Kibrick, Anne, "NLN: Nursing's Voice in Community Health," in *Nursing Outlook,* 19 (July 1971) 455.

Klein, Donald C., *Community Dynamics and Mental Health.* New York: John Wiley and Sons, Inc., 1968.

Knight, Jeane H., "Applying Nursing Process in the Community," in *Nursing Outlook,* 22 (November 1974) 708-11.

Leavell, Hugh R., and E. Gurney Clark. *Preventive Medicine for the Doctor in His Community.* New York: McGraw-Hill, 1965.

Milio, Nancy, *The Care of Health in Communities,* Riverside, N.J.: Macmillan, 1975.

National League for Nursing, *Maintaining Health—An Adventure in Transition.* New York: NLN Publication 52-1472, 1973.

Paul, Benjamin, *Health, Culture, and Community.* New York: Russell Sage Foundation, 1955.

Perlman, Robert, and Arnold Gurin, *Community Organization and Social Planning.* New York: John Wiley and Sons, Inc., 1972.

Ruybal, Sally E., Eleanor Bauwens, and Marie-Jose Fasla, "Community Assessment: An Epidemiological Approach," in *Nursing Outlook,* 23 (June 1975) 365-68.

Saba, Virginia K., *Management Information Systems for Public Health/Community Health Agencies.* New York: National League for Nursing, 1974

Sanders, Irwin T., "Public Health in the Community," in Howard Freeman, Sol Levine, and Leo Reeder, *Handbook of Medical Sociology.* 2nd ed. Englewood Cliffs, N.J.: Prentice-Hall, 1972.

Schulberg, Herbert C., Alan Sheldon, and Frank Baker, *Program Evaluation in the Health Fields.* New York: Behavioral Publications, 1969.

Sheldon, Alan, Frank Baker, and Curtis P. McLaughlin, *Systems and Medical Care.* Cambridge: MIT Press, 1970.

Shumway, Sharon M., and Doris E. Wisehart, "How To Know a Community," in *Nursing Outlook,* 17 (September 1969) 63-64.

Simmons, H.J., "Community Health Planning—With or Without Nursing?" in *Nursing Outlook,* 22 (April 1974) 260-64.

Tinkham, Catherine W., and Eleanor V. Voorhies, *Community Health Nursing Evolution and Process.* New York: Appleton-Century-Crofts, 1972.

Vail, M. David, "Planning for a Coordinated Community Health Service," in *Community Health—Strategies for Change.* New York: National League for Nursing (Pub. no. 21-1493), 1973.

UNIT V
THE PROBLEM-ORIENTED SYSTEM AND THE NURSING PROCESS

Chapter 14
The Problem-Oriented
System in Nursing

"Nursing is concerned with helping patients solve health problems. It is, therefore, a problem-solving process related to health."[1]

INTRODUCTION

Nursing is an applied science, the practice of which requires a substantial theoretical framework, synthesized from the biological, physical, and social sciences. Operating within this framework, you must learn to think critically and to utilize the scientific or problem-solving method. In an earlier chapter, we drew your attention to the basic steps in problem-solving (see p. 60). The problem-solving process is an essential component of nursing practice, without which nursing becomes routinized and stagnant. In your efforts to improve the quality of patient care, you will find that the scientific method helps you to proceed in an orderly and logical way, and provides you with the mechanism for investigation and research.

Research is one of the essential components that differentiates professional from vocational or technical practice. The professional nurse must develop a commitment to research in clinical practice. (See p. 44.) Everyday problems should be investigated with an inquiring mind.

Example

You are the coordinator of a stroke program that has always been well attended since its inception. You notice that the attendance begins to fall off.

Why? Has the teaching been so beneficial that the stroke victims and their families achieved optimum results and require no further contact? Or is it possible that some of the families are having difficulty getting to the program because of a breakdown in transportation? Or has the program become routine, monotonous and repetitious, and lost its meaning? How do you handle this type of problem?

Consider the following problem in which an elderly person, recently discharged from a nursing home, requests your service for "therapy" and assistance in ambulation. You implement a plan of action that has been effective in similar situations. However, this time your plan does not produce the expected results—it becomes apparent that the patient does not follow through when left on his own. Why? Is it possible that the patient is unable to follow your suggestions because he really does not understand the plan? Or does he have other needs that you have not as yet identified? What is your next step?

These are the everyday problems that arise in the practice of community health nursing. Together with your colleagues, you use the scientific method to identify these problems and to seek alternate approaches for their resolution.

Within the last few years frequent references to the problem-oriented system in health care settings have appeared in medical and nursing literature. The problem-oriented system, the core of which is the problem-solving process, provides a method for clarifying, communicating, and documenting health care activities performed by any member of the health team on behalf of patients/clients. In this chapter, we will describe the development of the problem-oriented system and explain its relevance to nursing practice in today's society.

Before we begin, we would like to point out that, long before the problem-oriented system achieved its present popularity, problem-solving methodology had been recognized as an inherent part of nursing. Its application to professional practice has been described in detail by well-known leaders and educators in nursing. We find that the work done by Abdellah et al. provides a solid foundation for the problem-solving approach in nursing. She has described the steps that nurses (essentially in hospital settings) most frequently use in identifying problems:

STEPS MOST FREQUENTLY USED BY NURSES IN IDENTIFYING NURSING PROBLEMS

(1) Learn to know the patient:
   (a) Explore available data, e.g., medical and social history prior to admission.
   (b) Observe the patient on admission.
   (c) Socialize with the patient. "When did he learn of his illness?" "What are

his symptoms?'' ''What problems does he bring to the hospital?'' ''What clues to his problems does he present?''

(d) Socialize with family or friends of patient.

(e) Discuss the patient's problems at a daily nursing conference (e.g., conference with team leaders).

(f) Discuss the patient's problems at a weekly or biweekly multi-discipline conference (i.e., with doctors, social workers, dietitians, etc.).

(2) Sort out relevant and signficant data.

(3) Make generalizations about available data in relation to similar nursing problems presented by other patients. ''What nursing principles do you need to keep in mind when caring for this patient?'' ''Why does this patient react the way he does?''

(4) Identify the therapeutic plan. ''Is surgery involved?''

(5) Test generalizations with patient and make additional generalizations, e.g., Mrs. Jones is to have a mastectomy—''Does she present the same physical, emotional, and rehabilitative problems as other patients for whom you have cared with similar nursing problems?''

(6) Validate patient's conclusions about his nursing problems with your own. Indicate what generalizations are relevant and significant today.

(7) Continue to observe and evaluate the patient over a period of time to identify any attitudes and clues affecting his behavior, e.g., ''What is the patient's reaction to his diagnosis?''

(8) Explore the patient's and family's reaction to the therapeutic plan and involvement of them in the plan.

(9) Identify how ''I'' (the nurse) feel about this patient's nursing problems. ''Do you expect this patient to feel as you do about his nursing problems?''

(10) Discuss and develop an overall nursing care plan.

Reprinted with permission of Macmillan Publishing Co., Inc. from Patient-Centered Approaches to Nursing by Faye G. Abdellah, Irene L. Beland, Almeda Martin, and Ruth V. Matheney. Copyright ©1960 by Macmillan Publishing Co., pp. 13-14.

On the basis of Abdellah's work, Mrozek has taken these ''steps most frequently used by nurses in identifying nursing problems,'' and assembled them into a format that reflects the five areas of the nursing process—assessment, planning, intervention or implementation, evaluation, and revision. These five areas are not viewed as being discrete and separate; indeed, they overlap with continuous feedback from one to another. You will find that this approach is very useful in understanding the problem-oriented system for planning and documenting patient care.

THE NURSING PROCESS AS A PROBLEM SOLVING METHOD

(A) Assessment

(1) Learn to know the patient:
   (a) Explore available data, e.g., medical and social history prior to admission.

(b) Observe the patient on admission.

(c) Assess the patient as soon as possible after admission. "When did he learn of his illness?" "What are his symptoms?" "What problems does he bring to the hospital?" "What clues to his problems does he present?"

(d) Interact with family or friends of patient.

(e) Discuss the patient's problems at a daily nursing conference (e.g., conference with team leaders).

(f) Discuss the patient's problems at a weekly or biweekly multi-discipline conference (i.e., with doctors, social workers, dietitians, etc.).

(2) Sort out relevant and significant data.

(3) Identify the problems as the patient sees them and as you see them by numbering them by priority.

(B) Planning

(1) Make generalizations about available data in relation to similar nursing problems presented by other patients. "What nursing principles do you need to keep in mind when caring for this patient?" "Why does this patient react the way he does?"

(2) Develop the therapeutic plan with directives to team members as to specific approach to use.

(3) Plan for short-term and long-range goals.

(C) Intervention or Implementation

(1) Nursing action done to, for, or with the patient.

(2) Test generalizations with patient and make additional generalizations, e.g., Mrs. Jones is to have a mastectomy—"Does she present the same physical, emotional, and rehabilitative problems as other patients for whom you have cared with similar nursing problems?"

(D) Evaluation

(1) Validate patient's conclusions about his problems with your own. Indicate what generalizations are relevant and significant today.

(2) Continue to observe and evaluate the patient over a period of time to identify any attitudes and clues affecting his behavior, e.g., "What is the patient's reaction to his diagnosis?"

(3) Explore the patient's and family's reaction to the therapeutic plan and involvement of them in the plan.

(4) Identify how "I" (the nurse) feel about this patient's nursing problems. "Do you expect this patient to feel as you do about his nursing problems?"

(E) Revision

(1) Always an ongoing continuous process. You must accept or reformulate your nursing action.

(2) Discuss, develop, and revise an overall nursing care plan.

An Educational Resource from the Western Pennsylvania Regional Medical Program developed by Ruth Mrozek, R.N., Nurse Consultant.

THE PROBLEM-ORIENTED SYSTEM

The problem-oriented system of patient care, introduced by Lawrence L. Weed, with his Problem-Oriented Medical Record (POMR), has gained wide recognition throughout the country. Weed's concept embodies more than just another method of recording the patient's condition or progress. Originally conceived as a method for teaching medical students, the system can be applied to many areas in the delivery of health care—the various health disciplines, clinical specialties, and health care settings. In its approach to patient care, the system emphasizes that all professional health care workers must learn how to identify problems—one by one—and organize them for solution. Students in the health sciences—nursing, medicine, social work, physical therapy, occupational therapy, and so on—are encouraged to become familiar with this method in their first clinical courses.

The Weed system provides for ongoing auditing of services rendered. The system of recording makes it possible to evaluate a patient's progress by comparing it with the predicted outcome of a specific plan developed for the resolution of an identified problem. In this way it serves as a tool to measure the quality of care. Instructors can identify areas of deficiency and direct their students toward a positive program for improving skills and knowledge. Agency supervisors can assist staff personnel to improve their proficiency. Home health agencies can document their services more clearly for third party payment sources.

The basic components of the Problem-Oriented Medical Record are illustrated in Figure 14-1.

Briefly, the system operates as follows: the data base is collected; the problems are identified; each problem is given a number. A plan is developed for each problem. Each plan is designated by a number which is identical with the number of its target problem. Outcomes of each plan may be evaluated from the progress notes, which are recorded in numerical order according to the problem list. The discharge summary becomes more meaningful as its content is expressed in terms of the resolution of specific numbered problems for which specific numered plans have been developed. These points will be illustrated more fully in subsequent chapters as we describe the steps involved in the system.

THE PROBLEM-ORIENTED SYSTEM AND
ITS RELATION TO THE NURSING PROCESS

The concept of the problem-oriented approach to patient care and its application to nursing have been the subject of much investigation by Mrozek and others from the Western Pennsylvania Regional Medical Program. In cooperation with the University of Pittsburgh's School of Nursing, and the

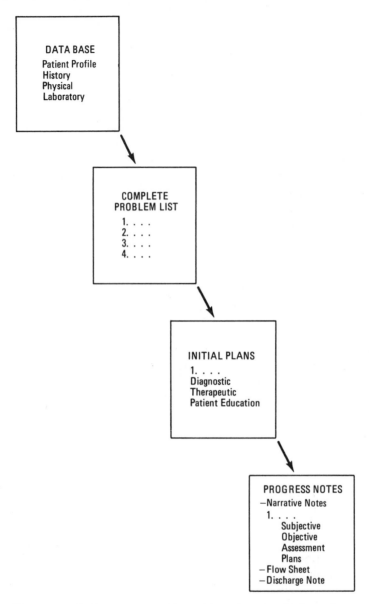

Figure 14-1 Basic components of the problem-oriented medical record.

Source From <u>Medical Records, Medical Education, and Patient Care</u> by L.L. Weed. Copyright © 1970 by Year Book Medical Publishers, Inc., Chicago. Used by permission.

Presbyterian-University Hospital's Nursing Service Department, Mrozek and her colleagues have identified the relationship of the nursing process and the problem-oriented charting system to scientific methodology. (See Figure 14-2.) They have incorporated elements from the nursing process and the problem-

Nursing Process	Scientific Method	Problem Oriented Charting System
	A. Problem finding	
Assessment	1. Gathering information 2. Examining information 3. Interpreting information 4. Identify the problem 5. Stating the problem	Data base Problem list
Plan	B. Problem Solving 1. Developing alternatives 2. Making a decision 3. Deciding on a plan of action	Plan
Intervention Evaluation Revision	4. Executing the plan 5. Evaluating the results 6. Redefine change	Progress notes

Figure 14-2   The relationship of the nursing process and problem-oriented charting to scientific methodology

Source   An Educational Resource from the Western Pennsylvania Regional Medical Program and the University of Pittsburgh School of Nursing. From H.K. Walker, J.W. Hurst, and M.F. Woody, Applying the Problem-Oriented System. ©1973 by Medcom, Inc., New York. Reproduced with permission.

oriented method as shown in Figure 14-2 and have devised a format for problem-oriented charting of patient progress notes. (See Figure 14-3.) In addition to being useful as a framework for record keeping, this format provides you with an orderly and logical methodology for the application of the basic steps in the nursing process. Although this format originally was worked out and implemented in hospital settings, problem-solving principles are basic to nursing practice in any setting.

ADAPTING THE PROBLEM-ORIENTED RECORD IN COMMUNITY NURSING

The burden on community nursing agencies increases as health care activities continue to expand outside the traditional institutional settings. For example, the growing trend of early hospital discharge has created a situation that intensifies the demand for skilled nursing services. Patients are being sent home with acute clinical problems, many of which require comprehensive nursing measures once considered possible only within the hospital setting. The nurse who enters the home must be prepared to analyze the total family situation quickly and efficiently. She must scientifically identify the problems that call for nursing intervention for which she will ultimately be held accountable by the consumer. For these reasons community nurses and nursing agencies are searching out and testing new methods to document, communicate, evaluate, and audit their services.

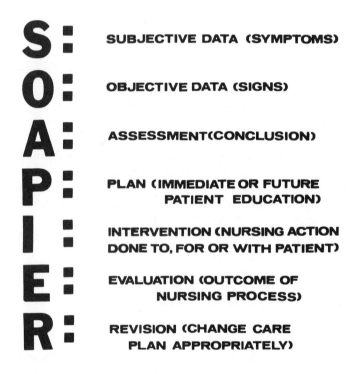

FORMAT

PROBLEM ORIENTED CHARTING
PATIENT PROGRESS NOTES

#:   Name of Problem:

S: SUBJECTIVE DATA (SYMPTOMS)

O: OBJECTIVE DATA (SIGNS)

A: ASSESSMENT(CONCLUSION)

P: PLAN (IMMEDIATE OR FUTURE
              PATIENT EDUCATION)

I: INTERVENTION (NURSING ACTION
          DONE TO, FOR OR WITH PATIENT)

E: EVALUATION (OUTCOME OF
              NURSING PROCESS)

R: REVISION (CHANGE CARE
              PLAN APPROPRIATELY)

Figure 14-3.

Source An Educational Resource from the Western Pennsylvania Regional Medical Program
and the University of Pittsburgh School of Nursing. Reprinted by permission.

Community nurses, in seeking better methods for organizing and recording their activities, will find that their national organizations have been active in establishing guidelines, resource materials, and consultant services. The American Nurses' Association, in *Standards of Community Health Nursing Practice,* has listed as Standard I "The collection of data about the health status of the consumer is systematic and continuous. The data are accessible, communicated, and recorded." The statement goes on to point out that data collection "is prerequisite to a realistic assessment for providing comprehensive care," and it offers a suggested outline for factors in assessment. The National League for Nursing has been active in promoting workshops for the implementation of the problem-oriented system in community nursing agencies. The League has developed a record system for the problem-oriented approach in community nursing. (See Appendix C.)

Let us look at the experience of a group of nurses in New England who developed their own method of adapting the problem-oriented record in community nursing. Nurses from voluntary and official community agencies in Vermont and New Hampshire worked together with the nursing staff from the area medical center to explore the advantages and disadvantages of adapting the Weed system (Problem-Oriented Medical Record) to community health nursing. They devised a record, which provides a mechanism for identifying family health problems, outlining the plans for resolving or modifying these problems, and monitoring the effectiveness of the planned intervention to meet family health needs.[2]

Our own experience with the problem-oriented system has come through a pilot study to introduce the problem-oriented record into a voluntary community nursing agency. The Community Nursing Service of Chester, Pennsylvania, with an active and ongoing staff-education program, is a small agency where the nursing students from Widener College (Chester) come for their field work. The pilot program was first introduced to the staff nurses who looked upon it with enthusiasm as a learning experience. Their overall approach to the study itself was a problem-solving one. Each step was a new challenge, posing "problems" to be investigated and resolved. "What is a defined data base and how do we go about formulating one? How much and what kind of information is necessary to include in the data base? How do we go about determining criteria? How do we identify 'patient' problems? How do we describe and record these problems in meaningful terms?" The group pooled their expertise and jointly explored ways to resolve these questions. Throughout this total process, the staff and students soon became aware that they were continuously sharpening and refining the problem-solving skills they used in everyday practice. This was one of the most valuable outcomes of the study, along with the data collection tools the nurses developed for their own use in the agency.

In the remaining chapters, we shall describe the steps involved in the problem-oriented system as it relates to the nursing process. In so doing, we shall draw from the experiences of the nursing staff and students who took part in the study, which was made possible by a grant from the Greater Delaware Valley Regional Medical Program. We will present the criteria and data collection tools developed by the participants in this study. Through selected case material, we shall also present examples of how these tools may be used.

REFERENCES

1. Faye G. Abdellah, Irene L. Beland, Almeda Martin, and Ruth V. Matheney, *Patient-Centered Approaches to Nursing* (New York: Macmillan Co., 1960), p. 80.

2. Sara P. Thompson, "Utilizing the Problem-Oriented System in Home Health Care," in H. Kenneth Walker, J.W. Hurst, and M.F. Woody, *Applying the Problem-Oriented System* (New York: Medcom Press, 1973), pp. 145-61.

ADDITIONAL READINGS

Aradine, Carolyn R., and Margaret Guthneck, "The Problem Oriented Record in a Family Health Service," in *American Journal of Nursing,* 74 (June 1974) 1108-12.

Atwood, Judith, and Stephen R. Yarnall, Symposium on "The Problem-Oriented Record," in *The Nursing Clinics of North America,* 9 (June 1974) 215-302.

Becknell, Eileen Pearlman, and Dorothy M. Smith, *System of Nursing Practice.* Philadelphia: F.A. Davis Co., 1975.

Berni, Rosemarian, and Helen Readey, *Problem-Oriented Medical Record Implementation.* St. Louis: C.V. Mosby Co., 1974.

Birk, Peter, "Problem-Oriented Medical Record." *Shop Talk,* New York State Medical Record Association, 10 (October 1970) 10.

Bloom, Judith T., et al., "Problem-Oriented Charting," in *American Journal of Nursing,* 71 (November 1971) 2144-48.

Bonkowsky, Marilyn L., "Adapting the POMR to Community Child Health Care," in *Nursing Outlook,* 20 (August 1972) 515-18.

————, et al., *The Problem-Oriented Health Care Record.* Dartmouth, New Hampshire: PROMIS Laboratory, 1974.

Cadmus, Marcia G., "Problem-Oriented Gynecology," in *Journal of OB-GYN Nursing,* 1 (June 1972) 45-48.

Cross, Harold, and John Bjorn, *The Problem-Oriented Private Practice of Medicine—A System for Comprehensive Health Care.* Chicago: Modern Hospital Press, 1970.

Elsass, Phyllis J., "Development of the Nurse's Role in Problem-Oriented Patient Care," a paper presented to the Third Annual Symposium at Naval Hospital Boston, Chelsea, Mass., May 1972, 18-19.

Field, Frances W., "Communication between Community Nurse and Physician," in *Nursing Outlook,* 19 (November 1971) 722-25.

Gane, Donna, "The Nurse's View of the Problem-Oriented Record," in Hurst, J. Willis and H. Kenneth Walker, eds., *The Problem-Oriented System.* New York: Medcom Press, 1972.

Gortner, Susan R., "Scientific Accountability in Nursing," in *Nursing Outlook,* 22 (December 1974) 764-68.

Graves, Stuart, "Better Records: First Step to Better Quality," in *Modern Hospital,* 116 (April 1971).

Hurst, J. Willis, and H. Kenneth Walker, eds., *The Problem-Oriented System.* Proceedings of a National Conference, September 10, 1971. New York: Medcom Press, 1972.

Hurst, J.W., "Ten Reasons Why Lawrence Weed Is Right," in *New England Journal of Medicine,* 284 (1971) 51-52.

Kane, Rosalie A., "Look to the Record," in *Social Work,* 19 (July 1974) 412-19.

Krismer, John R., and Jerome F. Cordes, "Problem-Oriented Record Begins with Patient," in *Modern Hospital* (November 1970).

Mitchell, Pamela Holsclaw, "A Systematic Nursing Progress Record: The Problem-Oriented Approach," in *Nursing Forum,* 12:2 (1973) 187-210.

Mrozek, Ruth, "Incorporating the Nursing Process into the Problem-Oriented Record," in Walker, H.K., et al., *Applying the Problem Oriented System.* New York: Medcom Press, 1973.

Schaefer, Jeannette, "The Interrelatedness of Decision Making and the Nursing Process," in *American Journal of Nursing,* 74 (October 1974) 1852-55.

Schell, Pamela L., and Alla T. Campbell, "POMR—Not Just Another Way To Chart," in *Nursing Outlook,* 20 (August 1972) 510-14.

Thoma, Delores, and Karen Pittman, "Evaluation of Problem-Oriented Nursing Notes," in *The Journal of Nursing Administration,* 11 (May-June 1972) 50-58.

Walker, H. Kenneth, J. Willis Hurst, and Mary F. Woody, *Applying the Problem-Oriented System.* New York: Medcom Press, 1973.

Weed, Lawrence L., "Medical Records That Guide and Teach," in *The New England Journal of Medicine,* 278: Part I, March 14, 1968; Part II, March 21, 1968.

———, *Medical Records, Medical Education, and Patient Care.* Cleveland, Ohio: Press of Case Western Reserve University, 1971. (Distributed by Year Book Medical Publishers, Inc., Chicago.)

Woody, Mary, and Mary Mallison, "The Problem-Oriented System for Patient Centered Care," in *American Journal of Nursing,* 73 (July 1973) 1168-75.

Woolley, F. Ross, Myrna Warnick, Robert Kane, and Elaine Dyer, *Problem-Oriented Nursing.* New York: Springer, 1974.

Chapter 15
Compiling the Family
Data Base

"But if you cannot get the habit of observation one way or other, you had better give up the idea of being a nurse, for it is not your calling, however kind and anxious you may be."[1]

INTRODUCTION

The language may sound quaint and archaic, and the gentle admonishment may strike you as decidedly mid-Victorian, but the meaning of the above excerpt from Nightingale's *Notes on Nursing* is every bit as pertinent now as it was when it was first printed over one hundred years ago. Equally as relevant today are some of her other precepts: "What you want are facts, not opinions . . . The most important practical lesson that can be given to nurses is to teach them what to observe—how to observe—what symptoms indicate improvement—what the reverse—which are of importance—which are of none—which are the evidence of neglect—and of what kind of neglect."[2]

Observing and assessing are basic skills, the warp and woof that go into the weaving of the nursing process. The problem-oriented approach in nursing is built around these skills. Your ability to make relevant assessments will depend largely upon your astuteness in making valid observations. On the basis of your observation and assessment, you collect the data to identify the problems, you develop a plan for each problem, and then translate your plan into action. You continue to monitor the response of the patient and family and to measure the effectiveness of your actions in accordance with standard nursing practice. These steps, which are the essence of the problem-oriented approach, are interwoven and interdependent, and may be summarized as follows:

(1) formulation of the data base;
(2) identification of the problems;
(3) development of plan for each problem;
(4) implementation of each plan;
(5) evaluation of the results.

In this chapter we will discuss the compilation of the family data base. You will see that your skills of observation and assessment are required in order to gather the essential information. We will describe the criteria for formulating a family data base, and we will present a tool or format to help you in organizing the collection of data.

THE REFERRAL AS A SOURCE OF INFORMATION

How do you begin to gather information for the family data base? An important first step is a review of the referral upon which the request for service was initiated. Requests to agenices for nursing service may originate in various ways. Formal, structured referrals may come from hospitals, other health and social agencies, private physicians, or others, either in writing or by telephone. Other requests may be less formal and come to the agency from families, neighbors, or the patients themselves. Many requests come about informally to a nurse when she is "highly visible" in the community. The "curbstone conference," for example, often yields information enabling the nurse to identify health problems in the community that might otherwise be overlooked.

From the referral source, you may expect to receive certain basic details such as name, address, directions to the home, and reason for referral. Incomplete referrals may require that you check back to the referral source with a phone call for information needed to plan the initial visit. You should try to get a description of existing health needs and socially related problems, a diagnosis of illness, the name of the physician and how he may be reached, the medical regimen, and so on. A carefully constructed referral form developed by the agency nursing staff, with input from the billing and statistical department, would be a valuable aid to the nurse in the district. Properly organized, it should include the information cited above, as well as prognosis and therapeutic goals. This tool would help to avoid unnecessary duplication and repetition. The form in Figure 15-1 is offered as an example. Along with the completed referral form that we present here, we include a copy of the plan of treatment signed by the patient's physician. (See Figure 15-2. These forms are also found in Appendix A.)

The referral may offer many cues to help you prepare for your first contact with the patient and family. For example, you may find it necessary to review the pathophysiology related to the disease process cited in the referral.

Community Nursing Service   REFERRAL FORM

Call Received by

_C. M. T._   _7/29/74_
Name   Date

_7 / 31 / 74_   _/_   _/_   _/_   _/_
Admitted   Readmitted   Discharge Date   Reason

Patient _Doe_   _Jane_   _400 757_
Last Name   First   (I.)   Record #

Address _8 Main St._
Number and Street   Apt. #   Home Care #

Anytown, USA   _/_   _US 9-0000_   _000-00-0000B_
City   Zip   Phone #   H.I. Claim #

_3-21-05_   _Cau._   _F_   _Widow_
Date of Birth   Race   Sex   Marital Status   M.A. #

_/_   _57_   _309_
Gov't Unit   Fee Status   Program   # of Visits   ( ) P. T.   ( ) H.H.A.   D. P. A. #
                                                ( ) Nursing

Daughter   _Elizabeth Jones_   _Daughter_
Referral Source   Responsible Person in Home   Relationship

Physician _Dr. R.S. MD_   Phone # _US 1-0000_

Address _100 Market St._   _Anytown_   _USA_   _19000_
Number & Street   City   State   Zip

General Hospital - Anytown, USA   _6-10-74_ / _7-3-74_
Hospital or E.C.F.   Address   Admission - Discharge Date

Diagnosis _Metastatic carcinoma - diabetes_

(Ca is inoperable - radiation therapy in hospital)

Prognosis _Poor_   Therapeutic Goals _Train bladder;_

improvement in ambulation

Medication _DBI-TD 50 daily; Percodan tab. ÷ q 3 to 4 hrs. prn._

Orders _Personal care prn - Teach daughter care of patient._

SS. Enema prn   P.T. evaluation if indicated

Report to Doctor: _incontinence of urine_

Patient Visited By: _C. Johnson   RN_   Date: _7 / 31 / 74_

Nurse's District: _C. Johnson   RN_   1. Billing
                                               2. File

Other Information: _M.D. has informed patient's daughter_
that patient's illness is "terminal"   3. Patient's Folder

Figure 15-1

282

DR. R. S. _____

_____

_____

COMMUNITY NURSING SERVICE

NAME OF PATIENT Doe, Jane   ADDRESS 8 main St. Anytown, USA

INITIAL ORDER [X]   RENEWAL [ ]   CONFIRMATION [ ]   DATE LAST SEEN BY PHYSICIAN

NURSES PROGRESS NOTES Initial home visit made. Patient's daughter is unable to cope with her mother's care; is overwhelmed with problems at this time. Pt is a diabetic but not following a diet; is eating a great amt. of "Starches." Pt is incontinent of urine at times. Pulse Rapid - but Regular at 104 - both apical & radial. Respirations 28. B/P 100/60

DATE OF NEXT VISIT 8-6 74

DATE 7-31-74   _____ C. Johnson _____ RN
                                              SIGNATURE

PLAN OF TREATMENT — TO BE COMPLETED BY PHYSICIAN

DIAGNOSIS (PRIMARY AND SECONDARY — IN ORDER) metastatic ca. Diabetes
(Ca is inoperable - radiation therapy in hospital)

SURGICAL PROCEDURE_____ DATE_____

PROGNOSIS poor   PATIENT INFORMED: DIAGNOSIS YES [ ] NO [ ] PROGNOSIS YES [ ] NO [ ]
                                   FAMILY INFORMED: DIAGNOSIS YES [ ] NO [ ] PROGNOSIS YES [ ] NO [ ]

THERAPEUTIC GOALS train bladder - improve ambulation

MEDICAL SUPERVISION IN HOME BY R S. (m.D.)   TEL. NO._____

ADDRESS_____CITY_____ZIP_____

HOME HEALTH SERVICES ORDERED: NURSING [X]   PHYSICAL THERAPY [ ]   MEDICAL SOC. SER. [ ]   SPEECH THERAPY [ ]   OCC. THERAPY [ ]   HOME HEALTH AID [ ]

MEDICATIONS DBI - TD 50 daily - Percodan 1 tab q 3 to 4 hr prn

DIET 1500 cal.   —   Nutritional status - fair

ACTIVITIES ALLOWED as tolerated

TREATMENT AND SPECIAL EQUIPMENT Personal care prn — SS Enema prn
Bladder training program - PHN may insert foley catheter if bladder training fails and if pt continues to be incontinent

SPECIAL INSTRUCTIONS, REACTIONS TO BE REPORTED TO PHYSICIAN continued incontinence

PATIENT TO BE SEEN BY PHYSICIAN: DATE_____ HOME [ ]   OFFICE [ ]   OPD [ ]

THE HOME HEALTH SERVICES TO BE PROVIDED ARE NEEDED TO TREAT THE CONDITION(S) FOR WHICH THE PATIENT RECEIVED SERVICES DURING THE RELATED STAY IN A HOSPITAL OR EXTENDED CARE FACILITY.   YES [ ]   NO [ ]

WERE INPATIENT DAYS SAVED DUE TO AVAILABILITY OF HOME CARE SERVICE? YES [ ] NO [ ]. YOUR ESTIMATE OF NO. SAVED_____

I CERTIFY THAT THE PATIENT IS (1) HOMEBOUND, (2) REQUIRES THE HOME HEALTH SERVICES INDICATED ABOVE ON AN INTERMITTENT BASIS, (3) THE PATIENT IS UNDER THE CARE OF A PHYSICIAN WHO WILL REVIEW THIS PLAN OF TREATMENT PERIODICALLY.

8-9-74   _____ MD
  DATE   PHYSICIAN'S SIGNATURE   REG. NO.

                                   _____
                                   PHYSICIAN'S NAME — PLEASE PRINT

Figure 15-2

You might wish to review a specific treatment procedure. You may wish to assemble health literature and other teaching aids that would be relevant to a particular illness or condition. If the referral alerts you to existing socially related needs, you might give some thought as to how these needs could be met through the use of other community resources (see Chapter 13). Oftentimes your own agency's records will give you additional information, as the person or family may have been known to the agency for previous services rendered. Like a detective, even before you see the patient and family, you gather together all these pieces of information to form a skeletal outline of the family data base.

WHAT IS THE FAMILY DATA BASE?

You have prepared for your initial contact with the family by noting the information in the referral, reviewing your theoretical knowledge about a specific disease process (if necessary), and gathering additional preliminary data. You are now ready to make your appraisal of the family/patient health problems in the home setting in order to compile the family data base. At this point we ask that you give some thought to what is meant by a "family data base." Referring back to the Weed system of the Problem-Oriented Medical Record, you will note that the entire process is built upon a "defined" data base. In community health nursing, the data base is defined in terms of the family as the unit of service. Individual health problems are viewed within the context of the family. The family data base includes all of the essential information—demographic, economic, social, and medical—that will help you to develop a family health profile.

When working with a family you may never consider the data base to be "complete" because the conditions it describes are never static. Therefore, periodic refining and updating of information are essential, if you expect to maintain a viable family health profile. Other important points for you to keep in mind when you are compiling the family data base are accuracy, thoroughness, and proper interpretation of information. An inaccurate data base leads to faulty assessment and ineffective planning. Meaningful data collection requires self-discipline and strict attention to detail. You also need a set of guidelines and a structured form to help you in gathering and recording information.

CRITERIA FOR DEVELOPING THE FAMILY DATA BASE

What are the criteria or guidelines for the compilation of a family data base? What kinds of information should you be looking for during the family/patient interview and assessment process? Some family needs may be more easily identified and more readily resolved than others. For example, certain physical problems may be alleviated through the immediate application of personal care or specific treatments such as colostomy irrigations, catheterizations, application of ointments or dressings. Other problems may not be so readily identified unless you have established criteria to guide you in gathering appropriate information for the family data base.

Who sets up these criteria in a community nursing agency? How are they determined? The formulation of such guidelines requires the combined efforts of the total staff, particularly of those nurses who are involved in direct patient care. All members of the staff contribute ideas culled from the observations and assessments that are part of their daily practice. Their experiences are translated into a workable formula that reflects the thinking of the total group. In this way, the group arrives at a set of guidelines, which should help the nurse to develop a comprehensive data base revealing the family health picture. In utilizing these criteria the nurse continues to employ her observation and assessment skills as she identifies health problems through her scientific appraisal of the patient, the family, and the home setting.

The following criteria for the family data base were developed during the pilot study:

Chief Complaint or Reason for Service

This should be a brief statement from the viewpoint of the family/patient concerning the health problem or the disease condition that prompted the request for service.

Present Conditions, Illnesses, Health Problems

When was the condition, illness, or health problem first noted? What were the first indications that a problem existed, e.g., presenting signs and symptoms? What happened after the first signs and symptoms appeared? What measures, if any, were taken to cope with the problem? What is the family's understanding of the health problem, the course of illness, treatment?

Family Profile

What specific demographic, social, and economic factors characterize this family? What is their source of health care? What is the source and extent of the family income? How does the family spend its average day? What are the family dynamics—role relationships, communication, behavior and attitude toward each other, commitment, etc.? (See Chapter 12.) What are the emotional strengths and weaknesses of the family group? What is the relationship of the family to the community? Do they take an active role in community activities?

Environmental Factors

What is the physical condition of the family dwelling? How many rooms are there? What are the living arrangements? What are the accommodations for activities of daily living—sleeping, eating, toileting, bathing, dressing, working, socializing? Are there household pets? Is the house clean and free of vermin, other insects, and rodents? Are there adequate safety and security measures? Are there provisions for emergencies—e.g., telephone and transportation? How effective are the heating, lighting, ventilation? What is the noise level?

Family Health History

What specific illnesses, chronic conditions or impairments, serious injuries, or hospitalizations has the family faced in the past? What measures are utilized by the family to meet these problems? What are the family practices with respect to the use of prescriptions and "over-the-counter" medications? How well do they understand the administration, dosage, and effects of the drugs they use? What are the ages and causes of death of parents, grandparents, siblings, children? Is there a history of allergy, cancer, stroke, heart disease, hypertension, renal disease, tuberculosis, alcoholism, drug abuse, diabetes, venereal disease, or mental illness? What measures has the family taken to prevent illness? Are their immunizations current?

Nutritional Needs and Dietary Habits

On visual inspection, how would you rate the general, overall nutritional status of the family members? What information have you gathered from the diet recall? (See pages 104-105 for diet recall guide.) How does this information coincide with the actual practices you observe (e.g., the diet recall indicates that each child drinks a quart of milk a day, but you never see milk in the home)? Is any member of the family on a special diet? If so, does he adhere to the diet? Do other members of the family understand and support this individual?

Level of Functioning

Do family members exhibit any major defects in speech, hearing, vision, motor movement and coordination? Has there been any interruption in normal growth and development as a result of genetic factors, congenital defects, birth trauma, or other accidents? What are the strengths and weaknesses in the family? Do they work together as a family unit?

Physical Assessment

An important activity in the compilation of the data base is the physical assessment which you perform. For this portion of the data base you focus on the family member(s) with the most acute health problem(s). Guidelines for establishing the nursing baseline assessment are suggested in Table 15-1. Knowledge of normal human anatomy and physiology is a prerequisite for the use of these guidelines, which should help you in identifying individual strengths and weaknesses. From this baseline assessment, you estimate the patient's level of performance and determine the appropriate nursing action.

METHODOLOGY FOR COLLECTING THE DATA: THE STRUCTURED FORM

In applying any set of criteria for developing a data base, you will need a structured form to help you focus on the collection of essential material. When you use structured forms, you view them merely as working tools that can facilitate data collection. It is your observation and assessment skills during the family/patient interview that move the activity of gathering data from a routinized task of "filling out a form" to a meaningful step in the problem-solving process.

The data collection tool should be conceived within the framework of community needs and agency policies. Ideally, the form should be developed, evaluated, implemented, and revised by agency nursing staff. The items contained in the form should be concise, organized, easy to read, and free of extraneous details. Numerous examples of data collection forms are in existence today, and are available commercially. Others are being developed, as home health agencies continue to move toward a more systematized approach to patient care. In Figures 15-3 and 15-4 we offer as examples the data collection tools developed by our group and show how these forms are being used. These figures also appear in Appendix A.

REFERENCES

1. Florence Nightingale, *Notes on Nursing,* Facsimile Reprint of the First Edition of Florence Nightingale's *Notes on Nursing* Published in 1860 by Harrison and Sons, Printers in Ordinary to Her Majesty, St. Martin's Lane, London (Philadelphia: University of Pennsylvania Printing Office, 1964), p. 63.
2. Ibid., p. 59

ADDITIONAL READINGS

Abdellah, Faye I., et al., *Patient-Centered Approaches to Nursing.* New York: Macmillan Co., 1960.

Bates, Barbara, *A Guide to Physical Examination.* Philadelphia: J.B. Lippincott Co., 1974.

Bates, Barbara, and Joan Lynaugh, "Teaching Physical Assessment," in *Nursing Outlook,* 23 (May 1975) 297-302.

Table 15-1   Guidelines for Establishing the Nursing Baseline Data

Overall appearance	*Body structure:* lean? obese? flabby? plump? emaciated? *Posture and bearing:* erect? stooped? slouched? Are there any obvious deformities?
General condition	Is the individual confined to bed? Is he fatigued, nervous, perspiring, short of breath? Is there any frank bleeding? Is there obvious edema of any body area—face, neck, chest, abdomen, extremities? Are there signs and symptoms such as vomiting, vertigo, fever, pain, nausea?
Skin	*Color:* pink? jaundiced? cyanotic? flushed? pallid? gray? hyperpigmented? *Condition:* smooth and regular? thin and transparent? irregularities in contour or surface? moles? eruptions: macules? papules? vesicles? pustules? acne? blackheads? excessive oil? scaling? dryness? rashes? petechiae? signs and symptoms of dermatitis, scleraderma, psoriasis, impetigo, ringworm, vermin? *Temperature:* cool? warm? clammy? hot? *Turgor:* flabby? firm? loose? tense?
Head	*Size and shape:* regular? micro- or macrocephalic? presence of tumors, cysts? *Hair:* presence or absence? condition: clean, dirty, dandruff, head lice? *Scalp:* ringworm? other lesions?
Eyes	*Appearance:* shape and size? conjunctiva: color and clarity? eyelids: edema? ptosis? granulation? infection? pupils: dilated? contracted? opaque? *Gross vision:* normal with corrective lenses? blind?
Nose	*Appearance:* gross size and shape? presence of moles, cysts, warts? Are there any obvious deformities? deviated septum? distorted nares?
Mouth	*Lips:* cracked? swollen? lesions? fissures? harelip? *Teeth and gums:* missing teeth? mouth hygiene? tender, swollen, bleeding, receding gums? lesions or abscesses of gums? sordes? *Buccal mucosa:* leukoplakia? canker sores or other lesions? *Tongue:* dry? smooth? leukoplakia? fissures? coated? abnormal color or pigmentation? lesions? *Throat:* redness? inflammation? enlarged or abscessed tonsils? *Hard and soft palate:* deviations? fissures? lesions? discoloration? cleft palate? perforated palate?
Neck	What is the general appearance? Have you noted any edema? tumors? enlarged thyroid? displacement of trachea? Have you tested for range of motion? Have you palpated for enlarged cervical glands? Have you asked to see the patient swallow? Have you lowered his head toward his chin without difficulty?
Chest	*Size and shape:* shrunken? pigeon-breast? barrel-shaped? distorted? Any abnormalities such as tumors? cysts? lesions? *Respiration:* discomfort on moving or breathing? Is inspiration/expiration cycle completed with a normal rhythmic pattern? Does patient assume a fixed position using his shoulder muscles to aid respiration? *Auscultation:* Is breathing stertorous? restricted? obstructed? painful? are rales present?
Breasts	*Size and shape:* enlarged? pendulous? flat? tumors? lesions? absence of breast(s)? *Nipples:* cracked? inverted? lactating? bleeding? Is there crusting or erosion? *Palpation:* freely moving masses? palpable nodes? Has the patient been instructed in breast self-examination?
Heart and blood vessels	*Auscultation:* This most useful technique to determine cardiac rate and rhythm requires a carefully selected, well-fitting stethoscope; an effort must be made to eliminate as much extraneous noise as possible. Is the heart rate regular? slow? fast? Are there other sounds in the chest impeding the verification of the heart rate? Is the rhythm intermittent, galloping, alternating, fluttering, spasmodic, regular, or irregular?

Radial beat: Is the rate full and bounding? Is it slow? fast? Is it small and barely palpable? Does the rate fall off rapidly? Is there a double impulse? Is the rhythm of the pulse regular or irregular? Is it weak or thready? Is the pulse wave low and flat? Is the rhythm peaked or unsustained? What is the pulse tension? volume? Is it full, bounding, or moderate? small or feeble, flickering or thready?

Apical beat: Note rate, rhythm, volume; how do they compare with the same observations of the radial pulse? What is the pulse deficit, if any?

Blood pressure: On the first assessment, the blood pressure should be examined in both arms and in the standing and recumbent positions; if you continue to monitor the blood pressure on subsequent visits, and the patient is not taking antihypertensive drugs, the recumbent position is adequate.

Circulation: Note presence or absence of pulsation in pedal, femoral, carotid areas; skin temperature in extremities, particularly the lower extremities, is a good monitor of the adequacy of circulation.

Abdomen	*Size and shape:* flat? distended? depressed?
	General appearance: scars? tumors? lesions? "-ostomy"? herniation? umbilical or inguinal incision?
	Palpation: Is there evidence of pain? tenderness? sensitivity? rigidity?
	Auscultation: Are bowel sounds present?
Genitalia	*Female:*
	Labia and surrounding area: ulcers? lesions? swelling? tenderness? discoloration? protrusion of tissue? uterine prolapse?
	Vaginal discharge: bloody? purulent? serous? malodorous? burning? itching?
	Note history of menses, date of last menstrual period and Pap test.
	Male:
	Penis, scrotum, and surrounding area: phimosis? ulcer? lesion? edema? tumors or abnormal masses? venous congestion?
	Penile discharge: bloody? purulent? serous? malodorous? burning? itching?
	Note history of prostatitis, urinary tract infection, difficulty in voiding.
Extremities	*Size and shape:* Are the limbs contorted? contracted? paralyzed? flaccid? spastic? withered? wasted? amputated?
	General appearance and condition: cleanliness? irritation? bruises? fissures? tumors? lesions? ulcers? varicosities? color? temperature? absence of pedal pulse? prostheses?
	Joints: Can full range of motion be completed? Have you checked for tenderness? swelling? rigidity?
Activities of daily living	*Mobility level:* Can the patient ambulate? How far? Does he require assistance? Is he capable of stair climbing? Can he dress himself? Does he need assistance? How much? Is he responsible for his own personal care? Does he need help? How much?
	Sleeping habits: Does the patient sleep through the night? Does he require medication for sleeping? Does he complain about early morning waking? Does he have nocturia?
	Elimination: What is his bowel pattern? Does he require the assistance of a laxative or enema on a regular basis? What is the extent of his urinary function? Does he depend on artificial help? indwelling catheter? Is he incontinent? totally or just at night?
Nutritional Status	*Twenty-four-hour diet recall:* Does the diet contain most of the nutrients required by the patient? Is it grossly lacking in even minimal requirements? Is there a particular therapeutic diet prescribed for the patient? How closely does he adhere to the diet? What is his fluid intake? Is it adequate for his particular needs?
Ability to communicate and understand	Can the patient communicate and make his needs known? If he has a speech problem, is he able to communicate through signs, writing? Can he read and comprehend written communication? Can he convey his understanding of the written material to others? Have you made sure that lack of communication is not due to a foreign language barrier?
State of orientation	Is the patient oriented to time, place, and other persons? Is his affect appropriate? flat? inappropriate? Does he exhibit vagueness? lapse of memory? echolalia?

PATIENT IDENTIFICATION

Name _Doe, Jane_

Address _8 Main ST._

Anytown, U.S.A.

Directions _West on 9th ST. - Rt. on K street -_
Rt. on Main ST. house on Rt.

Phone _US 9-0000_

CNS _400757_

HC _____

HI _000-00-0000 B_

MA/DPA _____

BC/BS _____

Classification _309_

Age _69_ Birthdate _3-21-05_ Sex _F_ Race _Cau._

Ethnic Group _Italian_ Marital Status _Widow_

Education _7th grade_ Occupation _—_

Religious Preference _Catholic_

Income: Employment _—_ Pension $58.00 SS $200.00

Expenses: Housing _____ Food _____ Other _____

FEE STATUS

Date	Fee	Date	Fee
7/31/74	57		

DATES OF SERVICE

Adm.	Disch.	Adm.	Disch.
7/31/74			

Friend or Relative to Notify in Case of Emergency:

Name _A. Brown_ Relationship _daughter_

Phone _US 8-0000_ Address _4 Maple ST. Anytown, U.S.A._

Friends or Relatives Outside Home Involved in Care:

Name	Address	Phone	Relationship

Doctor (Family) _Dr. R. S_ Phone # _US1-0000_

Address _100 Market ST. Anytown, U.S.A._ _19000_

Doctor (Consultant) _____ Phone # _____

Address _____

Pharmacy _Central Drug_ Phone # _US2-0000_

Ambulance Service _Allied_ Phone # _US3-0000_

Other Agencies Involved	Contact	Phone

Equipment in home (Itemize): _Hospital Bed - Side Rails - Commode_

Services presently involved (check in pencil): Nursing _✓_ P. T. _____

O. T. _____ S. T. _____ H. H. A. _____ H. M. _____

Med. SW _____ Other _____

Figure 15-3

290

FAMILY IDENTIFICATION

Family Name *Doe, Jane*   Pt's Rel. to HH *Head of house*

Members in Household	Sex	Birth Date	Marital Status	Rel to HH	Education	Occupation	CNS Record #	Open
Jane Doe	F	3-21-05	Widow	HH	7TH Gr.	—	400757	✓
Elizabeth Jones	F	3-1-25	Separated	dtr.	12TH Gr.	P.T. Clerk House wife		
Mary Jones	F	8-19-63	Single	G	5TH Gr.	student		

Family Economic Profile: *Pt. lives on income from Social Security and pension. Pt. owns house.*

Home Evaluation *Single-frame dwelling - fair condition*

Type & Condition of Home *Single-frame - 2 story*

No. of BR *1* Pt. prox. to BR *next to bedroom* Heating *Hot air - gas*

Pt. Sleeping Accom. *has own room* Kitchen Facilities *adequate*

Pt. prox. to family activity *Pt. stays upstairs* Housekeeping *done by dtr.*

Other pertinent info. *Household in disarray - daughter not very organized*

Family Health History

Family Member	TB	Cancer	Ht. Dis.	Diabetes	Renal Dis.	Epilepsy	Mental Dis.	Alcohol	VD	Other (allergy, surgery, injury, etc.)
Jane Doe	NO	yes	yes	yes	Ca. Kidney	NO	No	No	No	hyst. at age 26 allergic to Penicillin
Eliz. Jones	No	No	No	yes	No	No	No	No	No	C. section allergic to Tetanus
Mary Jones	No	No	No	No	No	No	No	No	No	allergic to Penicillin

Family dietary habits (include ethnic factors, meal times, etc.): *No special food preferences - Regular meal time*

Family medication habits (include usual remedies for constipation, headaches, nervousness, etc.)

Aspirin for headaches

Pt. is on Percodan ÷ Tab q3 to 4 hrs prn and DBI-TD 50 ÷ daily

Family dynamics (include significant family interpersonal relationships): *Mother and daughter devoted; get along well but daughter is now overwhelmed with care of mother - Is having difficulty coping with situation* C. Johnson R.N.

Figure 15-3 (continued).

NURSING BASELINE ASSESSMENT

Patient _Doe, Jane_   Age _69_   Ht. _4' 11"_   Wt. _94 lbs._

Diagnosis _Metastatic ca. — diabetes_

General Physical Appearance _Thin — Pale — Weak_

General Mental Condition _Oriented to Time and Place — quiet — stoic._

Physical Assessment		Not Exam.	Norm	Abnorm	Describe or Measure
SKIN	Color			X	Pale
	Condition		X		
	Temperature		X		
	Turgor			X	loose skin
HEAD	Hair		X		
	Shape		X		
EYES	Appearance			X	Conjunctiva pale
	Vision			X	wears glasses
	Pupils		X		
EARS	Appearance		X		
	Hearing		X		
MOUTH	Teeth & Gums			X	Most of teeth are missing
	Throat		X		has 1 tooth on bottom — wears
	Tongue		X		dentures — gums pale
NOSE			X		
NECK	Appearance		X		
	Mobility		X		
CHEST	Configuration		X		
	Auscultation		X		
	Respiration		28		
BREASTS	Appearance			X	Flabby
	Self Exam.				
HEART	Auscultation		X		Rapid - Regular Rate and
	Apical Pulse			104	Rhythm
	Radial Pulse			104	
	Blood Pressure		100/60		
	Circulation		X		
EXTREMITIES	Upper		X		
	Lower			X	Edema of both feet.
	Joints		X		
ABDOMEN	Shape			X	Flabby
	Bowel Sounds		X		
	Palpation			X	Mass R.U.Q.
GENITALIA	Menstruation				Had hysterectomy at age 26
	Last Pap Test				Never had Pap Test done
	Prostate				

Figure 15-4

292

FUNCTIONAL ASSESSMENT

		Not Exam.	Norm	Abnormal (Specify)
ACTIVITIES OF DAILY LIVING	Ambulation			Weak - Pt. can walk from bedroom To bathroom - otherwise Remains in bed.
	Stairs			
	Dressing		x	
	Feeding		x	
	Household Activity			Unable to perform any household activities.
	Personal Care			Able to do part of sponge bath-dtr. assists
SLEEP			x	
HABITS	Alcohol		x	Does not use any alcohol, Tobacco, or drugs
	Tobacco		x	
	Drugs		x	
	Other		x	
ELIMINATION	Bowel Function		x	Nocturia
	Urinary Function			Unable to hold urine until she gets To B.R.
NUTRITIONAL STATUS	Food		x	
	Fluid		x	
ABILITY TO COMMUNICATE & UNDERSTAND	Speech		x	
	Read		x	
	Understand		x	
ORIENTED			x	
AFFECT			x	

Adjustment to Illness   Very stoic - does not complain

Describe Patient's Usual Day:

Morning: _Breakfast at 10 AM — then listens to radio._

Afternoon: _Lunch at 2 PM - rests in bed - sleeps or listens to radio._

Evening: _Dinner at 6 PM - listens to radio - asleep about 10 PM_

24 Hour Diet Recall:

Breakfast _Fried potatoes - 1 fried egg - tea_

Lunch _Macaroni - salad - water_

Dinner _Meat - Mashed potatoes - corn_

Snacks _Fruit between meals_

HISTORY:

Medical _Diabetic for past 6 or 7 years - "Heart Trouble" - Ca. Kidney_

Surgical _Hysterectomy at age 26_

Figure 15-4 (continued)

Beland, Irene L., *Clinical Nursing.* 2nd ed. New York: Macmillan Co., 1970.

Brunner, Lillian, and Doris Suddarth, *Lippincott Manual of Nursing Practice.* Philadelphia: J.B. Lippincott Co., 1974.

Buckingham, William B., Marshall Sparberg, and Martha Brandfonbrener, *A Primer of Clinical Diagnosis.* New York: Harper and Row, 1971.

Burnside, John W., *Adams' Physical Diagnosis.* Baltimore: Williams and Wilkins Co., 1974.

Carlson, Sylvia, "A Practical Approach to the Nursing Process," in *American Journal of Nursing,* 72 (September 1972) 1589-91.

Cauffman, Joy G., et al., "A Study of Health Referral Patterns," in *American Journal of Public Health,* 64 (April 1974) 331-55.

Chambers, Wilda, "Nursing Diagnosis," in *American Journal of Nursing,* 62 (November 1962) 102-4.

Chinn, Peggy L., and Cynthia J. Leitch, *Child Health Maintenance: A Guide to Clinical Assessment.* St. Louis: C.V. Mosby Co., 1974.

Durand, Mary, and Rosemary Prince, "Nursing Diagnosis: Process and Decision," in *Nursing Forum,* 5(4) (1966) 50-64.

Fowkes, William, and Virginia K. Hunn, *Clinical Assessment for the Nurse Practitioner.* St. Louis: C.V. Mosby Co., 1973.

Fuller, Dorothy, and Janet Allan Rosenaur, "A Patient Assessment Guide," in *Nursing Outlook,* 22 (July 1974) 460-62.

Garant, Carol, "A Basis for Care," in *American Journal of Nursing,* 72 (April 1972) 699-701.

Gragg, Shirley H., and Olive M. Rees, *Scientific Principles in Nursing.* 6th ed. St. Louis: C.V. Mosby Co., 1970.

Hobson, Lawrence B., *Examination of the Patient.* New York: McGraw-Hill, 1975.

Jones, Mary C., "An Analysis of a Family Folder," in *Nursing Outlook,* 16 (December 1968) 48.

Komorita, Nori, "Nursing Diagnosis," in *American Journal of Nursing,* 63 (December 1963) 83-86.

Lehman, Sr. J., "Auscultation and Heart Sounds," in *American Journal of Nursing,* 72 (July 1972) 1242-46.

Littman, D., "Stethoscopes and Auscultation," in *American Journal of Nursing,* 72 (July 1972) 1238-41.

Lynaugh, Joan, and Barbara Bates, "Physical Diagnosis: A Skill For All Nurses?" in *American Journal of Nursing* 74 (January 1974) 58-60.

McCain, R. Faye, "Nursing by Assessment—Not Intuition," in *American Journal of Nursing,* 65 (April 1965) 82-84.

McPhetridge, L. Mae, "Nursing History: One Means to Personalize Care," in *American Journal of Nursing,* 68 (January 1968) 68-75.

Marriner, Ann, *The Nursing Process: A Scientific Approach to Nursing Care.* St. Louis: C.V. Mosby Co., 1975.

Matheney, Ruth V., et al., *Fundamentals of Patient-Centered Nursing.* St. Louis: C.V. Mosby Co., 1968.

Mayers, Marlene G., "A Search for Assessment Criteria," in *Nursing Outlook,* 20 (May 1972) 323-26.

Miller, Marian, and Marvin L. Sachs, *About Bedsores.* Philadelphia: J.B. Lippincott Co., 1974.

Moreland, Helen J., and Virginia C. Schmitt, "Making Referrals Is Everybody's Business," in *American Journal of Nursing,* 74 (January 1974) 96-97.

Murray, Ruth, and Judith Zentner, *Nursing Assessment and Health Promotion through the Life Span.* Englewood Cliffs, N.J.: Prentice-Hall, 1975.

———, *Nursing Concepts for Health Promotion.* Englewood Cliffs, N.J.: Prentice-Hall, 1975.

"Patient Assessment: Taking a Patient's History," a Programmed Instruction. *American Journal of Nursing,* 74 (January 1974) 293-324.

"Patient Assessment: Examination of the Abdomen" a Programmed Instruction. *American Journal of Nursing,* 74 (September 1974) 1679-1702.

"Patient Assessment: Examination of the Eye" (Part 1), a Programmed Instruction. *American Journal of Nursing,* 74 (November 1974) 2039 ff.

"Patient Assessment: Examination of the Ear" a Programmed Instruction. *American American Journal of Nursing,* 75 (January 1975) 105 ff.

"Patient Assessment: Examination of the Ear," a Programmed Instruction. *American Journal of Nursing,* 75 (March 1975) 457 ff.

"Patient Assessment: Examination of the Head and Neck" a Programmed Instruction. *American Journal of Nursing,* 75 (May 1975) 839 ff.

"Patient Assessment: Urological Examination" (Part 1), a Programmed Instruction. *American Journal of Nursing,* 75 (September 1975).

"Patient Assessment: Urological Examination" (Part 2), a Programmed Instruction. *American Journal of Nursing,* 75 (November 1975).

Ryder, Claire F., William F. Elkin, and Dana Doten, "Patient Assessment, an Essential Tool in Placement and Planning of Care," in *HSMHA Health Reports,* 86 (October 1971) 923-32.

Seedor, Marie M., *The Physical Assessment.* New York: Teachers College Press, 1974.

Sherman, Jacques, and Sylvia K. Fields, *Guide to Patient Evaluation.* Flushing, N.Y.: Medical Examination Publishing Co., Inc., 1974.

Smith, Dorothy M., "A Clinical Nursing Tool," in *American Journal of Nursing,* 63 (November 1968) 2384-88.

Smith, Dorothy, Carol P. Hanley Germain, and Claudia D. Gips, *Care of the Adult Patient.* 3rd ed. Philadelphia: J.B. Lippincott Co., 1971.

Wong, Donna M., "Providing Experience in Physical Assessment for Students in Basic Programs," in *American Journal of Nursing,* 75 (June 1975) 974-75.

Yura, Helen, and Mary Walsh, *The Nursing Process: Assessing, Planning, Implementing, and Evaluating.* New York: Appleton-Century-Crofts, 1973.

Chapter 16
Formulating
the Problem List

"A problem is defined as something that 'concerns' the patient and/or any member of the health team"[1]

INTRODUCTION

In Chapter 15 we emphasized the importance of the "defined" data base, we discussed the rationale for developing a family health profile, and we identified our criteria to help structure the format for the family/patient interview during the home visit. We presented an example of a data base on the Doe family as compiled by a staff nurse on her initial visit. The information on that record included data from the referral as well as the nurse's observations in the home. When a data base is compiled it becomes a vital source of information for the identification of family/patient health problems. In this chapter we will show how you proceed with the data base to identify health problems and formulate the problem list. The problem-oriented system is predicated upon the development of viable communication links between the nurse, physician, and other members of the health team. As you record and interpret the family/patient data, you correlate your findings with those of the physician and other members of the health team. You incorporate their information with the data you have compiled. The identification of problems requires an analytical approach, careful attention to detail, and an ability to determine which information is relevant. The success of the problem-oriented system hinges upon the formulation of an accurate problem list.

Once identified, problems are numerically listed, and the nursing management of the health needs of the family/patient should always be related to these problems. The problem list, which serves as the table of contents to the family health record, is divided into two basic parts—active and resolved/inactive problems. When listing the problems, you should record the date of onset and the date of resolution. As each problem is identified, it is numbered and added to the list. Whenever problems are resolved or consolidated, their numbers are retained and are not used again on that record; new numbers are assigned as additional problems are identified. Our own experience with the problem-oriented system has convinced us that the standardized recording of problems assists both staff and students to develop and improve their ability to resolve these problems and evaluate the effectiveness of their actions. Problems may fall into several categories:

(1) nursing and/or medical diagnoses—present or past;
(2) signs and symptoms observed by the nurse and/or expressed by the family/patient;
(3) laboratory and radiology findings;
(4) demographic or environmental factors;
(5) socioeconomic problems;
(6) psychosocial problems.

IDENTIFYING THE PROBLEMS

While the preceding discussion describes the mechanics of drawing up the problem list, it does not explain how you identify and state the problems. During our pilot study the nursing staff and students posed many questions, as they were attempting to master this important step in the application of the problem-oriented system, for example: "How do I proceed in stating the problems? Do I list the given medical diagnosis as a problem? Do I record signs and symptoms as problems? Have I identified socioeconomic needs? How should they be listed as problems? I have found disabilities and deficiencies that have resulted from the pathophysiological process—how are they listed as problems? Are there identifiable problems in the family relationships? Where do I begin and end in listing problems?"

In responding to these questions, we suggest that each situation must be handled on an individual basis. However, we recognize that several key points, which emerged during our study, might serve as general guidelines in identifying problems, as follows:

(1) To begin with, the identification of problems depends on a careful review and analysis of all available data.
(2) In formulating the problem list you are concerned with those situations or conditions that affect the well-being of the family/patient—as perceived by them or noted by you.
(3) If a diagnosis of clinical pathology has been established, you would consider

that diagnosis in terms of disabilities and deficiencies (generated by the pathological condition) that affect the family's/patient's level of performance. These disabilities and deficiencies would be subsumed under the given diagnosis.

(4) If a diagnosis is not available, you would list as problems the signs and symptoms which you have identified and include as one of your problems "incomplete data base—clinical diagnosis not available."

(5) You list those problems that are amenable to nursing intervention, keeping two essential points in mind: (a) you state problems in terms that help you conceptualize nursing care plans; (b) you state plans for nursing intervention in terms of expected outcomes that can be measured in patient progress.

BEGIN WITH THE FAMILY'S CONCERNS

We would like to cite a few concrete examples in order to illustrate some of the points we have outlined here. For instance, in formulating the problem list, we find that a good place to begin is with the chief complaint posed by the family/patient—with whatever they perceive as the greatest threat to their life style or health status. This could be a manifestation of obvious physical or mental pathology, lack of food, poor housing and sanitary facilities, ineffective family relationships, inadequate financial resources, or any combination of these or other conditions or circumstances.

EXAMPLE

Let us say that you are the nurse assigned to Mrs. Doe, whose family/patient data base was presented in Figures 15-3 and 15-4. As you review the available information, you find that she lives with her daughter and young granddaughter in modest but comfortable circumstances. The patient has returned home from the hospital where she had received a series of radiation treatments for "Inoperable Metastatic Carcinoma." The initial referral indicates that the patient's prognosis is poor, and the treatment plan calls for bladder training, improvement in ambulation, and personal care. You might therefore expect to find certain problems, such as generalized weakness, limited activity, urinary incontinence, pain, and mental depression. Your observation and assessment during the initial home visit confirm some of these problems you have anticipated. However, you pick up more urgent cues as the daughter anxiously reiterates: "I don't know how I am going to manage with my mother. She needs so much care and attention. I can't give up my job—I've got to work to pay the bills. I have no one to stay with my mother. She needs someone to keep her dry. Someone has to feed my mother because she won't eat." Your ability to understand the immediacy of the daughter's needs and her concern for her mother would prompt you to translate this meaningful information into a carefully stated problem: "daughter of patient overwhelmed with care of mother." From your analysis of the situation, it becomes obvious that this problem is perceived as the greatest threat to the family/patient and must be given immediate consideration.

HOW TO USE THE MEDICAL DIAGNOSIS

In identifying problems, you would certainly direct your attention to the given medical diagnosis. The question inevitably arises, "Do I list the medical diagnosis as one of the numbered 'patient problems' that require planned nursing intervention?" To answer this question, you must review your available data. If the information indicates that the pathophysiology has generated the disabilities or deficiencies that affect the family's/patient's level of performance, the diagnosis becomes a numbered problem. The disabilities or deficiencies you identify may then be subsumed under the diagnosis. In this way you can group those conditions which are better resolved by an overall strategy of planning. Let us say that you have been assigned to a middle-aged victim of a cerebrovascular accident (CVA). You are able to identify the following conditions that affect the patient's physical/mental status: urinary incontinence, right-sided paralysis, slurred speech, difficulty in chewing and swallowing. The available data clearly indicate that these problems are directly related to the clinical diagnosis—CVA. Your problem list might read as follows:

(1) Cerebrovascular accident
   (1a) urinary incontinence
   (1b) right-sided paralysis
   (1c) slurred speech
   (1d) difficulty in chewing and swallowing

Not all deficiencies and disabilities are as clearly related to the pathophysiology of the given diagnosis. In such situations the listing of the diagnosis as a problem may not be especially relevant for the immediate formulation of nursing plans.

EXAMPLE

Let us consider the case of Mrs. Jennings, a 45 year old woman, recently widowed, with three school age children. You receive a referral from Miss Smith, one of the school nurses, requesting a home evaluation on this family. Miss Smith has informed you that she is "worried about these children. They don't look too well, and they are often absent from school. When I've questioned them, they tell me that their father just died, their mother is sick, and they have to stay home with her. The only other thing I could find out was Mrs. Jennings has been spending a lot of time in bed since she got out of Blank Hospital a few months ago." In checking with the hospital, you learn that Mrs. Jennings had been treated in the past for "primary pernicious anemia," a condition that had been under control with appropriate medical care. However, about three months ago, complications set in following an episode of excessive premenopausal bleeding, which necessitated immediate hospitalization. The control of the hemorrhaging required several weeks of intensive therapy, including bed rest, multiple blood transfusions, a high protein diet, and special medications. She made a satisfactory recovery, and upon discharge from the hospital, was advised to return to the hematology clinic for a checkup in three weeks. A call to the clinic revealed that the patient had never kept her appointment. On your initial visit you are able to identify the following disabilities as "problems" which may or may not be attributed to the pathophysiology of the stated diagnosis—"primary pernicious anemia."

(1) generalized weakness
(2) acute depression
(3) patient confined to bed
(4) anorexia

Continuing with your assessment of the overall situation, you recognize other family problems and list those as well, for example:

(5) strained relationships between the patient and her eldest daughter, age 16
(6) inadequate finances to cover recently incurred medical expenses
(7) economic loss due to husband's death
(8) hazardous environmental conditions due to excessive accumulation of papers, trash, and garbage.

Your ability to recognize and tabulate specific problems such as these, would facilitate your plans for appropriate nursing intervention.

STATING PROBLEMS IN TERMS WHICH HELP CONCEPTUALIZE A NURSING CARE PLAN

When you formulate the problem list, you should try to state each problem in terms that can be translated into a plan for nursing intervention. This plan must reflect "expected outcomes" that are measurable in terms of family/patient progress.

EXAMPLE

You receive a request to visit a sixty-eight-year-old man who has been discharged from the local hospital where he had been diagnosed and treated for "Diabetes Mellitus." Throughout his hospitalization, attempts were made to instruct the patient in the technique of self-administration of insulin. However, he resisted all efforts to help him become independent with this procedure. Family members did not visit regularly and hospital staff members were unsuccessful in enlisting their assistance. Therefore, while still dependent on others, the patient was sent home with instructions to take "60 Units of NPH insulin daily." As this medication requires parenteral administration, the patient would obviously need assistance. In this situation, you might ask "How do I state the problem in realistic terms?" Certainly the fact that he has diabetes is a problem; also, the fact that he requires 60 Units of NPH insulin daily is a problem. However, when you attempt to construct the problem list in terms that can be translated into a plan for nursing intervention, you might aptly describe the problem as follows: "Patient unable to administer insulin." From this description, you can immediately recognize the implications for planning and "expected outcomes" that could be measured in patient progress. Thus your initial plan for this problem might read as follows: "(1) administer insulin daily until patient is ready to learn; (2) provide emotional support to patient while encouraging him to accept responsibility for self-administration; (3) set up a teaching plan for guiding the patient at his level of learning and acceptance; (4) involve a family member, neighbor, or friend, in the event that the patient becomes incapacitated and is unable to administer his insulin."

SUMMARY

In summary we would like to refer back to the case of Jane Doe, which appears earlier in this chapter (see page 298) to illustrate more fully the methodology of problem identification. In Figures 15-1, 15-2, 15-3, and 15-4 you will find the identifying data about the family/patient, that is, the initial referral, the plan of treatment, and the data base. As the nurse analyzes and synthesizes the available data, the following picture emerges:

Mrs. Doe, a sixty-nine-year-old woman with a diagnosis of "Inoperable Metastatic Carcinoma," has been discharged from the local hospital. Her daughter, having received instructions from the family physician for palliative care, has called the visiting nurse for assistance in the management of her mother's urinary incontinence and gradually debilitating condition. The patient is a small, thin person who appears listless and pale. The daughter has been informed by the physician that "your mother's illness is terminal." Mrs. Doe has generalized weakness which limits her ambulation and prevents her from moving freely about the house. Most of the time, she stays in bed. She is incontinent frequently during the day because of her inability to get to the bathroom in time. The patient is also troubled with nocturnal frequency. Mrs. Doe's dependence on others is increasing and her ability to become independent in activities of daily living is unlikely unless intervention is timely and specific.

The socioeconomic picture is one of growing concern. The patient owns her home. However, financial resources are limited, she does not have comprehensive medical or hospital coverage, and she may be facing a long and costly period of illness. She is dependent on her daughter for financial needs, personal care, and emotional support. The daughter holds a full time job and must continue to work in order to meet the mounting financial obligations. As a consequence of the patient's strained economic status, which requires this financial support from her daughter, a growing element of stress is introduced into their relationship. On one hand the daughter is sincerely devoted and concerned for the safety and welfare of her mother. On the other hand she realizes that without her continued income, she will not be able to provide food and shelter for herself, her ailing mother, and her school-aged daughter.

As to Mrs. Doe's mental status, she is oriented to time, place, and other persons. She responds to verbal stimuli with appropriate affect. The daughter describes her mother as a very stoic person who rarely complains of pain or discomfort. Overall, the patient seems "accepting" of her condition.

Through the eyes of the nurse who has worked with this family, we see the picture she has pieced together as she initiates and continues interaction with the family. Her contact with the family, the climate that is established when she first enters the home, and the therapeutic relationship that evolves all enable her to identify the problems and plan appropriate intervention. In other words the analysis and synthesis of data for the identification of problems involves more than just a review of information recorded on a structured form.

In Figure 16-1 we present the initial problem list formulated by the nurse working with this family. (This form also appears in Appendix A.)

REFERENCES

1. Ruth Mrozek, "Incorporating the Nursing Process into the Problem-Oriented Record," in H. Kenneth Walker, J. Willis Hurst, and Mary F. Woody, *Applying the Problem-Oriented System* (New York: Medcom Press, 1973), pp. 355-62.

ADDITIONAL READINGS

Bloch, Doris, "Some Crucial Terms in Nursing: What Do They Really Mean? in *Nursing Outlook,* 22 (November 1974) 689-94.

Burrill, Marjorie, "Helping Students Identify and Solve Patients' Problems," in *Nursing Outlook,* 14 (February 1966) 46-48.

Carrieri, Virginia, and Judith Stizman, "Components of the Nursing Process," in *Nursing Clinics of North America,* 6 (March 1971) 115-24.

Francis, Gloria N., "This Thing Called Problem Solving," in *The Journal of Nursing Education,* 67 (November 1967) 27-30.

Gebbie, Kristine, and M.A. Lavin, *Classification of Nursing Diagnoses.* St. Louis, C.V. Mosby, 1975.

PROBLEM LIST

Patient's Name **Doe, Jane** MD Name **Dr. R.S.**

Address **8 Main st. Anytown, U.S.A.** MD Phone # **US1-0000**

Phone # **US9-0000**

Date Entered	Problem #	Active Problems	Date Onset	Date Resolved	Resolved Or Inactive Problem
7-31-74	1	Daughter of Pt. over-whelmed with care of mother.			
7-31-74	2	Pt. incontinent of urine.	7-31-74	8-20-74→	inactive
8-6-74	3	Pitting edema of both feet	8-2-74		
8-16-74	4	Inadequate diet	7-31-74		
8-16-74	5	Limited financial Resources for continued health care	7-31-74		
8-16-74	6	Strain in family relationships due to stressors of illness	8-1-74		

Figure 16-1

303

_____, "Classifying Nursing Diagnoses," in *American Journal of Nursing,* 74 (February 1974) 250–53.

Hurst, J. Willis, "The Art and Science of Presenting a Patient's Problems," in *Archives of Internal Medicine* (September 1971).

Mundinger, Mary O., and Grace Jauron, "Developing a Nursing Diagnosis," in *Nursing Outlook,* 23 (February 1975) 94-98.

Murray, Jeanne B., "Self-Knowledge and the Nursing Interview," in *Nursing Forum,* 2 (1963) 69-78.

Roy, Sister Callista, "A Diagnostic Classification System for Nursing," in *Nursing Outlook,* 23 (February 1975) 90-93.

Schwartz, Doris, "Toward More Precise Evaluation of Patients' Needs," in *Nursing Outlook,* 13 (May 1965) 42-44.

Tayrien, Dorothy and Amelia Lipchak, "The Single Problem Approach," in *American Journal of Nursing,* 67 (December 1967) 2523-27.

Woody, M., and M. Mallison, "The Problem-Oriented System for Patient-Centered Care," in *American Journal of Nursing,* 73 (July 1973) 1168-75.

Chapter 17
Developing, Implementing, and Evaluating the Plan of Care

"I strongly believe that [problem-oriented recording] offers nursing an opportunity to define its practice and to communicate with other professions in a sophisticated, logical and very patient-centered way."[1]

INTRODUCTION

Now that we have discussed the methodology of problem identification, we would like to move on to the next step—planning appropriate nursing intervention for the resolution of problems. The formulation of nursing care plans is an integral part of nursing practice in any setting, and should represent the nurse's response to the needs of the family/patient. However, under prevailing patterns of practice, we often find that nursing care plans are stated in terms that reflect "nursing needs" and "nursing goals" rather than family/patient problems. Furthermore they are frequently presented in the form of specific tasks responding only to the physician's plan of treatment. The problem-oriented system with its emphasis on family/patient problems offers an alternative approach. Under this system members of the health team work collaboratively to develop a course of action aimed at resolving family/patient problems. In this chapter we will discuss the development and implementation of nursing care plans within the framework of the Weed System. Using actual case histories, we will present examples of the Initial Plan, the Progress Notes, the Flow Sheet, and the Discharge Summary. We will conclude with some comments on how the evaluation process is facilitated through the application of the problem-oriented system.

THE INITIAL PLAN

To begin with, after you have identified specific problems, you must formulate an initial plan of nursing action for each problem. Plans are numbered and titled according to the problem list, and must include the following components:

(1) Plans for additional data;
(2) Plans for treatment or management;
(3) Plans for family/patient education.

How is the Initial Plan formulated? It is important to remember that in the problem-oriented system each "problem" must be considered individually. The Initial Plan for a problem is based on careful assessment. This assessment involves both subjective and objective observation, which you record within a structured format designated by the acronym, S O A P:

S = subjective observation
O = objective observation
A = assessment
P = plan

Subjectively, you should consider all symptoms or complaints presented to you by the family/patient, quoting the patient's own words whenever possible. Objectively, you must observe, measure, and record the signs of disequilibrium related to the problem you have identified. Your next step is to make an assessment of the problem on the basis of all available data and draw up a plan for resolving the problem.

To illustrate the formulation of an Initial Plan for a given problem, we offer the following example.

Let us say that you received a request for service from the family of Mr. A.V. three weeks after his discharge from the hospital. When Mrs. A.V. called you, she stated, "My husband has cancer . . . there's a tube in his stomach . . . it's all sore and red around the tube . . . it hurts him . . . we're having an awful time with the tube feedings . . ." In checking with the hospital you learned that on July 7, 1974, a gastrostomy procedure was performed on Mr. A.V. for "Inoperable CA of the Esophagus." The patient was sent home a week later with instructions for tube feeding. During your first home visit (August 4, 1974), you discovered that the patient and family were having some difficulties with the care of the gastrostomy site as well as with the management of the tube feeding. You might state the problem and structure it in the SOAP format as follows:

August 4, 1974

Problem No. 1—Difficulty in Managing Gastrostomy

Subjective

In this category, you would note symptoms or complaints made by the patient himself, his family, or other persons close to him. You would also record statements obtained from the hospital and other health or social agencies in the community that are involved in the patient's care and treatment. For example:

Patient: "I have not been able to swallow solid food for over a year. Now I've got this tube in my stomach, and it's all sore around there. I spend all my time trying to get food into it."

Family: Mrs. A.V. states, "We had to take him to the hospital quite often so they could feed him by vein before this operation. Now he gets his food through that tube in his stomach, but it takes us all day to keep up with the feedings. The tube rubs against his stomach. The opening around the tube is irritated and he complains of burning there. There's a lot of yellow drainage leaking out around the tube; it stains the bedclothes. The whole thing has him so weak he hardly ever gets out of bed any more."

Information from the Hospital: "Patient hospitalized June 30, 1974, to July 13, 1974. There was a large tumor mass in the esophagus. A biopsy confirmed 'Squamous Cell Carcinoma of Esophagus.' Due to advanced infiltration of the tumor mass, surgical excision of the affected area was not possible. A gastrostomy procedure was performed on July 7, 1974. The prognosis is poor."

Objective

In this category you would observe the visible signs of physical and emotional distress. Information recorded here should be based on a measurement or a professional observation. Thus, you might record your findings as follows:

There is a reddened, excoriated area on the abdomen surrounding the gastrostomy site. The inflamed surface is approximately 2 to 3 cm. in size and very sensitive to stimuli. There is a moderate amount of mucopurulent drainage exuding from the area. The gastrostomy tube itself is causing friction on the skin surface. The patient is visibly distressed by this condition. When he attempts to prepare for his gastrostomy feeding, he gasps with pain. When the tube is moved even slightly, a large amount of mucopurulent drainage spills over his abdomen. The patient becomes more apprehensive as he tries to manage the tube feeding equipment.

Mr. A.V. demonstrates that he is able to take some fluids my mouth, e.g., water and diluted fruit juice. His skin turgor indicates that presently there is no problem with dehydration. The patient is maintaining prescribed daily nutritional intake of 2500 calories supplied through 250 cc of sustagen plus 50 cc of water in 6 equal feedings. Other family members assist with the procedure, but Mrs. A.V. assumes the major responsibility.

Assessment

In this category, you state your conclusions about the problem, based on the subjective and objective data. Your assessment must reflect your professional judgment, and for this problem, it might be expressed as follows:

The excoriation on the abdomen is due primarily to the irritation of the tube. In addition, the patient and his wife were overwhelmed by the magnitude of the problem, and were ill-prepared to care for the gastrostomy. The area should improve with a nursing regimen of daily cleansing and protective measures to maintain skin integrity. The family's willingness to care for the patient can be the major factor in maintaining comfort and safety measures throughout the terminal stages of illness. However, the patient and family will need continued support to help them cope realistically with the overall situation.

Plan

This phase calls for a plan of action to respond to the foregoing conclusions made through your careful assessment of the problem, and should include the following:

(Plans for additional data)

(a) Obtain additional data—summary of progress while in hospital including extent of instruction offered to family/patient.

(Plans for treatment or management)

(b) Cleanse gastrostomy site and surrounding affected area with a solution of equal parts of hydrogen peroxide and sterile water, apply vaseline gauze and a dry dressing; place a cushioning collar around gastrostomy tube to reduce irritation and pressure on affected area. Continue treatment on a daily basis until drainage is reduced and excoriation begins to heal. Reevaluate in one week.

(c) Assist wife and patient to develop a daily schedule that will permit Mr. A.V. to resume previous activities as often as possible.

(d) Encourage Mr. A.V. to ambulate and get dressed in street clothes at least part of the day.

(Plans for family/patient education)

(e) Instruct patient and family in the care of the tube site and the surrounding area of excoriation. Stress importance of avoiding further contamination. Use appropriate visual aid materials. Help Mr. A.V. understand the gastrostomy and the use of the special feedings.

PROGRESS NOTES AND FLOW SHEETS

After the Initial Plan for each problem is formulated and entered into the patient's record, "follow-up" information on subsequent nursing intervention and patient progress is recorded in Progress Notes and Flow Sheets.

Progress Notes should describe how the family/patient is responding to your plan of care. You begin with the problems you have already identified and "SOAP-ed." Each entry into the Progress Notes should be related to one of these problems, numbered accordingly, and presented in the SOAP format. Information should be recorded in terms of the Initial Plan and its continued effect on that identified problem. There should be an easy flow from the problem to the Initial Plan to the Progress Notes, so that you are able to determine the family/patient's progress at any given point.

What types of information should be entered into the Progress Notes? Certainly you would note changes in the patient's condition (improvement or decline) as they relate to a specific problem. You would record nursing intervention activities under the problem for which they are intended. You would also record laboratory findings, results of treatments and medications, unexpected side effects or unusual occurrences in the course of therapy, changes in family structure or relationships, changes in family/patient behavior that may come about through health teaching. The following example illustrates the way in which a part of the Progress Notes might appear for the problem cited above.

Progress Notes

August 5, 1974—No. 1 Difficulty in Managing Gastrostomy.

    S: "My wife can't do this dressing, nurse." "He's right, I don't think I can ever learn to do it myself."

    O: Dressings on abdomen are encrusted with drainage. Excoriated area has not been cleansed or dressings changed since last treatment by nurse 24 hours earlier. Mrs. A.V. attempted to cleanse the irritated area and apply a clean dressing, but she became very apprehensive about carrying out the procedure.

    A: Mrs. A.V. understands the procedure but she needs more support in order to gain confidence in carrying out the treatment.

    P: Continue to assist Mrs. A.V. in caring for gastrostomy site until she is more comfortable with the procedure. Reassure both husband and wife of the nurse's continued support and understanding.

August 6, 1974

    S: "Nurse, I'm really going to try today because I know I have to learn to do this to help my husband."

    O: Mrs. A.V. removed dressing and cleansed site with assistance. Drainage less purulent today. Mrs. A.V. replaced collar on tube with nurse's help.

    A: Irritated area surrounding stoma responding to treatment. Mrs. A.V. is becoming more comfortable with procedure.

    P: Continue to encourage Mrs. A.V. and suggest that she take over the procedure on next visit.

August 7, 1974

    S: "Nurse, I still feel very nervous about this. I'm afraid I won't do it right, and I don't want to hurt my husband."

    O: Mrs. A.V. completed care of gastrostomy site with assistance. Excoriated area is beginning to show improvement, and drainage is decreasing.

    A: Mrs. A.V. still needs assistance and encouragement with procedure.

    P: Continue to supervise and assist Mrs. A.V. with care of gastrostomy site.

August 11, 1974.

    S: "My wife's really getting pretty good at taking care of me—see how much better this looks now. And I'm doing pretty good with my tube feedings."

O: Mrs. A.V. has taken over care of gastrostomy site and is comfortable with the procedure. Excoriated area less than 1 cm. and drainage has almost completely subsided.

A: Mrs. A.V. is able to assume full responsibility for care of gastrostomy site. Abdominal excoriation almost completely healed.

P: Reduce visits to 3 times weekly; continue to monitor condition of wound. Call physician to report progress of patient, and follow up with written report.

The above Progress Notes, which respond to the overall plan for Problem No. 1 "Difficulty in Managing Gastrostomy," serve to illustrate the immediacy of the patient's and his wife's need for emotional support, instruction, and prompt implementation of the prescribed treatment. Additional Progress Notes related to this and other problems could be recorded in the same format. However, it is not necessary to record all follow-up information in narrative form. You might wish to plot specific parameters of care for this patient on a *Flow Sheet.*

Flow Sheets are specially designed Progress Notes built around preestablished parameters of care which you identify during the assessment process. For example, parameters of care associated with specific pathophysiology might include items such as fluctuations in vital signs, the effect of insulin on the glucose level in the blood or urine of a diabetic patient, the change in a patient's prothrombin time as a result of anticoagulant therapy, and so on. A sample Flow Sheet is presented in Figure 17-1. For additional examples, see Appendix B. Flow Sheets will help you to document patient progress logically and succinctly. Parameters of care defined on the Flow Sheet graphically illustrate changes in the condition of the family/patient, and thereby help you to measure the effectiveness of nursing intervention. Through the use of Flow Sheets your plan of action and the expected outcomes of your nursing intervention may be readily discerned by other members of the health team who are working with the family/patient. The record itself becomes more comprehensible because you have defined exactly what you plan to monitor with regard to the patient's condition or family situation. You will find that the actual exercise of defining parameters of care will help you to increase your total knowledge because this activity encourages you to seek additional data about the disease process, family socioeconomic conditions, other agencies involved in the care, and so on.

Items on the Flow Sheets must be properly coded so that any member of the health team can interpret the information and understand the rationale for your approach. When you use Flow Sheets, it is important that you identify all abbreviations, word symbols, and other indications of change in the given parameters. Entries must be dated as well as coded because the time sequence is an important factor in the recording of changes on a Flow Sheet.

FLOW SHEET – DIABETES MELLITUS

Name _____

ADA Diet _____
Insulin: type/dosage _____
System Involvement:
Eye _____ Renal _____
C–V _____ Skin _____
P–V _____ Neuro _____

PARAMETERS	Date of Visit 19____															
Weight																
Temperature																
Pulse																
Respiration																
Blood pressure																
Urine glucose A. M. / P. M.																
Blood glucose																
Skin appearance																
Peripheral pulse																
Peripheral temperature																
Peripheral sensation																
Eye appearance																
Frequency of urination (# x's/day)																
Nocturia																
Appearance of mucous membranes																
*Mental status																
Initials																

Code: C – Care   D – Discussion   *1. Lethargic   *5. Apprehensive
       I – Instruction   S – Supervision   *2. Stuporous   *6. Restless
       N – Narrative   E – Evaluation   *3. Unconscious   *7. Memory loss
                                                 *4. Comatose   *8. Alert

Figure 17-1

311

PARAMETERS	Date of Visit 19___																
Disease Process																	
Drug: Oral agent																	
Insulin																	
type																	
administration																	
rotation of sites																	
storage of insulin																	
care of syringe																	
reaction: hyperglycemia																	
hypoglycemia																	
Instruction in diet																	
Use of Exchange List																	
Menu planning																	
Role in treatment																	
Exercise: effects on blood sugar																	
First aid																	
Skin care																	
observe for boils, furuncles																	
avoid mechanical, chemical, thermal trauma																	
Personal hygiene																	
Perineal and foot care																	
Initials																	

Figure 17-1   (continued)

312

Let us go back to the situation of Mr. A.V., the patient with the problem of "Difficulty in Managing Gastrostomy" to demonstrate how a Flow Sheet was used to record the nursing intervention and to monitor the family/patient progress. Careful study of the information on the form shown in Figure 17-2 will demonstrate that, initially, the nurse gave direct care. She then instructed the family to perform the treatment, supervised the wife in the procedure, and evaluated the outcome of the actions she had taken. In time sequence, the nurse visited daily for eight days, during which she observed desired results from her intervention. Her evaluation of the problem at the end of that time period showed improvement in the patient's condition and the wife's ability to handle the treatment regimen. A Progress Note written in the SOAP format on the date that the Flow Sheet indicated E (evaluation) sums up the outcome of the nursing care plan for this particular problem.

DISCHARGE SUMMARY

The Discharge Summary is, in essence, the final Progress Note, and should be problem-oriented. Summaries or final Progress Notes should reflect the status of the family/patient in relation to each active problem. The information on each problem should present a clear picture of the level of resolution attained, and should explain or justify the discharge of a family/patient from the agency service. The Data Base (particularly those areas that have changed since service was initiated) and the Problem List should be reviewed and brought up to date. Since the Discharge Summary may be regarded as the final entry on the Progress Notes, it is important to review the Initial Plan for each problem before developing the Discharge Summary. Flow Sheets should be checked and clarified, as they illustrate graphically the main events that have occurred during the period of service to the family/patient. Furthermore Flow Sheets provide a quick reference for any member of the health team who might wish to review the record at the time of discharge, recertification, or reinstitution of service. When service to a family includes input from other disciplines, the nurse should abstract essential information from progress reports and include it as part of the general summary at the time of discharge.

In preparing a Discharge Summary you should present the data in the SOAP format. This approach lends itself best to situations where the outcomes of active problems may be succinctly described within the framework of the SOAP acronym. For example, let us return to the case or Mr. A.V. The Discharge Summary (or final Progress Note) for the problem "Difficulty in Managing Gastrostomy" might be recorded as in Figure 17-3. This example lends itself very well to the SOAP format. In using this format you would respond to each problem in a similar manner. However, one drawback we discovered in our pilot study was that some final Progress Notes became very lengthy and cumbersome in the SOAP outline. Therefore, we found it ap-

FLOW SHEET

Name Mr. A. V.

PARAMETERS	Date of Visit 19 74																
	8/4	8/5	8/6	8/7	8/8	8/9	8/10	8/11									
Care of Gastrostomy site		C	C	C	C	C	C	E									
a. Cleanse with H_2O_2 & H_2O in equal parts																	
b. apply vaseline gauze and dry dressing																	
Instruct wife in the care of gastrostomy site		N	N	N	S	S	S	N									
*Condition of gastrostomy site																	
1. drainage		U	S1 ↓	↓	↓	↓	↓	↓									
2. excoriation		U	U	S1 ↓	↓	↓	↓	↓									
Gastrostomy feeding 6 x daily:		C	C	C	C	C	C	C									
250 cc Sustagen & 50cc H_2O																	
Instruct pt & wife in technique of tube feeding		D	D	I	I	I	S	S									
Instruct wife in preparation of Sustagen feeding		D	D	D	I	I	S	S									
Initials		cf	cf	cf	cf	cf	cf	cf	cf								

(Left margin vertical text: INITIAL PLAN)

CODE: C — Care
           I — Instruction
           N — Narrative

D — Discussion
S — Supervision
E — Evaluation

* Code if Desired
↑- Increased
U- Unchanged
↓- Decreased

Figure 17-2

314

Patient's Name __Mr. A. V._____

Date	P.#	Problem Title - Subjective, Objective, Assessment, Plan
8/24	1	Difficulty in Managing Gastrostomy.

Difficulty in Managing Gastrostomy.

S - "My dressings have. been dry for the last three days. I have not felt pain or irritation for a week. I can move around, nurse. I'm going out on the porch now. I feel so much better."

O - Abdominal excoriation around gastrostomy site has healed. Dressings are clean and intact. There is no evidence of drainage since last visit. Patient is now on first floor most of day. He is finally resuming some of his previous activities. There is less evidence of fatigue.

A - Although illness is terminal, patient has made a remarkable recovery from effect of wound infection and accompanying fatigue. He is able to cope with gastrostomy tube and wife is more confident in assisting him in maintaining skin integrity as well as management of gastrostomy tube feeding procedure. No further services from nursing agency should be required at this time.

P - Call MD and report patient's progress. Inform physician of discharge plans. Discharge with appropriate written instructions to family for continued care and future contact with nursing service.

C. Johnson, RN

Figure 17-3

propriate, in some situations, to summarize the problems in narrative form, and we offer the following example:

Mrs. E.H. was referred to the community nursing agency from the Home Care Program of the local hospital, following her discharge on 9/3/75. The patient's condition at that time was deteriorating. She was in an advanced stage of generalized carcinoma with metastasis to the skeletal and central nervous systems. Mrs. E.H., bedridden and mentally confused most of the time, was incontinent of bowel and bladder. Seven problems had been identified by the nurse in the course of her service to the family. The final Progress Notes reflect the state of resolution for each problem. (See Figure 17-4.)

EVALUATING THE PLAN OF CARE

One of the noteworthy features of the problem-oriented system is the fact that it offers a built-in mechanism for periodic evaluation of the quality of patient care. Indeed, as you work with the system, you will find that evaulation is an inherent part of its overall approach to patient care. Subtly and almost imperceptibly, the process of evaluation is intertwined throughout the component parts of the system. Outcomes associated with any phase of activity must be measured before you can proceed from one step to the next. For example, let us say that you have identified a particular patient problem—"unsteady gait." Your plan of action would call for physical therapy evaluation. Before you initiate a referral, you must check the Data Base for information regarding the extent of the problem—how is the patient's ambulation affected? Does he require the assistance of another person? Does he use an assistive device such as a quad cane, walker, or crutches? Is he limited in stair climbing? The referral to the physical therapist should include this type of descriptive information for each problem you have identified. In consultation with the physical therapist, you formulate a plan to alleviate the problem. As the system calls for measurement of expected outcomes, you would document the progress of the patient with specific observable events, such as, "patient now walks unassisted to bathroom" or "patient climbs stairs once a day with assistance." Thus, in noting these improvements, you are attesting to the effectiveness of your plan. If no improvement is noted in terms of measurable outcome, for instance, "patient still unable to ambulate to bathroom unassisted" or "patient is reluctant to climb stairs," your plan must be reviewed and revised if necessary.

The vitality of the system lies in the fact that the more you use it, the more you become involved, and you begin to look more critically not only at individual care plans but at the total process of nursing. In nursing we consistently strive to achieve excellence in service to the public. Implicit in the

PROGRESS NOTES

Patient's Name___Mrs. E. H._____

Date	P.#	Problem Title - Subjective, Objective, Assessment, Plan
10/17	1	COMMUNICATIONS: October 17, 1975. Telephone call from Home Care Department - patient expired during the night. INCONTINENCE OF STOOL Pt. was given Fleets and tapwater enemas periodically to attempt to control the incontinence, but this did not help and they were discontinued. Pt. took colace tab daily - stools remained soft and incontinence continued.
	2	IMMOBILITY: UNABLE TO PERFORM ADL Patient remained in bed continuously, in one position, unless she was moved. Skin was in good condition, no areas of breakdown when patient first visited. Family at first assumed all personal care for patient. Family taught importance of turning pt. q. 2 hours and use of lotion to soften skin. On 9/27 first areas of skin breakdown were noticed. VN resumed giving personal care to pt. on this day and continued to do so for remainder of visits. ROM was given along with instructions to family to keep pt's arms and legs from contracting. Joints became more rigid with continuing visits. Pt's skin became increasingly dry, family instructed to put lotion over areas frequently. Family not willing to follow through with ROM because pt. moaned when this was attempted.
	3	FOLEY CATHETER Catheter inserted on discharge from hospital. Foley began leaking - changed PRN, and irrigations started 2x daily. Husband was taught this procedure also. Pt's fluid intake continued to be adequate (2000 cc daily); urine was amber with sediment and mucus threads. Daily output 1800 cc.
	4	FAMILY ADJUSTMENT TO ILLNESS AND EVENTUAL DEATH OF PATIENT From the first visit, family members appeared to accept the eventual outcome of pt's illness. She had been ill for many months and the family had had time to accept the diagnosis and her eventual death. They have a 26-year-old retarded son who also understands his mother's illness and her eventual death. The family appeared encouraged by pt's ability to eat and drink so well throughout her illness. Retarded son, John, became disturbed when his mother moaned and groaned; he felt someone was hurting her.

Figure 17-4

317

PROGRESS NOTES

Patient's Name   Mrs. E. H.

Date	P.#	Problem Title - Subjective, Objective, Assessment, Plan
		Pt's family remained close and supportive of each other and gave the pt. as much care as they could.
	5	GENERALIZED PAIN

Pt. began complaining of pain when she was moved on 9/13/75 but moaned and groaned only when moved. Tylenol was ordered, PRN, for pain. On 9/27/75 she was having more pain than usual and Talwin was ordered. After that she slept through bath and complained of no pain when turned. Her pain tolerance appeared to change daily. During the last 8 visits she began to moan more frequently when touched. This also continued to upset the family. |
| | 6 | HUSBAND'S ATTITUDE RE: PATIENT'S MEDICATIONS

Pt. unable to swallow medications. This developed around 9/27 when husband began to have trouble administering medications. He questioned whether the medications were actually necessary to help her. Pt. was on Prednisone and Digitalis. Patient's MD stated medications could be omitted but family did continue to mash them and mix them with her foods. Throughout the rest of the visits the family was able to administer medications to the patient. |
| | 7 | PRESSURE ULCERS

When visits first started patient's skin was in good condition. Red pressure areas were occasionally noted. On 9/23 sacral area became reddened with a blister over coccyx. On 9/30 a decubitus had developed to the left of the coccyx. Family was not getting patient completely off her back when they tried to turn her. Peroxide was used first to cleanse the area, then a heat lamp, and finally Maalox was applied to the ulcer. This procedure was repeated 3 to 4 times daily. Ulcer increased in size, to about a half dollar. On 10/7 a blister was noted on the left heel. Heel booties were ordered for patient's feet and pillow used for positioning. Maalox was also used on this area. Ulcer on coccyx increased and a new area formed to left of first one. Red scabbed areas appeared on both ears. Continued to encourage family to apply lotion frequently. Pt's skin was so dry it peeled off when she was receiving care. Skin breakdown was progressing.

                                                    C. Johnson, RN |

Figure 17-4   (continued)

318

"contract" between the nursing profession and society are the consumer's right to high quality care and our responsibility for providing this care. We have a professional obligation to monitor our activities. This obligation increases with the growing public demand for accountability. If we are to continue to fulfill our professional responsibility to the public, we must find ways to monitor family/patient problems and document the appropriateness of our nursing intervention. As a result of our pilot study, we found that the problem-oriented record provides an effective means to carry out these activities.

REFERENCES

1. Sara P. Thompson, "Utilizing the Problem-Oriented System in Home Health Care," in H. Kenneth Walker, et al., *Applying the Problem-Oriented System* (New York: Medcom Press, 1973), p. 152.

ADDITIONAL READINGS

Benedikter, Helen, *The Nursing Audit—A Necessity. How Shall It Be Done?* Pub. No. 20-1501. Council of Hospital and Related Institutional Nursing Services. New York: National League for Nursing. 1973.

Brodt, Dagmar, "Obstacles to Individualized Patient Care," in *Nursing Outlook,* 14 (December 1966) 35-36.

Carlson, Carolyn E., *Behavioral Concepts and Nursing Intervention.* Philadelphia: J.B. Lippincott Co., 1970.

Donovan, Helen, "Determining Priorities of Nursing Care," in *Nursing Outlook,* 11 (January 1963) 44-45.

Harris, Barbara L., "Who Needs Written Care Plans Anyway?" in *American Journal of Nursing,* 70 (October 1970) 2136-38.

Little, Dolores, and Doris Carnevali, "The Nursing Care Planning System," in *Nursing Outlook,* 19 (March 1971) 164–67.

————, *Nursing Care Planning,* Philadelphia: J.B. Lippincott Co., 1969.

Mayers, Marlene, *A Systematic Approach to the Nursing Care Plan.* New York: Appleton-Century-Crofts, 1972.

Newman, Margaret, "Identifying and Meeting Patients' Needs in Short-Span Nurse-Patient Relationships," in *Nursing Forum,* 5(1) (1966) 76-86.

Palmer, Mary Ellen, "The Nursing Care Plan: A Tool for Staff Development," in *Journal of Nursing Administration,* 4 (May-June 1974) 42-45.

Pennsylvania Department of Health, *Guide for Preparing a Health Care Plan: A Multidisciplinary Approach.* Harrisburg, Pa: Bureau of Nursing Programs and Resources, Penna. Dept. of Health, 1972.

Phaneuf, Maria, *The Nursing Audit: Profile for Excellence.* New York: Appleton-Century-Crofts, 1972.

Wagner, Berniece M., "Care Plans: Right, Reasonable and Reachable," in *American Journal of Nursing,* 69 (May 1969) 986-90.

Yura, Helen, and Mary Walsh, *The Nursing Process: Assessing, Planning, Implementing, Evaluating.* 2nd ed. New York: Appleton-Century-Crofts, 1973.

Appendix A
Family Health Record on Jane Doe

Community Nursing Service   REFERRAL FORM

Call Received by

_____C. M. T._____   _7/29/74_
Name   Date

_7 / 31 / 74_   _/   /_   _/   /_   _____
Admitted   Readmitted   Discharge Date   Reason

Patient _Doe_____ _Jane_____ _____   _400 757_____
        Last Name   First   (I.)   Record #

Address _8 Main St._____   _____
        Number and Street   Apt. #   Home Care #

Anytown , USA   _/_   _US 9-0000_   _000-00-0000B_
City   Zip   Phone #   H.I. Claim #

_3-21-05_____   _Cau._   _F_   _Widow_____   _____
Date of Birth   Race   Sex   Marital Status   M.A. #

_/_   _57_____   _309_____   _____   ( ) P. T. ( ) H.H.A.   _____
Gov't Unit Fee Status Program   # of Visits   ( ) Nursing   D. P. A. #

_Daughter_____   _Elizabeth Jones_   _Daughter_
Referral Source   Responsible Person in Home   Relationship

Physician _Dr. R.S. MD_____   Phone # _US 1- 0000_

Address _100 Market St._   _Anytown_   _USA_   _19000_
        Number & Street   City   State   Zip

General Hospital - Anytown, USA   _6-10-74 / 7-3-74_
Hospital or E.C.F.   Address   Admission - Discharge Date

Diagnosis _Metastatic carcinoma - diabetes_____
          (Ca is inoperable - radiation therapy in hospital)

Prognosis _Poor_____   Therapeutic Goals _Train bladder;_
          improvement in ambulation

Medication _DBI-TD 50 daily; Percodan tab. ÷ q 3 to 4 hrs. prn._

Orders _Personal care prn - Teach daughter care of patient._
       SS. Enema prn   P.T. evaluation if indicated

Report to Doctor: _incontinence of urine_____

Patient Visited By: _C. Johnson   RN_____   Date: _7 / 31 / 74_

Nurse's District: _C. Johnson   RN_____   1. Billing
                                                      2. File
Other Information: _M.D. has informed patient's daughter_   3. Patient's Folder
                   that patient's illness is "Terminal"

Figure A-1 Referral Form.

322

DR. *R. S.*

_____

_____

COMMUNITY NURSING SERVICE

NAME OF PATIENT *Doe, Jane*   ADDRESS *8 main St. Anytown, U.S.A.*

INITIAL ORDER ☒   RENEWAL ☐   CONFIRMATION ☐   DATE LAST SEEN BY PHYSICIAN

NURSES PROGRESS NOTES *Initial home visit made. Patient's daughter is unable to cope with her mother's care; is overwhelmed with problems at this time. Pt is a diabetic but not following a diet; is eating a great amt. of "Starches." Pt is incontinent of urine at times. Pulse rapid - but regular at 104 - both apical + radial. Respirations 28. B/p 100/60*

DATE OF NEXT VISIT *8-6-74*

DATE *7-31-74*   _____ *C. Johnson* _____ RN
                                SIGNATURE

PLAN OF TREATMENT — TO BE COMPLETED BY PHYSICIAN

DIAGNOSIS (PRIMARY AND SECONDARY – IN ORDER) *metastatic Ca. Diabetes (Ca is inoperable - radiation therapy in hospital)*

SURGICAL PROCEDURE_____ DATE_____

PROGNOSIS *poor*   PATIENT INFORMED: DIAGNOSIS YES ☐ NO ☐ PROGNOSIS YES ☐ NO ☐
                     FAMILY INFORMED: DIAGNOSIS YES ☐ NO ☐ PROGNOSIS YES ☐ NO ☐

THERAPEUTIC GOALS *train bladder - improve ambulation*

MEDICAL SUPERVISION IN HOME BY *R S. (M.D.)*   TEL. NO._____

ADDRESS_____ CITY_____ ZIP_____

HOME HEALTH SERVICES ORDERED: NURSING ☒   PHYSICAL THERAPY ☐   MEDICAL SOC. SER. ☐   SPEECH THERAPY ☐   OCC. THERAPY ☐   HOME HEALTH AID ☐

MEDICATIONS *DBI - TD 5⁰ daily - Percodan + tab q 3 to 4 h. prn*

DIET *1500 cal.*   — *Nutritional status - fair.*

ACTIVITIES ALLOWED *as tolerated*

TREATMENT AND SPECIAL EQUIPMENT *Personal care prn — SS Enema prn Bladder training program - PHN may insert foley catheter if bladder training fails and if pt. continues to be incontinent*

SPECIAL INSTRUCTIONS, REACTIONS TO BE REPORTED TO PHYSICIAN *continued incontinence*

PATIENT TO BE SEEN BY PHYSICIAN: DATE_____ HOME ☐   OFFICE ☐   OPD ☐

THE HOME HEALTH SERVICES TO BE PROVIDED ARE NEEDED TO TREAT THE CONDITION(S) FOR WHICH THE PATIENT RECEIVED SERVICES DURING THE RELATED STAY IN A HOSPITAL OR EXTENDED CARE FACILITY.   YES ☐   NO ☐

WERE INPATIENT DAYS SAVED DUE TO AVAILABILITY OF HOME CARE SERVICE? YES ☐ NO ☐. YOUR ESTIMATE OF NO. SAVED_____

I CERTIFY THAT THE PATIENT IS (1) HOMEBOUND, (2) REQUIRES THE HOME HEALTH SERVICES INDICATED ABOVE ON AN INTERMITTENT BASIS, (3) THE PATIENT IS UNDER THE CARE OF A PHYSICIAN WHO WILL REVIEW THIS PLAN OF TREATMENT PERIODICALLY.

8-9-74   _____ *R__ S_____ M.D.* _____ *M.D.*
DATE   PHYSICIAN'S SIGNATURE   REG. NO.

PHYSICIAN'S NAME — PLEASE PRINT

Figure A-2   Plan of Treatment.

323

PATIENT IDENTIFICATION

Name _Doe, Jane_

Address _8 Main ST._

Anytown, U.S.A.

Directions _West on 9th ST. - Rt. on K street -_
Rt. on Main ST. house on Rt.

Phone _US 9-0000_

Age _69_ Birthdate _3-21-05_ Sex _F_ Race _Cau._

Ethnic Group _Italian_ Marital Status _Widow_

Education _7th grade_ Occupation _—_

Religious Preference _Catholic_

Income: Employment _—_ Pension _$58.00_ SS _$200.00_

Expenses: Housing _____ Food _____ Other _____

CNS _400757_

HC _____

HI _000-00-0000 B_

MA/DPA _____

BC/BS _____

Classification _309_

FEE STATUS

Date	Fee	Date	Fee
7/31/74	57		

DATES OF SERVICE

Adm.	Disch.	Adm.	Disch.
7/31/74			

Friend or Relative to Notify in Case of Emergency:

Name _A. Brown_ Relationship _daughter_

Phone _US 8-0000_ Address _4 Maple ST. Anytown, U.S.A._

Friends or Relatives Outside Home Involved in Care:

Name	Address	Phone	Relationship

Doctor (Family) _Dr. R. S_ Phone # _US 1-0000_

Address _100 Market ST. Anytown, U.S.A._ _19000_

Doctor (Consultant) _____ Phone # _____

Address _____

Pharmacy _Central Drug_ Phone # _US 2-0000_

Ambulance Service _Allied_ Phone # _US 3-0000_

Other Agencies Involved	Contact	Phone

Equipment in home (Itemize): _Hospital Bed - Side Rails - Commode_

Services presently involved (check in pencil): Nursing _✓_ P. T. _____

O. T. _____ S. T. _____ H. H. A. _____ H. M. _____

Med. SW _____ Other _____

Figure A-3 Patient/Family Identification.

324

FAMILY IDENTIFICATION

Family Name *Doe, Jane*   Pt's Rel. to HH *Head of house*

Members in Household	Sex	Birth Date	Marital Status	Rel to HH	Education	Occupation	CNS Record #	Open
Jane Doe	F	3-21-05	Widow	HH	7TH Gr.	—	400757	✓
Elizabeth Jones	F	3-1-25	Separated	dtr.	12TH Gr.	P.T. Clerk House wife		
Mary Jones	F	8-19-63	Single	G	5TH Gr.	student		

Family Economic Profile: *Pt. lives on income from Social Security and pension. Pt. owns house.*

Home Evaluation *Single-frame dwelling - fair condition*

Type & Condition of Home *Single-frame - 2 story*

No. of BR *1* Pt. prox. to BR *next to bedroom*   Heating *Hot air - gas*

Pt. Sleeping Accom. *has own room*   Kitchen Facilities *adequate*

Pt. prox. to family activity *Pt. stays upstairs*   Housekeeping *done by dtr.*

Other pertinent info. *Household in disarray - daughter not very organized*

Family Health History

Family Member	TB	Cancer	Ht. Dis.	Diabetes	Renal Dis.	Epilepsy	Mental Dis.	Alcohol	VD	Other (allergy, surgery, injury, etc.)
Jane Doe	NO	yes	yes	yes	Ca. Kidney	NO	No	No	No	hyst. at age 26 allergic to Penicillin
Eliz. Jones	No	No	No	yes	No	No	No	No	No	C. section allergic to Tetanus
Mary Jones	No	No	No	No	No	No	No	No	No	allergic to Penicillin

Family dietary habits (include ethnic factors, meal times, etc.): *No special food preferences - Regular meal time*

Family medication habits (include usual remedies for constipation, headaches, nervousness, etc.)

Aspirin for headaches

Pt. is on Persodan ÷ Tab q3 to 4 hrs prn and DBI-TD 50 ÷ daily

Family dynamics (include significant family interpersonal relationships): *Mother and daughter devoted; get along well but daughter is now overwhelmed with care of mother - Is having difficulty coping with situation   C. Johnson R.N.*

Figure A-3 Patient/Family Identification (continued).

NURSING BASELINE ASSESSMENT

Patient _Doe, Jane_ Age _69_ Ht. _4' 11"_ Wt. _94 lbs._

Diagnosis _Metastatic ca. — diabetes_

General Physical Appearance _Thin – Pale – Weak_

General Mental Condition _Oriented to time and place – quiet – stoic._

Physical Assessment		Not Exam.	Norm	Abnorm	Describe or Measure
SKIN	Color			X	Pale
	Condition		X		
	Temperature		X		
	Turgor			X	loose skin
HEAD	Hair		X		
	Shape		X		
EYES	Appearance			X	Conjunctiva pale
	Vision			X	Wears glasses
	Pupils		X		
EARS	Appearance		X		
	Hearing		X		
MOUTH	Teeth & Gums			X	Most of teeth are missing
	Throat		X		has 1 tooth on bottom – wears
	Tongue		X		dentures – gums pale
NOSE			X		
NECK	Appearance		X		
	Mobility		X		
CHEST	Configuration		X		
	Auscultation		X		
	Respiration		28		
BREASTS	Appearance			X	Flabby
	Self Exam.				
HEART	Auscultation		X		Rapid – Regular Rate and
	Apical Pulse			104	Rhythm
	Radial Pulse			104	
	Blood Pressure		100/60		
	Circulation		X		
EXTREMITIES	Upper		X		
	Lower			X	Edema of both feet.
	Joints		X		
ABDOMEN	Shape			X	Flabby
	Bowel Sounds		X		
	Palpation			X	Mass R.U.Q.
GENITALIA	Menstruation		.		Had hysterectomy at age 26
	Last Pap Test				Never had Pap test done
	Prostate				

Figure A-4 Nursing Baseline Assessment.

FUNCTIONAL ASSESSMENT

		Not Exam.	Norm	Abnormal (Specify)
ACTIVITIES OF DAILY LIVING	Ambulation			Weak- PT. can walk from bedroom To bathroom - otherwise Remains in bed.
	Stairs			
	Dressing		x	
	Feeding		x	
	Household Activity			Unable to perform any household activities.
	Personal Care			Able to do part of sponge bath-dtr. assists
SLEEP			x	
HABITS	Alcohol		x	Does not use any alcohol, Tobacco or drugs
	Tobacco		x	
	Drugs		x	
	Other		x	
ELIMINATION	Bowel Function		x	Nocturia
	Urinary Function			Unable to hold urine until she gets To B.R.
NUTRITIONAL STATUS	Food		x	
	Fluid		x	
ABILITY TO COMMUNICATE & UNDERSTAND	Speech		x	
	Read		x	
	Understand		x	
ORIENTED			x	
AFFECT			x	

Adjustment to Illness   Very stoic - does not complain

Describe Patient's Usual Day:

Morning: _Breakfast at 10AM — then listens to radio._

Afternoon: _Lunch at 2PM - rests in bed - sleeps or listens to radio._

Evening: _Dinner at 6PM - listens to radio- asleep about 10PM_

24 Hour Diet Recall:

Breakfast _Fried potatoes - 1 fried egg - tea_

Lunch _Macaroni - salad - water_

Dinner _Meat - Mashed potatoes — corn_

Snacks _Fruit between meals_

HISTORY:

Medical _Diabetic for past 6 or 7 years. "Heart Trouble" - Ca. kidney_

Surgical _Hysterectomy at age 26_

C. Johnson R.N.

Figure A-4 Nursing Baseline Assessment (continued).

PROBLEM LIST

Patient's Name ___Doe, Jane___ MD Name ___Dr. R. S.___

Address ___8 Main St.   Anytown, U.S.A.___ MD Phone # ___US1-0000___

Phone # ___US9-0000___

Date Entered	Problem #	Active Problems	Date Onset	Date Resolved	Resolved Or Inactive Problem
7-31-74	1	Daughter of Pt. overwhelmed with care of mother.			
7-31-74	2	Pt. incontinent of urine.	7-31-74	8-20-74→inactive	
8-6-74	3	Pitting edema of both feet	8-2-74		
8-16-74	4	Inadequate diet	7-31-74		
8-16-74	5	Limited financial	} 7-31-74		
		Resources for			
		Continued health care			
8-16-74	6	Strain in family relationships due	8-1-74		
		to stressors of illness			

Figure A-5 Problem List.

INITIAL PLAN

Patient's Name___Doe, Jane_____

Date	Prob. No.	Problem Title - Plans for: Additional data, Management, Pt. education
7/31	1	Daughter of pt. is overwhelmed with care of her mother. **Subjective:** "I don't know how I am going to manage with my mother. She needs so much care and attention. I can't give up my job - I've got to work to pay the bills. I have no one to stay with my mother. She needs someone to keep her dry. Someone has to feed my mother, because she won't eat."
		Objective: Daughter looks tired and distraught. House is topsy-turvy. Daughter has hair in curlers. Grooming is poor.
		Assessment: Daughter unable to cope with the many problems which are overwhelming her at this time. She needs advice and assistance.
		Plan: 1. Provide emotional support to patient's daughter.
		2. Advise daughter to contact local chapter of American Cancer Society for equipment and supplies.
		3. Instruct daughter in the care of a bed patient.
	2	Patient is incontinent of urine. **Subjective:** "My mother is unable to hold her urine, she wets on the way to the bathroom and as she is walking from bathroom to bedroom she dribbles."
		Objective: PHN observed that there were urine stains on the rug from the bedroom to the bathroom. Did not actually observe patient voiding on way to the bathroom.
		Assessment: On basis of dtr's information about mother being incontinent, and observing the urine stains, PHN feels pt. is probably incontinent of urine.
		Plan: 1. Instruct pt. & dtr. in a bladder training program by having pt. go to bathroom or use bed pan every two hours, gradually increasing period of time between voiding.
		2. Restrict fluids after 7 PM.
		3. If incontinence persists, telephone doctor and get order for Foley catheter.
		C. Johnson, RN

Figure A-6 Initial Plan.

329

Patient's Name___Doe, Jane_____

Date	Prob. No.	Problem Title - Plans for: Additional data, Management, Pt. education
8/6	3	**Pitting edema of both feet.** Subjective: Pt's daughter reports that pt. voided excessively yesterday, almost continuously, that she used 36 sheets changing pt's bed. And also, the urine has subsided a great deal today - pt. has not wet the bed all day. Objective: Noted that pt. has pitting edema of both feet. The edema is more than it was one week ago. Also noted the bed linens were dry today. Assessment: In view of the pitting edema of both feet, I feel this pt. may have a problem with electrolyte imbalance; or, this pt's daughter may be exaggerating about the excessive amount of urine the patient has voided. Plan: 1. Instruct pt's daughter to keep a strict intake & output, especially intake. It may be impossible for the daughter to keep a record of the output since pt. is incontinent, but will instruct her to try to do so. 2. Monitor pt's vital signs, especially blood pressure, to see if there is any rise in blood pressure or pulse. 3. Check pt. each visit for the amount of edema. 4. Call doctor and inform him of the increased edema of both feet. 5. Ask doctor for instructions regarding diet. C. Johnson, RN
8/16	4	**Inadequate Diet.** Subjective: Pt's daughter reports that her mother does not eat properly - eats mostly starches. Objective: PHN had done verbal diet recall and noted that pt's diet consisted mainly of starches. PHN also checked with Dr. S., who said that the pt. should be on a 1500 calorie diet, but he doubted that pt. would adhere to this and he felt it was futile to press diet, but said that PHN may attempt to instruct on 1500 calorie diet.

Figure A-6 Initial Plan (continued).

INITIAL PLAN

Patient's Name Doe, Jane_____

Date	Prob. No.	Problem Title - Plans for: Additional data, Management, Pt. education
8/16	4	**Assessment:** Pt's daughter needs instruction on 1500 calorie diet. **Plan:** Attempt to instruct daughter in 1500 calorie diet, and hope that she will follow the diet. C. Johnson, RN

Figure A-6 Initial Plan (continued).

331

FLOW SHEET

Name **Doe, Jane**

Date of Visit 19 **74**

PARAMETERS	7/31	8/6	8/9	8/12	8/13	8/16	8/20	8/23									
Instruct dtr. in Care of bed PT.	I	I			I	I	I	I									
Emotional support to Pt's dtr.	C	C			C	C	C	C									
Refer dtr. to acs	C																
Bladder Training Program	I	I		N													
Insert foley cath Size 16 & 5cc bag					C	C/N											
Instruct in irrigation of catheter					I	I	S/I										
Instruct Pt's dtr To keep strict intake and output record					I	I	N	N									
Edema of feet		E	E	E	E	E	E	E									
Apical pulse		104	100	108	100	96	104	108									
Radial pulse		104	100	108	100	96	104	108									
Respirations		28	32	24	26	20	24	28									
Blood Pressure		120/80	104/50	104/50	104/60	100/60	100/50	112/70									
Instruction in diet 1500 cal.						I	N										
Initials	cf	cf	cf	cf	cf	cf	cf	cf									

CODE:
C – Care   D – Discussion   N – Narrative
I – Instruction   S – Supervision   E – Evaluation

Figure A-7 Flow Sheet.

332

PROGRESS NOTES

Patient's Name Doe, Jane

Date	P.#	Problem Title - Subjective, Objective, Assessment, Plan
8/6		Tel. call to Dr. , regarding patient. Informed MD of patient's excessive voiding, also informed him of pitting edema of both feet, and asked for instructions regarding patient's diet. Dr. feels that the pitting of patient's feet is result of widespread cancer. According to MD, this patient should be on a 1500 calorie diet at this stage. The patient is obviously dying of cancer and MD feels that it is futile to press diet too much. He has instructed PHN to attempt to help patient's daughter and see if she will comply in any way to get her mother to follow the 1500 calorie diet. If the patient's incontinence persists, PHN may call Dr. for order for Foley catheter. C. Johnson, RN
8/9	1	S - O - Patient alone today - unable to determine when daughter will return, edema of feet is increasing. A - Daughter is still having difficulty caring for her mother, she needs much support and encouragement. P - 1. Continue with original plan of supportive therapy. 2. Continue to assist daughter with mother's care, but keep emphasis on teaching daughter how to keep mother comfortable. C. Johnson, RN
	3	S - O - Intake and output have not been kept, edema of feet is increasing - 4+ pitting edema today. Vital signs: apical and radial pulses both 100, respirations 32, blood pressure 104/50. A - Need for more careful monitoring of intake and output. P - Continue to emphasize time and amount of voiding. C. Johnson, RN

Figure A-8 Progress Notes.

Patient's Name___Doe, Jane_____

Date	P.#	Problem Title - Subjective, Objective, Assessment, Plan
8/12	2	S -
		O - Patient is still incontinent.
		A -
		P - Patient needs Foley catheter inserted tomorrow.
8/12	3	S -
		O - No intake/output record has been kept by patient's daughter. Edema of feet is less today than 3 days ago. Vital signs checked, apical and radial pulses both 108, respirations 24, blood pressure 104/56.
		A - Pt. showing signs of congestive failure.
		P - Call MD to request further orders. C. Johnson, RN
8/13	2	S -
		O - Pt. unable to hold urine, bed wet all the time.
		A - Pt. needs Foley catheter.
		P - 1. Insert Foley catheter, #16 - 5 cc bag.
		2. Instruct patient's daughter in the irrigation of Foley with normal saline.
		3. Change Foley catheter, p. r. n.

Figure A-8 Progress Notes (continued).

PROGRESS NOTES

Patient's Name   Doe, Jane

Date	P.#	Problem Title - Subjective, Objective, Assessment, Plan
8/13	3	S - O - Less pitting edema of both feet noted today. Vital signs taken, apical and radial pulses both 100, respirations 26, blood pressure 104/60. A - Patient is still not adhering to strict diet, eating mostly starches, daughter says obviously mother will eat only what she chooses. P - Call MD for further orders and to report findings.
8/13		Tel. call to Dr. _____ to report patient's condition. Informed MD that Foley catheter was being inserted and instructions to be given to patient's daughter. Also informed MD re: edema of feet and her vital signs.
8/16	2	S - O - Foley catheter draining well. Urine is clear amber. A - Daughter observed technique and will return demonstration on Tuesday, August 20. P - Continue to supervise daughter in irrigation of Foley catheter. C. Johnson, RN
	3	S - O - Feet somewhat less edematous today. Vital signs checked: apical and radial pulses 96, respirations 20, blood pressure 100/60. A - Daughter still insecure with some aspects of mother's care. P - PHN supervised daughter in monitoring intake and output. To date, daughter has not been able to follow through with this request. C. Johnson, RN

Figure A-8   Progress Notes (continued).

PROGRESS NOTES

Patient's Name Doe, Jane

Date	P.#	Problem Title - Subjective, Objective, Assessment, Plan
8/16	4	S - Daughter states her mother eats what she wants and doubts if she will be able to follow this diet. O - A - Daughter is trying; however, mother is unable to eat. P - Review 1500 calorie diet with daughter, and support her in her efforts to follow through with this. C. Johnson, RN
8/19		Tel. call from patient's daughter stating her mother's catheter was leaking. Patient's daughter instructed over phone to remove Foley catheter and nurse will visit tomorrow to check patient and possibly reinsert catheter.
8/20	2	S - O - Pt. still wetting bed since Foley catheter was removed yesterday. A - Pt. unable to follow bladder training program due to inadequate bladder control. Foley catheter should be reinserted. P - 1. Insert Foley catheter size #16 - 5 cc bag. 2. Since daughter has already been instructed in irrigation of catheter, observe her giving return demonstration today. 3. Change Foley catheter p.r.n. C. Johnson, RN

Figure A-8 Progress Notes (continued).

Patient's Name   Doe, Jane

Date	P.#	Problem Title - Subjective, Objective, Assessment, Plan
8/20	3	S -
		O - Edema of both feet noticed. Vital signs checked: apical and radial pulses both 104, respirations 24, blood pressure 100/50.
		A - Pt's dtr. still reluctant to keep intake and output.
		P - Continue to assist dtr. with pt's catheter and diet.
8/23	3	S - "I'm trying to keep track of Mother's fluids, but it is difficult."
		O - Patient has taken in 800 cc of liquid and put out about 500 cc yesterday. Apical and radial pulses are both 108. Respirations 28, blood pressure 112/70.
		A - Feet less edematous today. Dtr. seems to be taking more of an interest and gaining a little bit more cooperation with mother.
		P - Continue to encourage dtr. to follow plan for diet and intake and output monitoring. Offer more assistance with care of mother as pt. becomes progressively worse. Connie Johnson, RN

Figure A-8 Progress Notes (continued).

Appendix B
Sample
Flow Sheet
Forms

Arthritis
Cardiac Disease
Chronic Obstructive Pulmonary Disease (C.O.P.D.)
Urinary Catheter Care

FLOW SHEET – ARTHRITIS

Name _____

PARAMETERS	Date of Visit 19___																
Subjective																	
Pain:																	
location																	
type																	
severity																	
relieved by medications																	
Gastric irritation:																	
nausea/vomiting																	
diarrhea																	
Appetite																	
Elimination																	
Vision changes																	
Rest/Sleep																	
Objective																	
Temperature																	
Blood pressure																	
Pulse																	
Respirations																	
Affected joints:																	
swelling																	
inflammation																	
contractions limitations																	
Initials																	

CODE: C – Care   D – Discussion   N – Narrative
       I – Instruction   S – Supervision   E – Evaluation

Figure B-1 Arthritis.

PARAMETERS	Date of Visit 19 ___																			
Objective	Eyes: redness																				
	dryness																				
	secretions																				
	Skin: rash																				
	abrasions																				
	decubiti																				
	Nutritional status																				
	Emotional status																				
	Exercise regimen																				
	Transfer																				
	Ambulation																				
	ADL: feeding																				
	personal hygiene																				
Instruction	Safety hazards																				
	Disease process																				
	Balanced rest/activity																				
	Compliance with medication and exercise regimen																				
	Physical limitations																				
	Avoiding stress and emotional anxiety																				
	*Use of special aids																				
	Proper positioning																				
	Initials																				

*1. braces
*2. adaptive devices
*3. walker
*4. wheel chair
*5. quad cane
*6. commode

Figure B-1 Arthritis (continued).

341

FLOW SHEET – C A R D I A C   D I S E A S E

Name _____

PARAMETERS		Date of Visit 19___															
Subjective	Chest pain:																
	location																
	duration																
	severity																
	relieved by																
	Vertigo/Syncope																
	Palpitations																
	Shortness of breath (S.O.B.)																
	Dyspnea on exertion (D.O.E.)																
	Orthopnea																
	Fatigue																
	Diaphoresis																
	Cough: Productive																
Objective	Blood pressure																
	Apical pulse rate/rhythm																
	Radial pulse rate/rhythm																
	Respiration rate																
	Respiration quality																
	Breath sounds R/L																
	Weight																
	Initials																

CODE: C – Care   D – Discussion   N – Narrative
       I – Instruction   S – Supervision   E – Evaluation

Figure B-2 Cardiac Disease.

342

PARAMETERS		Date of Visit 19____																			
Objective	* Neck vein distension																					
	*Ascites																					
	Extremities:																					
	pulse R / L																					
	color R / L																					
	edema R / L																					
	temperature R / L																					
	*Cyanosis																					
	Apprehension/Anxiety																					
Instruction	Progression of activity																					
	Fluid restriction (I/O)																					
	Diet (specify)																					
	Avoid smoking																					
	Avoid heavy drinking																					
	Avoid caffeine																					
	Emotional coping																					
	Use of special equipment: Oxygen, IPPB																					
	Initials																					

*Presence or Absence (P or A)

Figure B-2   Cardiac Disease (continued).

FLOW SHEET – CHRONIC OBSTRUCTIVE PULMONARY DISEASE

Name ____________________

	PARAMETERS	Date of Visit 19____														
Subjective	Cough:															
	productive															
	frequency															
	when prevalent															
	Sputum:															
	color															
	amount															
	consistency															
	Chest pain															
	Activity tolerance															
	Shortness of breath (S.O.B.)															
	Dyspnea on exertion (D.O.E.)															
	Orthopnea															
	Nausea															
	Fatigue															
	Restlessness, apprehension															
	Confusion, lightheadness															
	Anxiety															
	Fluid intake (cc)															
Initials																

CODE: C – Care; I – Instruction; D – Discussion; S – Supervision; N – Narrative; E – Evaluation

Figure B-3 Chronic Obstructive Pulmonary Disease (C.O.P.D.).

PARAMETERS	Date of Visit 19 _____																		
Objective																			
Temperature																			
Pulse																			
Respiration: rate																			
depth																			
Use of accessory muscles																			
Blood pressure																			
Breath sounds * R ul/ml/ll																			
Breath sounds * L ul/ll																			
Rales ** R ul/ml/ll																			
Rales ** L ul/ll																			
Weight																			
Cyanosis: central ***																			
Cyanosis: peripheral ***																			
Signs of oxygen hunger																			
Nutritional status																			
Instruction																			
Disease process / Treatment																			
Special equipment – use and maintenance																			
Breathing exercises, postural drainage, fluids																			
Avoid smoking, drafts, respiratory irritants																			
Avoid overexertion and emotional stress																			
Preventive measures																			
Initials																			

CODE: *Breath Sounds   **Rales   ***Cyanosis
        1–full   1–coarse   P –Present
        2–moderate   2–medium   A–Absent
        3–diminished   3–fine
        4–absent

Figure B-3   Chronic Obstructive Pulmonary Disease (C.O.P.D.) (continued).

345

FLOW SHEET – URINARY CATHETER CARE

Catheter Size _____

Name _____

Reason for Catheter _____

	PARAMETERS	Date of Visit 19 ___																
Subjective	Pain/Discomfort at site																	
	Leakage around catheter																	
	Non-drainage of catheter																	
	Difficulty with catheter irrigation																	
	Fluid intake																	
Objective	Temperature																	
	Urine output: amount																	
	color																	
	Sediment *																	
	Mucus *																	
	Bladder distension *																	
	Perineal: irritation *																	
	excoriation *																	
	blistering *																	
	Closed system drainage *																	
Instruction	Perineal care																	
	Catheter care:																	
	equipment, maintenance and use																	
	irrigation solution preparation																	
	irrigation technique																	
	drainage bag cleansing technique																	
	Initials																	

CODE: C – Care   D – Discussion   N – Narrative
      I – Instruction   S – Supervision   E – Evaluation
* Present – P   Absent – A

Figure B-4 Urinary Catheter Care.

		Date of Visit 19 ____																	
PARAMETERS																				
Instruction	Safety precautions																			
	emergency removal of catheter																			
	securing catheter																			
	proper positioning of drainage bag																			
	increase fluid intake																			
	Initials																			

Figure B-4 Urinary Catheter Care (continued).

Appendix C
Selected Samples from the National League for Nursing Problem-Oriented Record System

Preadmission Request for Service
Interagency Care and Treatment Plan
Family Data and Problem Index
Patient Baseline Data (form)
Patient Baseline Data (guide)
Patient Problem Index
Patient Care Plan—Flow Sheet
Narrative Progress Notes

Selected samples from the Problem-Oriented Record System for Home and Community Health Service Agencies, developed by the Department of Home Health Agencies and Community Health Services, National League for Nursing. Reproduced by permission of the National League for Nursing.

DHHA/CHS Form 21-PRS
©1973 National League for Nursing

PREADMISSION REQUEST FOR SERVICE

NAME_____

ADDRESS_____

PATIENT STATUS

☐ ACTIVE   ☐ NEW PATIENT
☐ OLD CHART   ☐ NEW THIS YEAR

PHONE (_____)_____BIRTH DATE_____SEX: ☐ M ☐ F   ☐ READMISSION: ☐ Same DX ☐ New DX

PATIENT I.D. No._____

DIAGNOSIS_____   _____
(Date of onset
if known)   _____   _____

PHYSICIAN_____PHONE (_____)_____

ADDRESS_____

HOSPITAL_____   S.N.F._____

DATE: Adm._____Disch._____   DATE: Adm._____Disch._____

ORDERS	REMARKS

FEE STATUS/BILLING INFORMATION   Social Security No._____

☐ MEDICARE No._____   ☐ OTHER   NAME_____
☐ MEDICAID No._____   INSURANCE   No._____

BILL TO_____   ADDRESS_____

REFERRAL SOURCE: NAME_____   PHONE (_____)_____
☐ AGENCY   ☐ S.N.F.
☐ HOSPITAL   ☐ SELF/RELATIVE   ADDRESS_____
☐ PHYSICIAN   ☐ OTHER   From whom did you
learn of this service?_____

REQUEST TAKEN BY_____DATE_____TIME_____ AM/PM

DISPOSITION

☐ ADMITTED: By_____

☐ NOT ADMITTED: ☐ Adm. to hospital   ☐ Adm. to S.N.F.   ☐ Service not available   ☐ Agency policy (explain under other)

☐ REFERRED: To_____

☐ OTHER (explain):   _____
_____

PATIENT NAME_____   PATIENT I.D. No._____

FORM 21-PRS   ©1973 National League for Nursing

Figure C-1   Preadmission Request for Service.

DHHA/CHS Form 21 - ICTP/PS
©1974 National League for Nursing

INTERAGENCY CARE AND TREATMENT PLAN
(Physician's Section)

TO_____ FROM_____

_____ _____

_____ _____

Agency Provider No. _____

Patient Name _____

Address _____

Birth Date	Soc. Sec. No.
Medicare No.	Medicaid No.
Other Insurance	No.

MEDICAL PROBLEMS	MEDICAL PLANS

DIAGNOSES:

Primary—

Others (List)—

DIET AND MEDICATIONS, INCLUDING FREQUENCY AND DOSAGE

Diet: _____

PROGNOSIS: _____

FUNCTIONAL LIMITATIONS (motor or sensory deficits): _____

THERAPY

☐ H.H.A.   ☐ NURSING   ☐ P.T.   ☐ OTHER (Specify) _____

☐ M.S.W.   ☐ O.T.   ☐ S.T.   _____

Last seen by physician ___ Date: _____
Recertification due ___ Date: _____
Sent to physician ___ Date: _____

CERTIFICATION—RECERTIFICATION: I certify that the above-named patient (1) is under my care, (2) is homebound except when receiving outpatient services, (3) requires skilled nursing care on an intermittent basis or physical or speech therapy as specified in the original orders with the modifications listed above.
Is Recertification Statement pertinent to this patient? ☐ Yes ☐ No

EFFECTIVE DATES:

From _____ To _____

_____ _____
(Physician's Signature)   (Date)

FORM 21-ICTP/PS

Figure C-2   Interagency Care and Treatment Plan.

FAMILY NAME _____

FAMILY I.D. No. _____

FAMILY DATA
AND PROBLEM INDEX

DATE	ADDRESS	DIRECTIONS—C/O—NEAR	APT/FLOOR	TELEPHONE	HEALTH AREA

FAMILY ROSTER

NAME	RACE	BIRTH DATE	MARITAL STATUS
Man:			☐ S ☐ M ☐ W ☐ D ☐ Sep.
Woman: Maiden name:			☐ S ☐ M ☐ W ☐ D ☐ Sep.

Emergency contact: Address: Phone:

	FAMILY/HOUSEHOLD MEMBER	SEX	BIRTH DATE	RACE	COMMENTS relationship—occupation—education—etc.
1					
2					
3					
4					
5					
6					
7					
8					
9					
10					
11					
12					

RECORD OF SERVICE

NAME	DATE Adm.	Disch.	PRIMARY DIAGNOSIS	NAME	DATE Adm.	Disch.	PRIMARY DIAGNOSIS

FORM 21-FDPI   DHHA/CHS   © 1974 National League for Nursing

Figure C-3   Family Data and Problem Index.

OTHER AGENCIES ACTIVE					
DATE	FAMILY MEMBER	AGENCY	NAME OF WORKER	TELEPHONE NUMBER	DATE INACTIVE

FAMILY DATA BASE	
HISTORY	
physical, functional, nutritional, etc.	
Sign and date all entries.	

Figure C-3 Family Data and Problem Index (continued).

FAMILY PROBLEM INDEX

List all potential, current, or significant past problems that affect the family as a group. **Identify family member when appropriate.**
Include date of onset or identification and the date of resolution for each problem.

PROB. NO.	FAMILY MEMBER	FAMILY PROBLEMS POTENTIAL/CURRENT—ACTIVE	DATE OF ONSET	DATE RESOLVED	FAMILY PROBLEMS SIGNIFICANT PAST—INACTIVE

CONTINUE ON A NEW FORM

Figure C-3 Family Data and Problem Index (continued).

354

ENVIRONMENT

housing,
sanitation,
transportation,
safety,
etc.

Sign and date
all entries.

ADJUSTMENTS

social,
emotional,
cultural,
vocational,
religious,
etc.

Sign and date
all entries

_____   _____
(Date)   (Signature and title)

Figure C-3   Family Data and Problem Index (continued).

355

PATIENT
BASELINE DATA

PATIENT NAME_____

PATIENT I.D. No._____

Page_____

CODE: √ = Problem present   O = No problem present

PARAMETERS	DATE		SUBJECTIVE AND OBJECTIVE OBSERVATIONS PHYSICAL, FUNCTIONAL, EMOTIONAL, SOCIAL, AND SAFETY
AIR Source			
Inspiration-expiration			
O_2-CO_2 exchange			
O_2-CO_2 transport			
Cell utilization			
Other (describe)			
COMMUNICATION Language			
Speech patterns			
Organs of speech			
Non-verbal			
Comprehension			
Educational level			
Other (describe)			
ELIMINATION Bowel			
Bladder			
Other (describe)			
EXERCISE Pattern			
Strength			
Voluntary movement			
Involuntary movement			
Productivity			
Independence			
Equipment			
Other (describe)			
FOOD AND WATER Physical appearance			
Eating patterns			
Ability to ingest			
Ability to digest and absorb			
Ability to metabolize			
Aids			
Securing			
Storing			
Preparing			
Other (describe)			

FORM 21-PBD   DHHA/CHS   CONTINUE ON OTHER SIDE

Figure C-4   Patient Baseline Data (form).

356

	PARAMETERS	DATE		SUBJECTIVE AND OBJECTIVE OBSERVATIONS PHYSICAL, FUNCTIONAL, EMOTIONAL, SOCIAL, AND SAFETY
P S Y C H O S O C I A L	Life style and relationships			
	Religion			
	Coping mechanisms			
	Basic needs			
	Development stage			
	Other (describe)			
R E S T A N D S L E E P	Patterns			
	Meaning of rest			
	Interfering factors			
	Circadian rhythm			
	Adequacy			
	Aids			
	Other (describe)			
S A F E T Y A N D P R O T E C T I O N	Care of body			
	Clothing			
	Housing			
	Environment			
	Health maintenance measures			
	Allergic reactions			
	Other (describe)			
S E N S O R Y P E R C E P T I O N	Vision			
	Hearing			
	Touch			
	Taste and smell			
	Pain			
	Affect			
	Memory			
	Balance			
	Consciousness			
	Kinesthetic awareness			
	Other (describe)			
O T H E R				

Signature and title_____ Date _____

Signature and title_____ Date _____

Figure C-4   Patient Baseline Data (form) (continued).

Focus: Health Status and Self-Care System

GUIDE FOR SYSTEMATIC OBSERVATION
(PATIENT DATA BASE)
TO ACCOMPANY FORM 21-PBD

AIR

Source (Quality of environmental air, level of O_2 in a tent, etc.)
Inspiration-Expiration (Patency of airway (nasal, tracheal); breath sounds (wheeze, cough, bubbly), manner of tracheostomy care)
O_2-CO_2 Exchange (Pale conjunctiva, blue nail beds, Hgb level)
O_2-CO_2 Transport (BP, heart sounds, pulse rate and regularity)
Cell Utilization (Healing rate, energy level, metabolic rate)

FOOD AND WATER

Physical Appearance (Height, weight, skin dryness and turgor, etc.)
Eating Patterns (Usual type and amount of food and fluid intake, factors affecting appetite, etc.)
Ability to Ingest (Dental status, ability to swallow, etc.)
Ability to Digest and Absorb (Abdominal discomfort, history of G.I. related illness, e.g. ulcers, pancreatitis, etc.)
Ability to Metabolize (Healing rate, metabolic rate, energy level)
Aids (Special utensils, gastrostomy, etc.)
Securing (Financing, transporting, etc.)
Storing (Refrigeration, infestation, etc.)
Preparing (Cooking facilities, etc.)

EXERCISE

Pattern (Amount, type, timing, etc.)
Strength (Hand grasp, extremity vs. resistance, etc.)
Voluntary Movement (Gross, fine, joint range of motion)
Involuntary (Tremors, seizures, etc.)
Productivity (Work, recreation, other)
Independence (Of movement or assistance required)
Equipment (Cane, crutches, etc.)

REST AND SLEEP

Patterns (Amount, quality, etc.)
Meaning of Rest (What would individual consider restful)
Interfering Factors (Pain, noise)
Circadian Rhythm (Best hours for sleep, time least and most rest required, etc.)
Adequacy (Patient's subjective evaluation: fatigued, rested, etc.)
Aids (Pre-sleep rituals, medication)

ELIMINATION

Bowel (Patterns, characteristics, management, medication, equipment, etc.)
Bladder (Patterns, characteristics, management, medication, equipment, etc.)
Other (Wound drainage, perspiration, etc.)

SAFETY AND PROTECTION

Care of Body (Skin, mucous membrane, etc.)
Clothing (Adequacy for environment)
Housing (Adequacy for environment)
Environment (Sanitation, noise, infestation, etc.)
Health Maintenance Measures (Dental exams, medical exams, immunization, etc.)
Known Untoward Reactions (Allergies, hypersensitivities)

SENSORY PERCEPTION

Vision (Acuity, glasses, etc.)
Hearing (Acuity, aids, etc.)
Touch (Numbness, hypersensitivity)
Taste and Smell (Preferences, responses)
Pain (Presence, absence, where, when, etc.)
Affect (Appropriate, flattened)
Memory (Recent, remote)
Balance (Sitting, standing, turning)
Consciousness (Attention span, seizures)
Kinesthetic Awareness (Position, body parts)

PSYCHO-SOCIAL

Life Style and Relationships (Marital, social, etc.)
Religion (Type, relative importance, etc.)
Coping Mechanisms (Problem-solving methods, risk-taking, impulse control, etc.)
Basic Needs (Manner of meeting: love, security, control, esteem, etc.)
Developmental Stage (Adolescence, productivity—degree of task fulfillment, independence vs. dependence, job or life's work, reproductive phase, etc.)

COMMUNICATION

Language (Foreign, articulation, grammar)
Speech Patterns (Stutter, emissive aphasia)
Organs of Speech (Tongue, palate)
Non-Verbal (Vocalizations, gestures, writing)
Comprehension (Reading, hearing)
Educational Level (Eighth grade, Ph.D. in_____)

OTHER

Sources of Health Care (Physician, dentist, clinic or difficulties in obtaining health care)
Health History (Disease, injury, operations)
Diagnostic Results (Medical, psychological, vocational, etc.)
Patterns of Seeking Care (Regularly planned, emergency only, etc.)

FACTORS: Physical, Functional, Emotional, Social and Safety

DHHA/CHS

Figure C-5   Patient Baseline Data (guide).

PATIENT NAME				
PATIENT I.D. No.				

PATIENT PROBLEM INDEX

List all potential, current, or significant past problems that affect the patient. Include date of onset or identification and the date of resolution for each problem.

Page _____

PROBLEM NO.	PROBLEMS POTENTIAL/CURRENT—ACTIVE	DATE OF ONSET	DATE RESOLVED	PROBLEMS SIGNIFICANT PAST—INACTIVE

FORM 21-PPI   DHHA/CHS   CONTINUE ON OTHER SIDE

Figure C-6 Patient Problem Index.

359

PATIENT CARE PLAN–FLOW SHEET

INITIAL STATUS—Activities of Daily Living (Check): ☐0-Total Dependence ☐1-Severe Dependence ☐2-Moderate Dependence ☐3-Minimal Dependence ☐4-Total Independence

FLOW SHEET

DATE	PROB. NO.	PLAN, ACTIONS TO BE TAKEN, AND EXPECTED OUTCOMES

ENTER
Date Here ▶
Site of Visit Here ▶

PAYMENT
REVISIT DATE

Signature & Title

CONTINUE ON A NEW SHEET

FLOW SHEET CODES

PROBLEM STATUS

2—No change from previous visit

3—Change (see Narrative/Progress Notes)

4—Problem no longer present

CARE PROVIDED

C—Direct care

E—Evaluation

N—See Narrative/Progress Notes

Injection site codes—RD, LG, etc.

R—Referral

S—Supervision

T—Teaching or counseling

Figure C-7 Patient Care Plan—Flow Sheet

NARRATIVE/PROGRESS NOTES

PATIENT NAME _____

PATIENT I.D. No. _____

Begin entries pertaining to subjective findings (S), objective findings (O), assessment (A), and plans (P) in the column appropriately headed and write through remaining columns to the right margin. The signature and title of the recorder must appear after each entry.

Page _____

DATE	PROBLEM NO.	S	O	A	P	NARRATIVE/PROGRESS
		SUBJECTIVE	OBJECTIVE	ASSESSMENT	PLANS	

FORM 21-NPN   DHHA/CHS   CONTINUE ON OTHER SIDE

Figure C-8   Narrative/Progress Notes.

361

Index